Arthroscopy of the Knee

A **Slide Atlas of Arthroscopy of the Knee** based on the material in this book is available. Further information concerning the slide atlas may be obtained from:

Gower Medical Publishing
34–42 Cleveland Street
London W1P 5FB, UK

Arthroscopy of the Knee

A Diagnostic Color Atlas

David J. Dandy F.R.C.S.

Consultant Orthopaedic Surgeon
Addenbrooke's Hospital, Cambridge, U.K.
Newmarket General Hospital, Newmarket, U.K.
Associate Lecturer in the Faculty of Clinical Medicine
University of Cambridge, Cambridge, U.K.

Lea & Febiger · Philadelphia

Gower Medical Publishing · London · New York

Distributed in the USA and Canada by:
Lea & Febiger
600 Washington Square
Philadelphia, Pennsylvania 19106
USA

Distributed in all countries except USA, Canada and Japan by:
Butterworth and Co. (Publishers) Limited
Borough Green
Sevenoaks
Kent TN15 8PH
UK

Distributed in Japan by:
Maruzen Company Ltd.
3–10 Nihonbashi 2-chome
Chuo-ku
Tokyo 103, JAPAN

Project editor: Sharyn Wong

Design: Mehmet Hussein
Helen Leahy

Illustrator: Chris Furey

Cover design: Jeremy Rose

Library Cataloging in Publication Data:

Dandy, David J.
Arthroscopy of the knee.
1. Knee—Diseases—Atlases
I. Title
616.7'2 RC932

Printed in Singapore by Imago Productions (Far East) Pte. Ltd.

Preface

Arthroscopy and arthroscopic surgery have grown rapidly in the last ten years and have changed our approach to the knee. Some of the structures most obvious at arthroscopy do not appear at all in earlier anatomical texts. The magnification of the arthroscope has brought a new approach to pathology in the knee and both the normal and abnormal anatomy of the knee have been seen differently.

In this Atlas, an attempt is made to set down the arthroscopic appearance of the knee in health and disease. The observations and comments made are based on personal experience and are open to criticism. Although time and the experience of others will show many of these ideas to be incorrect, it is hoped that this Atlas will serve as a baseline for future work.

The omission of references is not intended to deprecate the excellent work of others, but the quotation of references can sometimes inhibit criticism and the body of knowledge relating to arthroscopic anatomy is still too small to be authoritative. Without references, the subject can be seen more clearly as a whole, and the content is offered for criticism at all points.

Acknowledgements

Many people have contributed to the preparation of this Atlas. I am particularly grateful to Mrs. Shirley French and Mrs. Caroline Sheehan for typing and re-typing the manuscript so frequently, to Miss Sharyn Wong of Gower Medical Publishing Ltd. for invaluable help with the final editing and design, and to Mr. Chris Furey, who was obliged to learn the arthroscopic anatomy of the knee himself in order to prepare the line diagrams that accompany the colour photographs.

Finally, I would like to record my deepest thanks to my wife, Jane, and to our children, James and Emma, for their patience and forbearance during a long and time-consuming project that occupied many weekends and evenings that would otherwise have been shared.

Contents

1

The Normal Knee

SUPRAPATELLAR POUCH

Most surgeons begin their arthroscopic examination of the knee in the suprapatellar pouch which, to the arthroscopist, is a dark cavern with smooth arched walls and roof and a slightly uneven floor. Photography in the pouch is more difficult than in other areas because light is not reflected as well from the red synovium as it is from white articular cartilage, and the space itself is larger than other parts of the knee so that the background is not as well illuminated as the foreground.

Articularis genu muscle

The upper limit of the pouch is marked by the insertion of the articularis genu muscle, the lowermost portion of the vastus intermedius muscle, which is attached to the synovial membrane at the apex of the suprapatellar pouch. The muscle insertion, which appears as a purplish-brown discoloration at the uppermost limit of the pouch, usually consists of several patches of muscle rather than a single bundle and is more marked in children than in adults. The muscle insertion is clearly seen in Fig. 1.1. The patient was a boy of ten with a discoid lateral meniscus.

Medial suprapatellar plica

On the medial side of the joint, approximately 2cm below its apex, lies the medial suprapatellar plica (also known as the plica synovialis suprapatellaris and plica suprapatellaris medialis) which appears as a fold running backwards and distally from the back of the extensor mechanism to the front of the femur. The crescentic lateral margin of the plica is often thick and fibrous (Fig. 1.2) and is covered by synovium.

The medial suprapatellar plica probably represents the embryonic or phylogenetic vestige of a synovial membrane that once separated the upper part of the synovial cavity from the rest of the knee. It is a normal feature of the knee but, as befits the functionless vestige of a once important anatomical structure, it is very variable in both shape and size.

In Fig. 1.3 the plica is larger than that seen in Fig. 1.2 and has a firm fibrous rim that extends anteriorly to leave a smaller than normal opening between its free lower margin and the synovium covering the anterior surface of the femur. The membrane can form a continuous ring around the entire circumference of the suprapatellar pouch (Fig. 1.4), giving the appearance sometimes known as a 'porta' in which a central opening seems to have been punched through a membrane that once stretched from side to side across the suprapatellar pouch, dividing it into two separate parts. In Fig. 1.4, the insertion of the articularis genu muscle can be seen through the porta as a brown stain at the apex of the synovial cavity.

The size of the opening in the suprapatellar membrane is very variable. Fig. 1.5 shows a medial suprapatellar

1.1

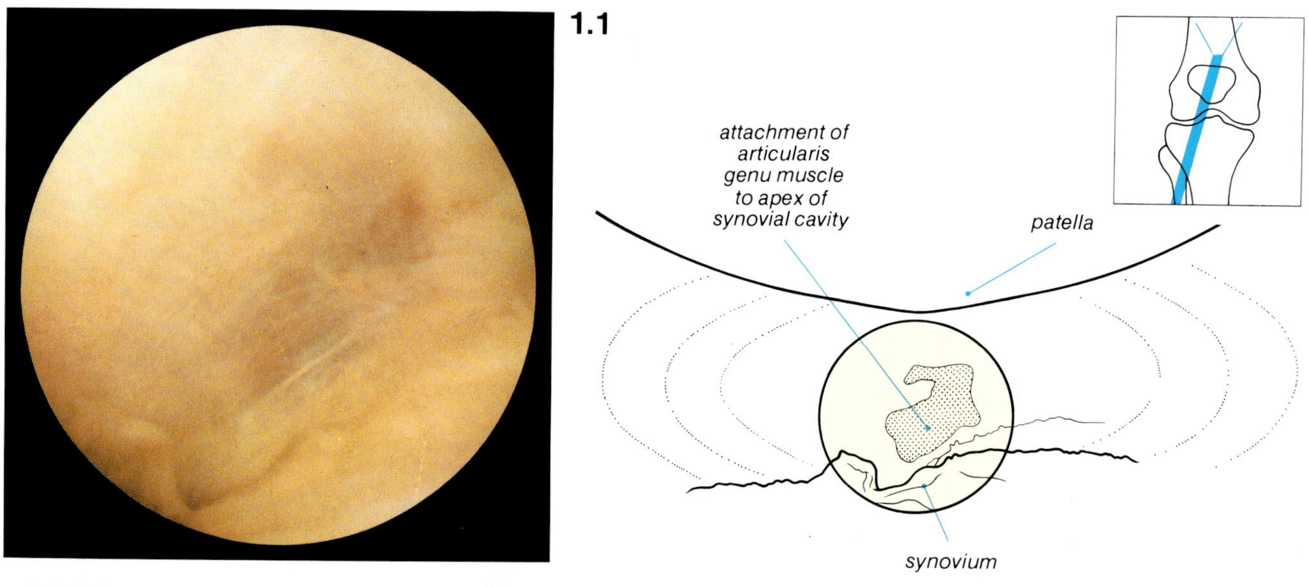

1.2

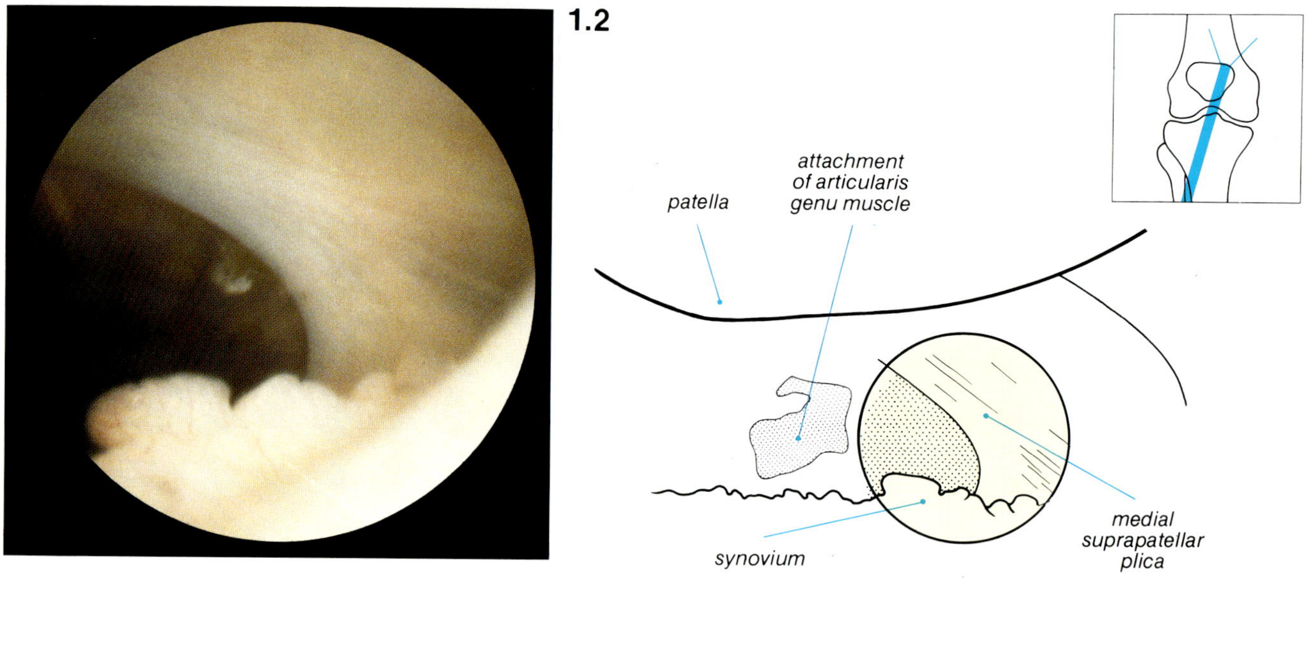

plica that is almost a complete suprapatellar membrane. The opening is much smaller than that seen in Fig. 1.4 and, indeed, is little more than a slit. Tense collections of synovial fluid are occasionally found in the upper part of the knee and may give rise to painful discomfort above the patella. A valve mechanism has been suggested as a cause of such loculated swellings of synovial fluid, and it is possible to imagine the structure in Fig. 1.5 acting as a non-return valve allowing synovial fluid to enter the closed space above the membrane while preventing its return to the rest of the knee.

Although there is no definite information to help in deciding whether a 'porta' is pathological or not, to divide a membrane such as that in Fig.1.5 under arthroscopic control is a simple procedure with negligible morbidity and may relieve symptoms.

1.3

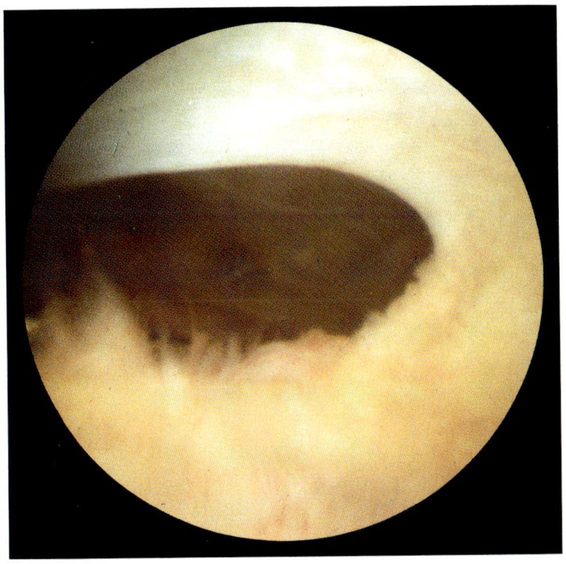

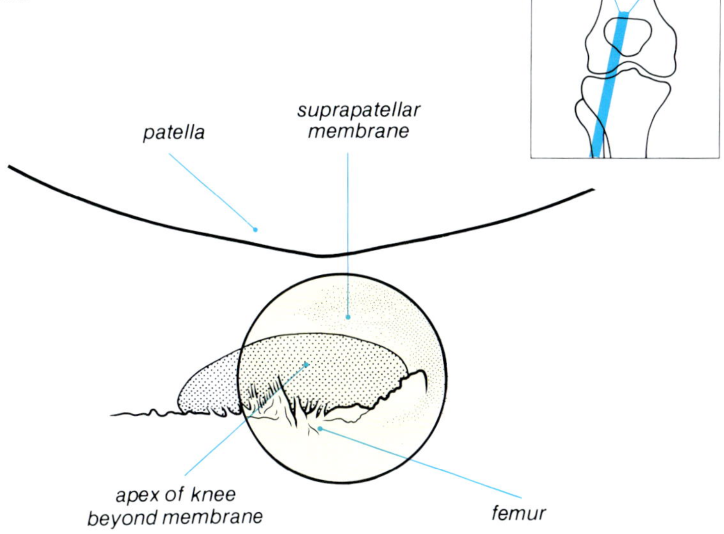

1.4

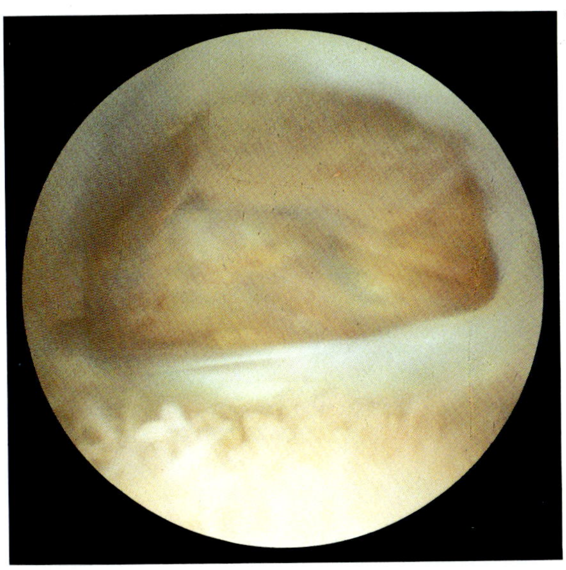

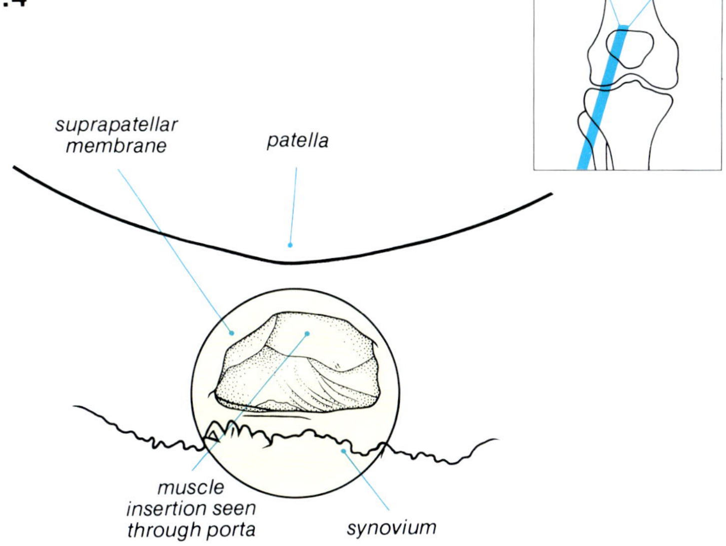

1.5

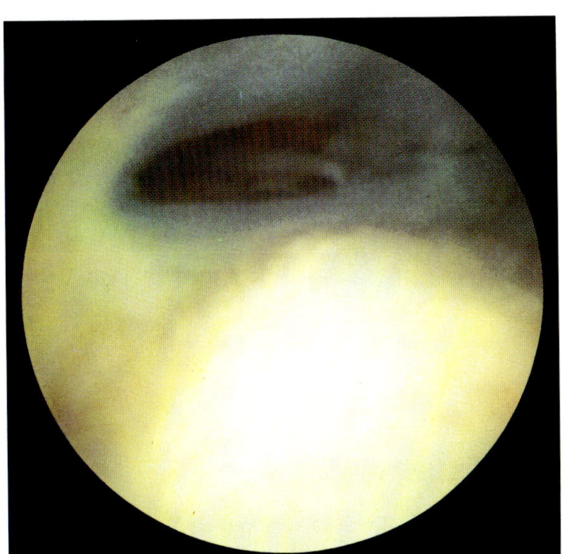

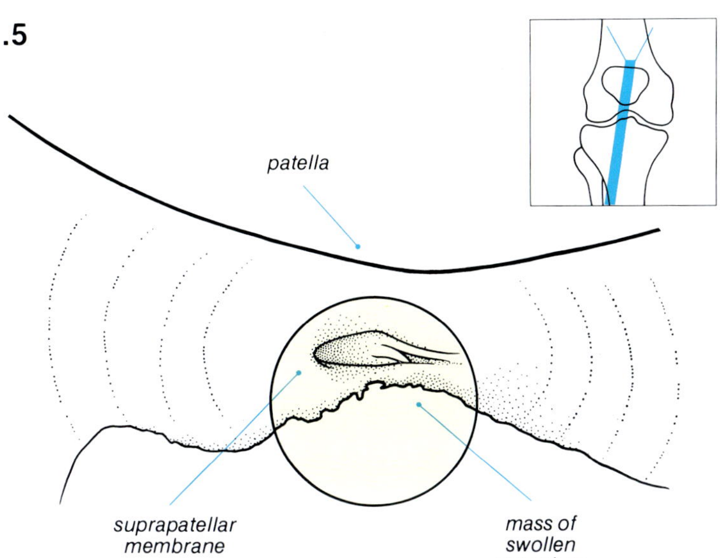

In some patients the suprapatellar membrane may appear to be complete with no opening between the space above and the rest of the knee. Before deciding that a suprapatellar plica is in fact a complete membrane, it should be carefully examined with a hook or needle to be certain that it is not simply a large plica. The plica in Fig.1.6 shows the typical slate blue appearance of a complete suprapatellar membrane, and it extends all the way down to the synovium overlying the anterior surface of the femur. The probing needle shows no space beneath the plica, but the lower margin of the plica is thick and fibrous, an appearance not seen in a complete suprapatellar membrane. In Fig.1.7, of the same knee as in Fig.1.6, the needle has been used to lift the fibrous edge of the plica, demonstrating a small arched opening beneath it. Like the slit shown in Fig.1.5, it is easy to imagine such a structure acting as a non-return valve.

Although many knees which at first sight seem to have a complete suprapatellar membrane are later found, on careful probing, to have only a large medial suprapatellar plica, complete suprapatellar membranes do occur and appear as slate blue membranes stretched across the entire width of the knee. Fig.1.8 shows such a membrane, pierced by the irrigation needle to demonstrate its flimsy nature, with a space beyond it. The space beyond the membrane is sometimes distended with synovial fluid. Such a membrane can be entirely asymptomatic and is sometimes recognized only at arthroscopy when, after the knee has been drained at the conclusion of the examination, a large tense swelling remains above the patella. If the arthroscope is reinserted and the knee reexamined, the membrane will be identified, presenting the downward bulge seen in Fig.1.9.

Because a complete suprapatellar membrane consists of normal synovium, there may be difficulty in distinguishing it from the apex of the synovial cavity. In this respect, the articularis genu muscle is a useful landmark. If the muscle can be seen, the apex of the knee has been reached and there cannot be an intact suprapatellar membrane unless it has been pierced by the arthroscope. Accordingly, if the medial suprapatellar plica cannot be seen on the medial side of the knee, special care should be taken to identify the articularis genu muscle so that a complete suprapatellar membrane is not overlooked.

Figs.1.8 and 1.9 show another characteristic of the medial suprapatellar plica. The synovium overlying the femur in Fig.1.8 is smooth and normal while that in Fig.1.9 is swollen and inflamed; yet the suprapatellar membrane presents the same smooth and even appearance in both. It is unusual to find the appearances

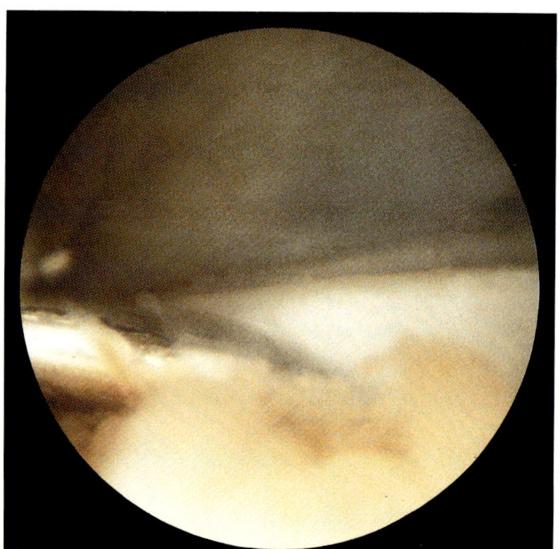

1.6

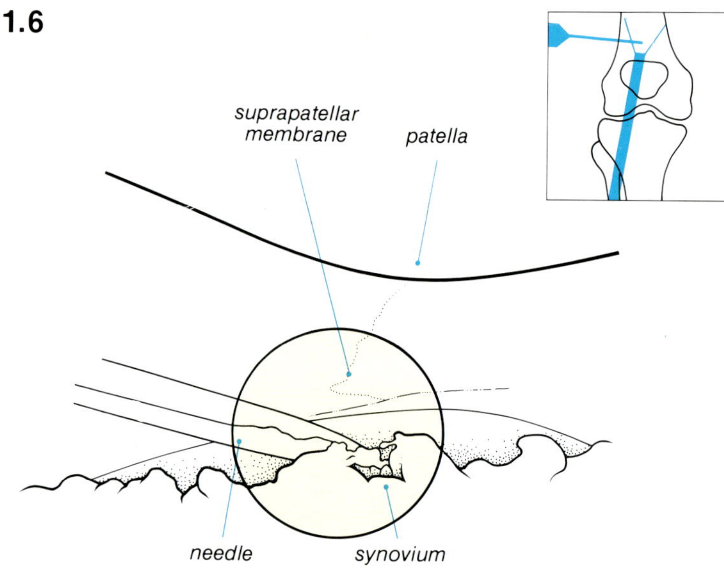

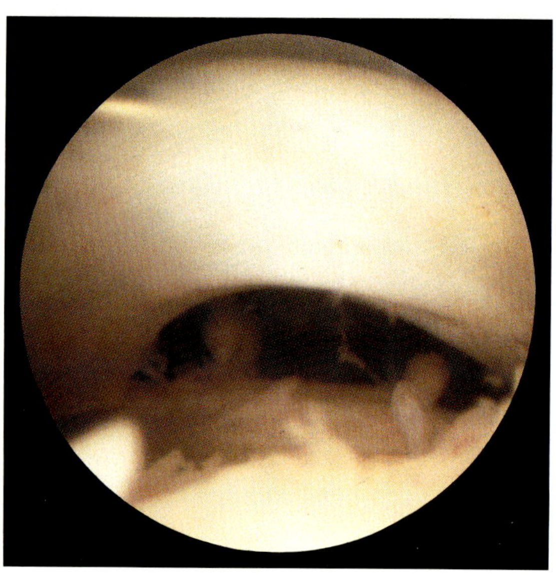

1.7

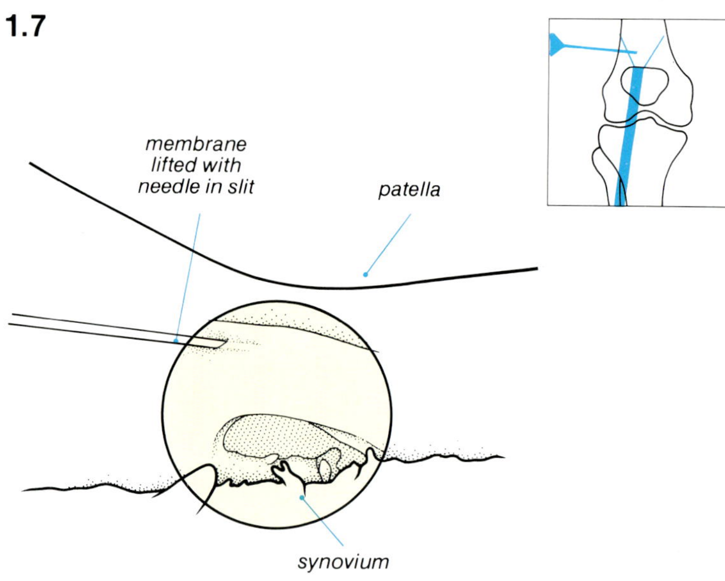

of synovitis on the suprapatellar membrane and there is no obvious explanation for this observation, unless perhaps the vascularity of the synovium overlying the femur and soft tissues supporting it causes the synovium to behave differently from that in the unsupported suprapatellar plica.

The medial suprapatellar plica usually appears as a crescentic fold of variable width on the medial side of the knee, but many other appearances are found. Fig. 1.10 shows a central pillar with an opening on either side. A needle has been passed behind the central pillar to demonstrate its position.

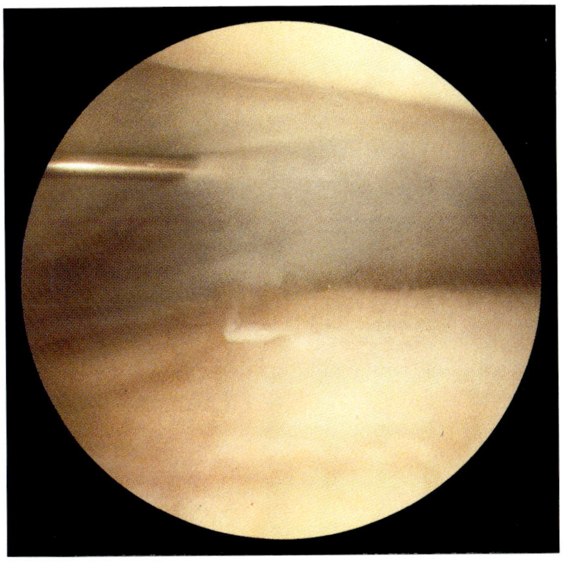

1.8

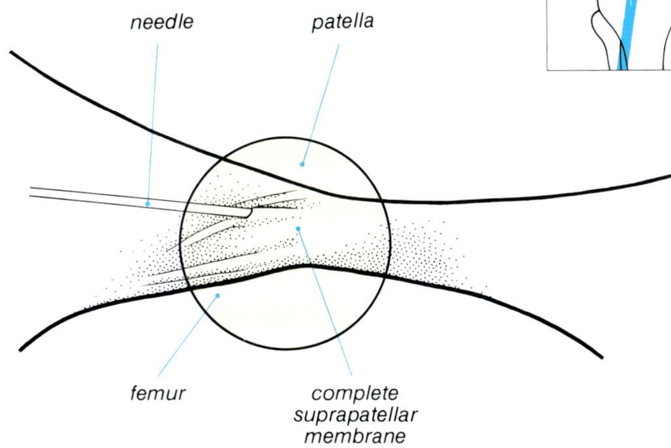

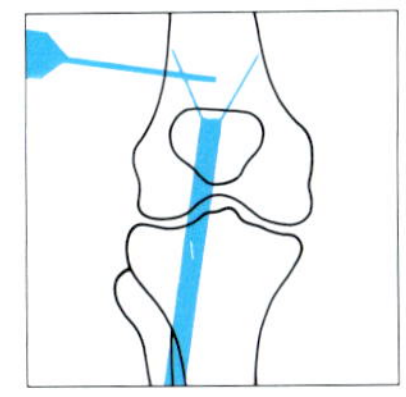

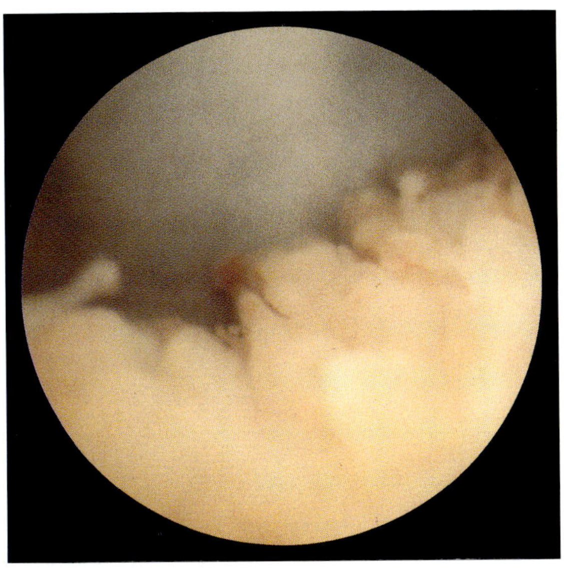

1.9

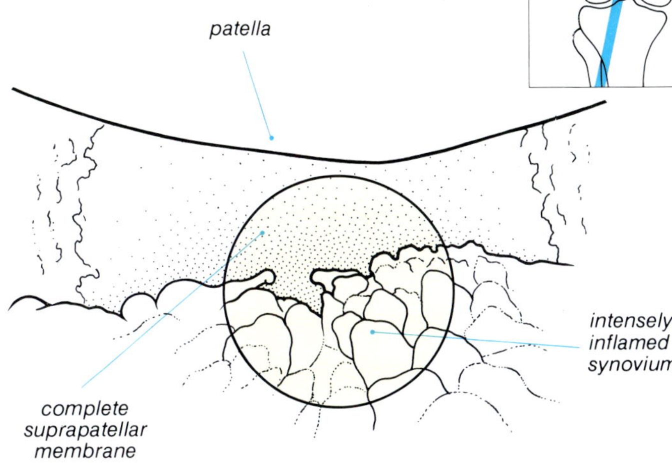

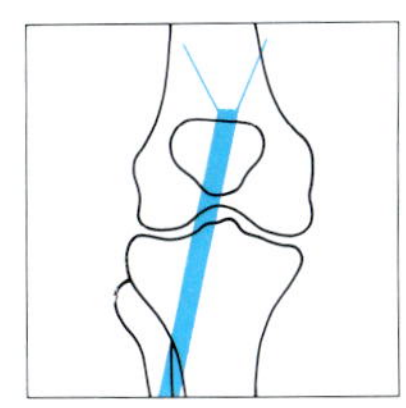

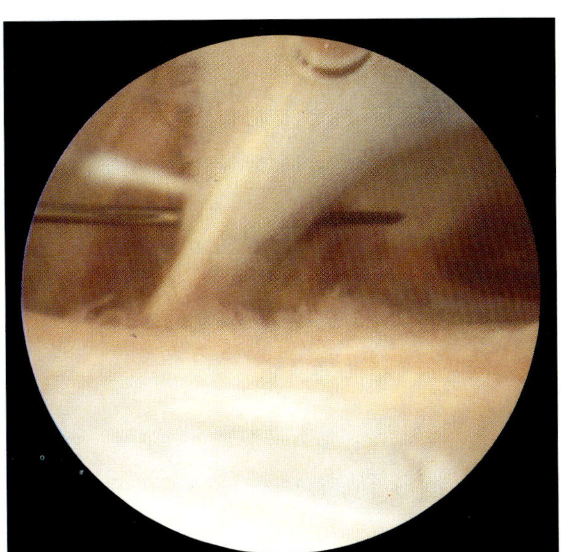

1.10

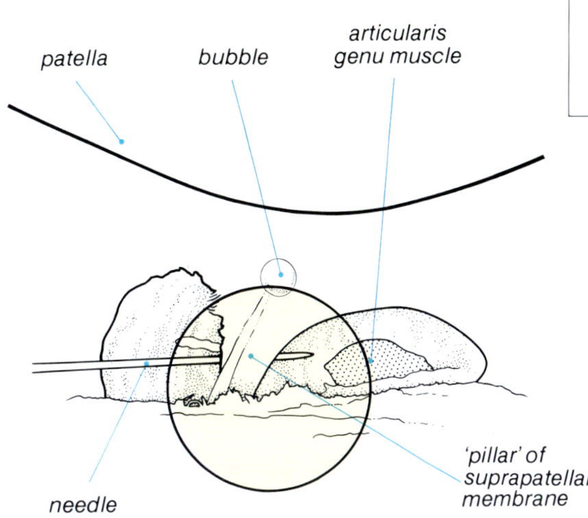

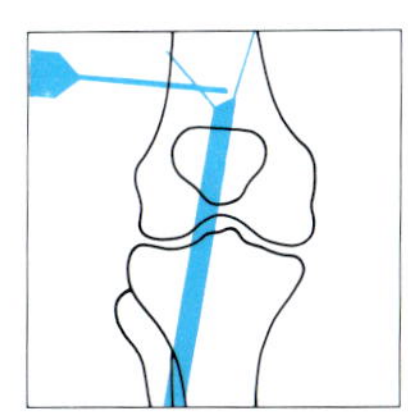

Fig.1.11 also shows a central strand of tissue, but in this knee the strand is lying in the space above the suprapatellar plica and runs into the insertion of the articularis genu muscle. This structure was not part of the medial suprapatellar plica, which was entirely normal, and there was no history of injury to suggest that the strand represented a post-traumatic adhesion.

There is no central strand of tissue in Fig.1.12; instead there is an additional fold of synovium on the lateral side of the knee as well as a stout fibrous edge to a large porta. These patterns each have many other variations.

Medial synovial shelf

The medial synovial shelf (also known as the plica synovialis mediopatellaris, Aoki's ledge and Iino's band) runs in the coronal plane from the medial side of the synovial cavity to the infrapatellar fat pad so that it sweeps over the medial femoral condyle when the knee is flexed, much as an eyelid sweeps over the orbit. Like the medial suprapatellar plica, the medial synovial shelf probably represents a phylogenetic or embryonic vestige that may once have divided the patellofemoral joint from the tibiofemoral. The medial synovial shelf is sometimes simply referred to as the 'plica', which is nothing more than the Latin for 'fold' and does not distinguish the medial synovial shelf from the medial suprapatellar plica, the infrapatellar fold or from any other folds of synovium in the knee. To avoid ambiguity and confusion it is preferable to refer to the plica synovialis mediopatellaris as the medial synovial shelf.

The medial synovial shelf is a normal structure of very variable appearance and may even be entirely absent. If the shelf is not present, its site is usually represented by a narrow ridge of synovium. In the knee in Fig.1.13 there are two ridges which indicate the course in which the shelf would have run if present.

In other knees, the shelf is represented by a very narrow strip of tissue. In Fig.1.14 the shelf is no more than 1mm wide but is quite definitely present. The shelf can be seen running into the infrapatellar fat pad anteriorly, and the patella can be seen above it with a small irregularity on its facet.

Unlike the medial suprapatellar plica, the medial synovial shelf is associated with symptoms. Many attempts have been made to determine the precise incidence of the medial synovial shelf and to distinguish

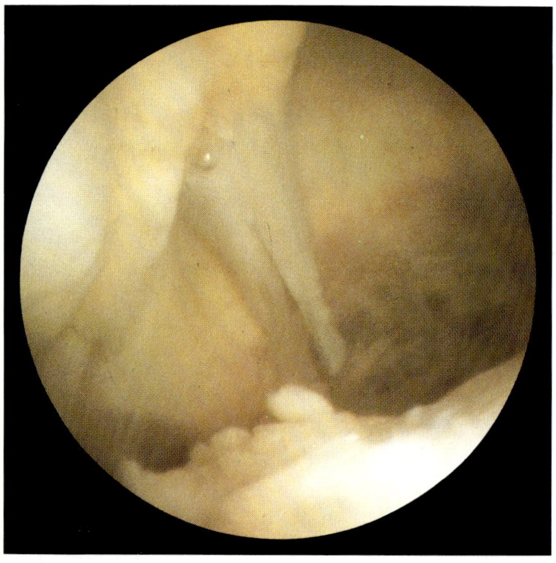

1.11

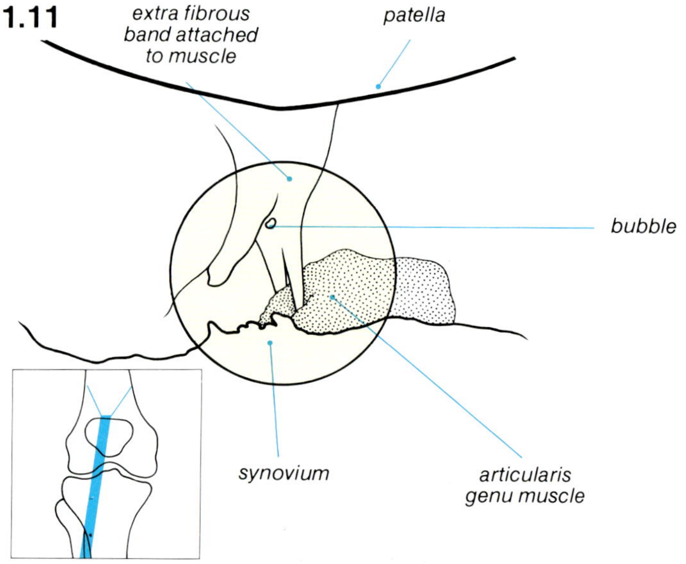

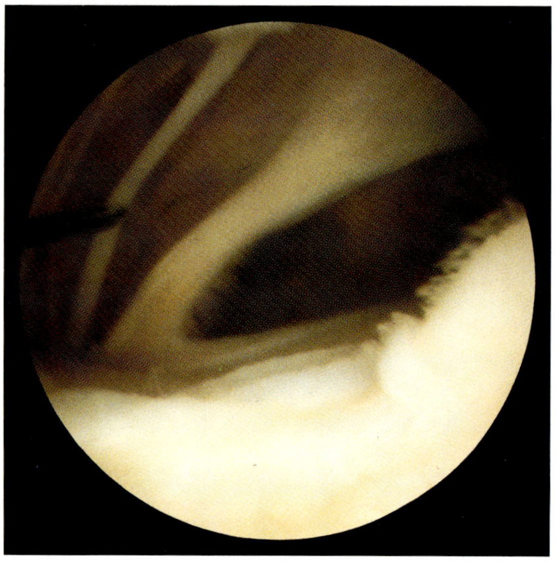

1.12

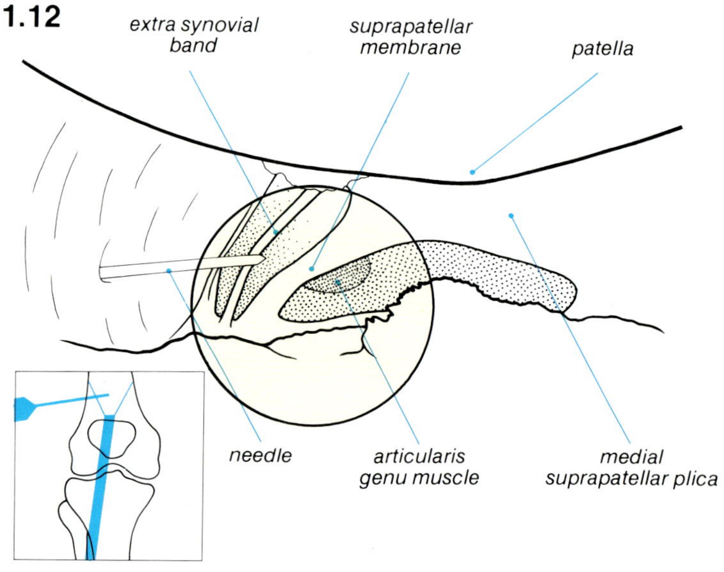

those which cause symptoms from those which do not. Unfortunately, the medial synovial shelf varies in appearance so much that it is not possible to classify shelves usefully on the basis of their size alone, although attempts have been made to do so on the assumption that the broadest shelves are the most likely to cause symptoms.

The shelf shown in Fig. 1.15 is unusually wide and has a sharp knife-like edge. The photograph was taken with the knee in almost full extension and the shelf lying lightly upon the medial femoral condyle. The femoral condyle is smooth and the shelf is neither inflamed nor fibrotic, but it is easy to imagine how such changes could cause irritation when the shelf is stretched as the knee is flexed.

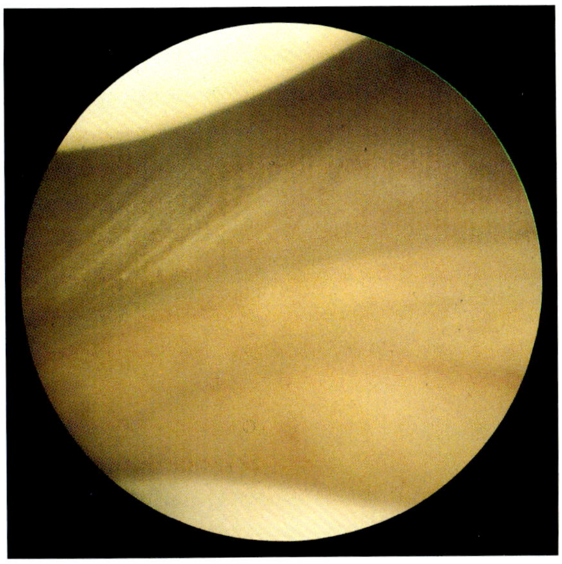

1.13

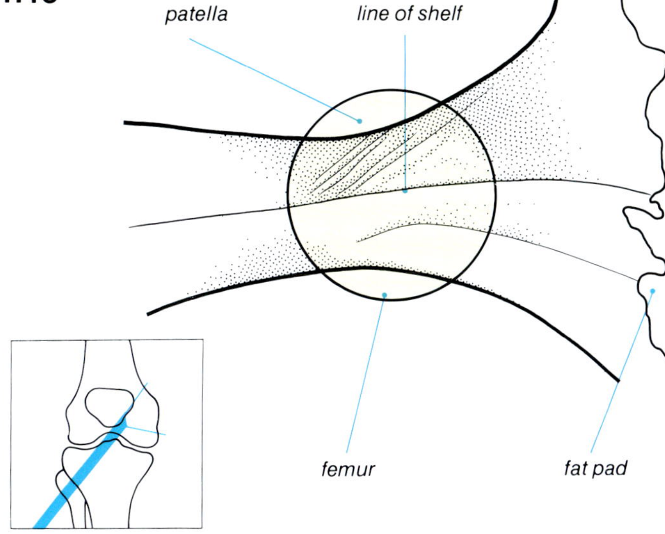

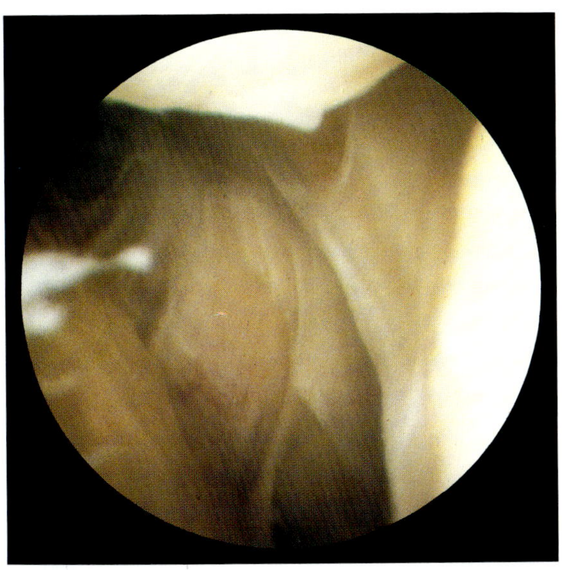

1.14

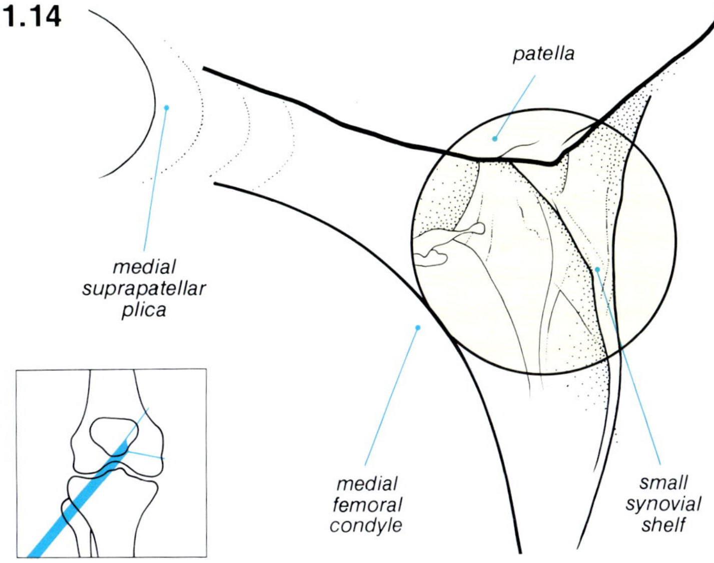

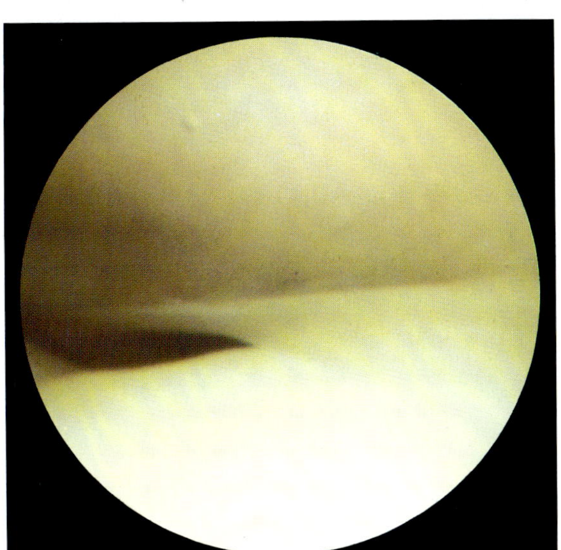

1.15

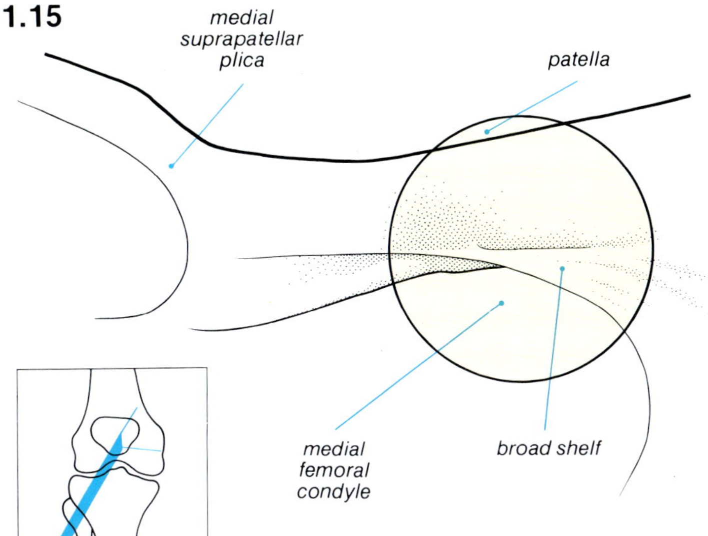

Fig.1.16 shows another shelf which is tightly stretched over the femoral condyle with the knee flexed to about thirty degrees. The shelf is thicker than in Fig.1.15 and its tension is readily apparent. It is not difficult to appreciate how an irregularity of the femoral condyle could give rise to a click or snap, or even to a painful arc of flexion when the tightly stretched shelf crosses over an irregularity in the femoral condyle.

Although the relationship of the synovial shelf to the medial femoral condyle can be understood from the anterolateral approach, it is most clearly seen from the lateral suprapatellar approach. Fig.1.17 shows a wide

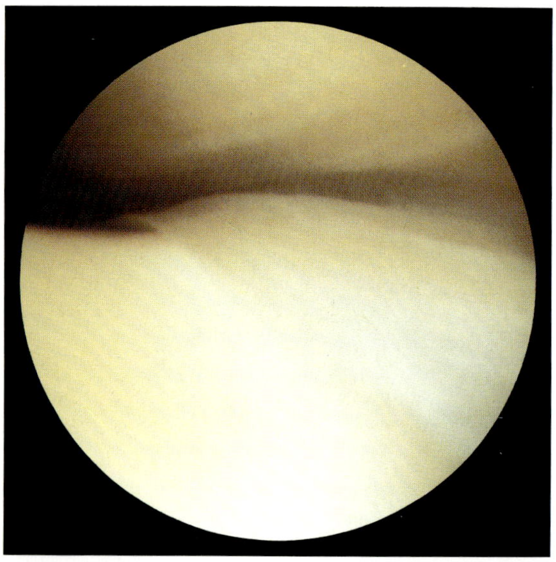

1.16

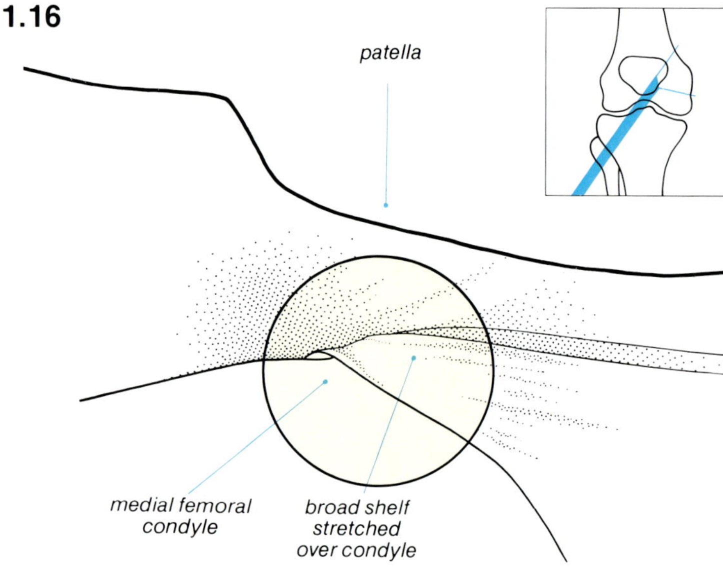

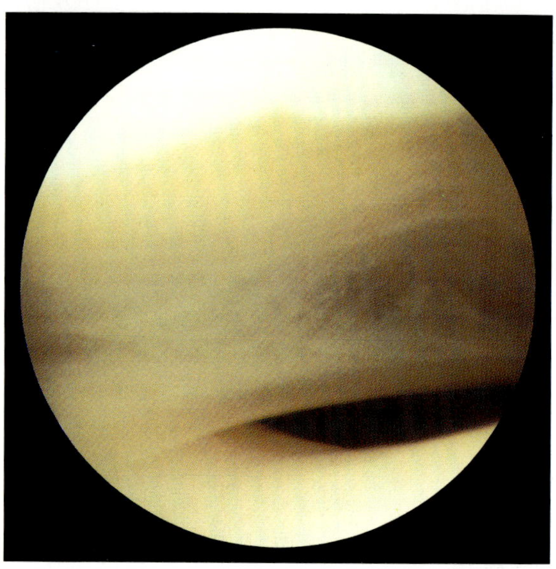

1.17

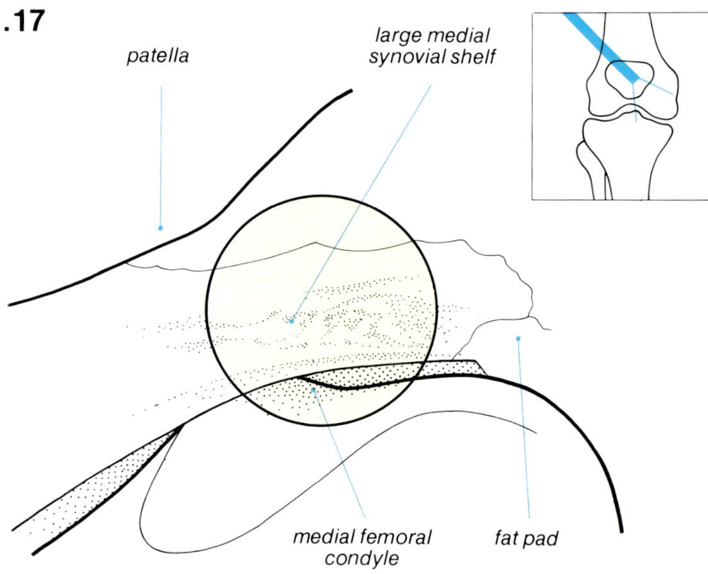

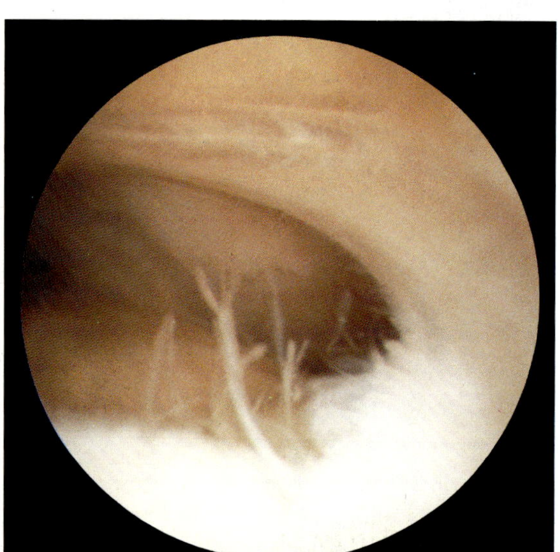

1.18

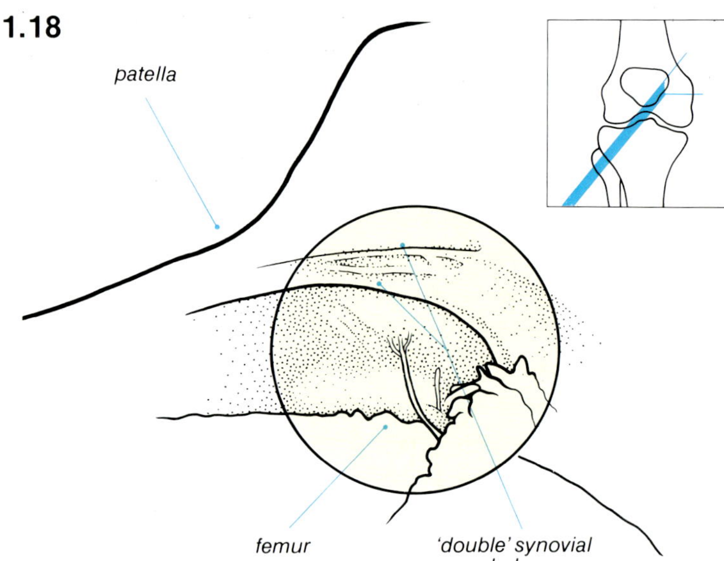

shelf with a marked fibrotic edge sweeping across the medial femoral condyle into the infrapatellar fat pad. This picture clearly demonstrates that the shelf does not insert into the anterior horn of the medial meniscus, as has sometimes been stated.

The anatomy of the medial synovial shelf, like that of the medial suprapatellar plica, is extremely variable. Not only may the shelf vary in width but it may also be reduplicated. In Fig.1.18 a 'double' shelf is present. The lower of the two shelves is the larger and above it can be seen a narrower shelf running parallel. When two shelves are present, the lower is invariably the larger of the two. Very rarely, three parallel shelves may be seen, diminishing in size with the lowest, or most posterior, the largest.

The shelf may also vary in position. While the shelf is usually placed in such a position that it will lie across the femoral condyle when the knee is extended (Figs.1.15 & 1.17), a much higher position is sometimes noted, as seen in Fig.1.19 in which the shelf is lying almost vertically, close to the medial margin of the patella. Such folds do not present a true shelf-like appearance but resemble a pocket and because of their situation, they cannot be stretched over the femoral condyle as the knee is flexed. The margins of such 'shelves' are usually tight and fibrotic and may be affected by synovitis. Vertical shelves of this type are so placed that they may be responsible for localized synovial irritation. In Fig.1.19 an area of pannus is seen extending across the inferomedial margin of the patella, perhaps due to repeated contact with the medial femoral condyle in full flexion. These vertical shelves are also in a position to trap small loose bodies, which can be caught behind the shelf and come to lie in the position of the bubble shown in Fig.1.19.

The shelf is sometimes perforated in such a way that only its firm fibrous edge remains intact. Such a perforated shelf is shown in Fig.1.20 in which the shelf is replaced by a tight fibrous band running straight across the femoral condyle. This pattern is sometimes referred to as a 'chorda'. Because the chorda is tethered only at each end and has no restraining influence on its medial side, it tends to run in a straight line rather than a curve and therefore lies more centrally on the femoral condyle. Because of this central position, a chorda is more likely to cause a click or snap on flexion than will an intact synovial shelf. In addition, the chorda may apply localized traction to the synovium which may result in localized synovitis on the chorda itself (Fig.1.20).

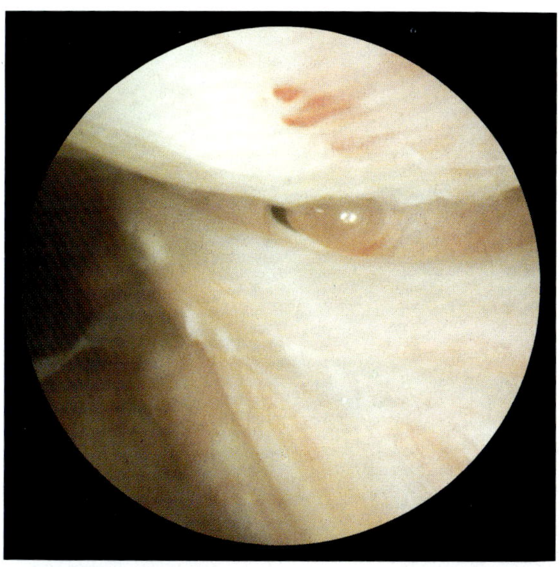

1.19

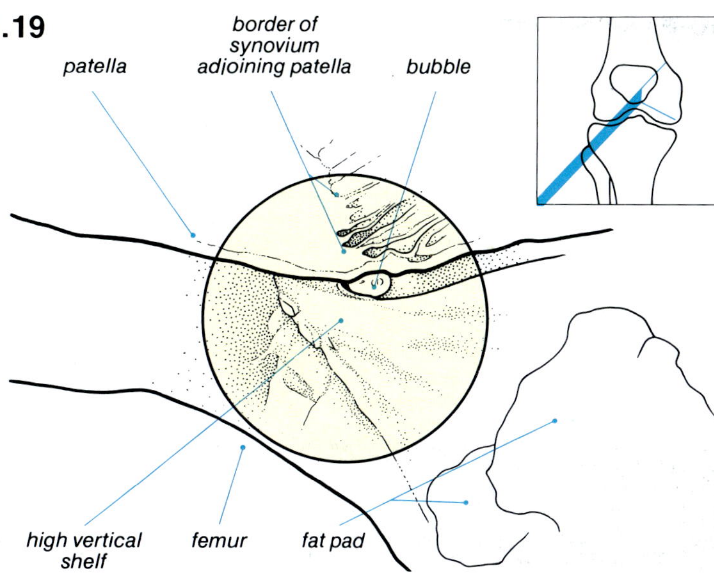

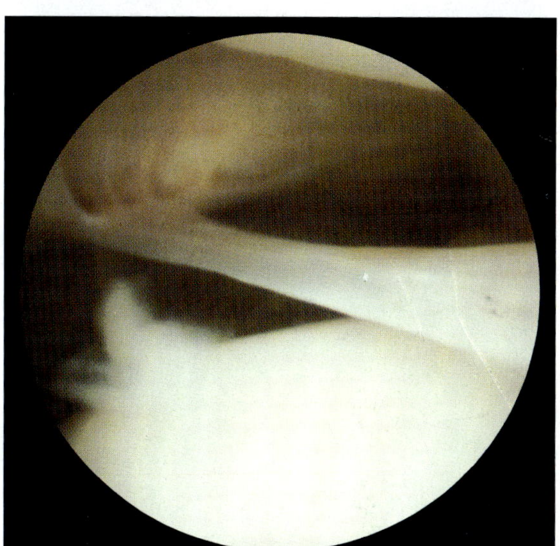

1.20

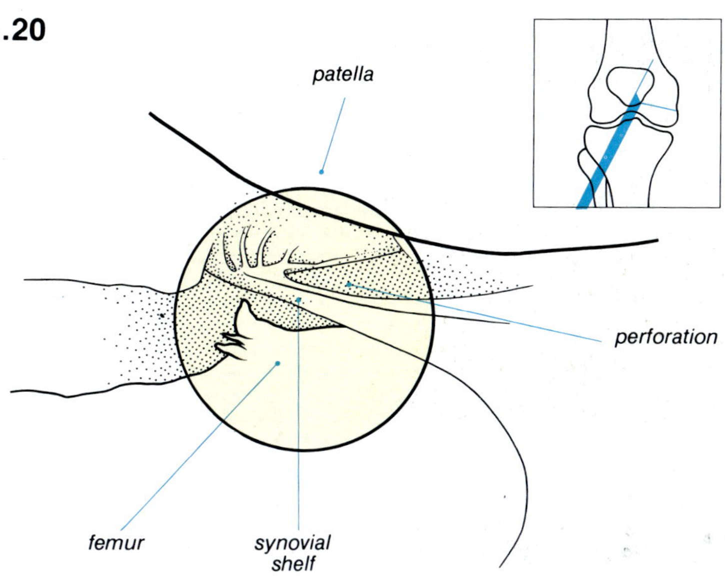

Not every chorda is represented by a tight fibrous band; some appear as a broader structure, often with a fringe of synovial fronds along the proximal border. Fig.1.21 shows a border which is less tight and flimsy and appears much softer and more synovial in character. These 'soft' shelves are perhaps more likely to cause the aching and tenderness of synovial irritation than the mechanical symptoms of the fibrous chorda in Fig.1.20. The more vertical shelves of the type shown in Fig.1.19 may also be fenestrated (Fig.1.22). This appearance is quite unusual and its relationship to symptoms is unclear. The patient suffered from anterior knee pain, had slight irregularity on the articular surface and was tender over the medial synovial shelf. The symptoms were not relieved by excision of the shelf.

Some authors have suggested that the medial suprapatellar plica and the medial synovial shelf are continuations of the same structure; although this configuration may exist, diligent search has as yet failed to find an example. A more common arrangement is for the two folds to cross each other more or less at right angles, as in Fig.1.23 where the uppermost end of the medial synovial shelf can be clearly seen as a separate structure beyond the medial suprapatellar plica, crossing the latter at approximately ninety degrees. This appearance is unusual and only seen if the medial synovial shelf is both broad and unusually long, but it does serve to demonstrate the relationship of these two quite distinct folds.

In Fig.1.24 the synovium above the suprapatellar plica is unusually smooth, but two parallel ridges are seen on the medial wall of the joint. The ridges bear a strong

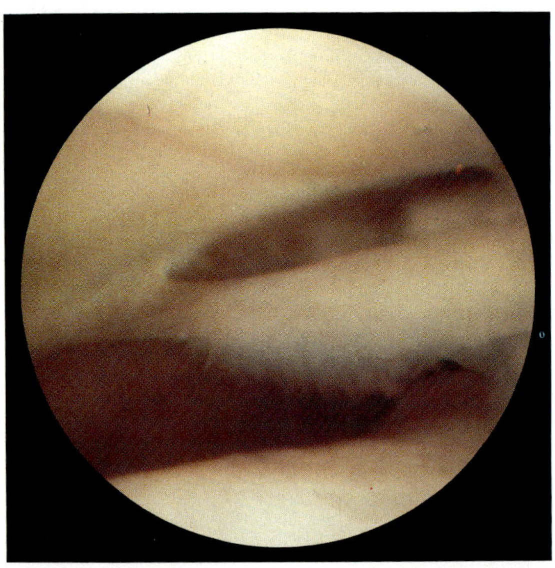

1.21

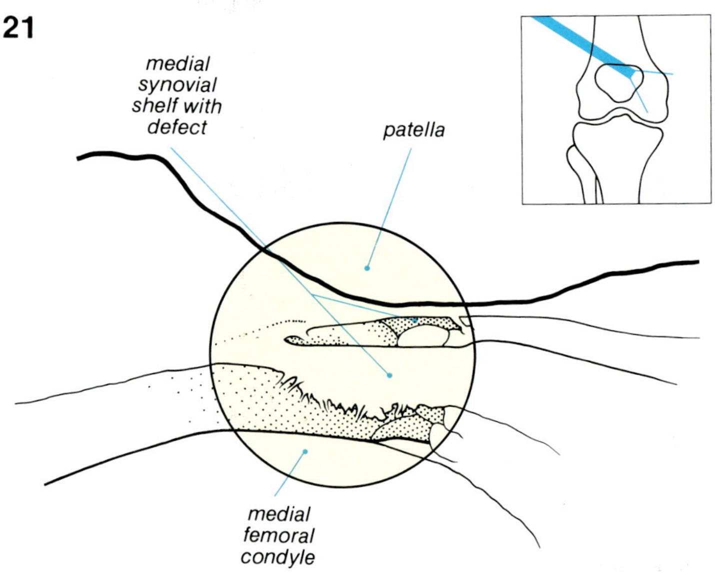

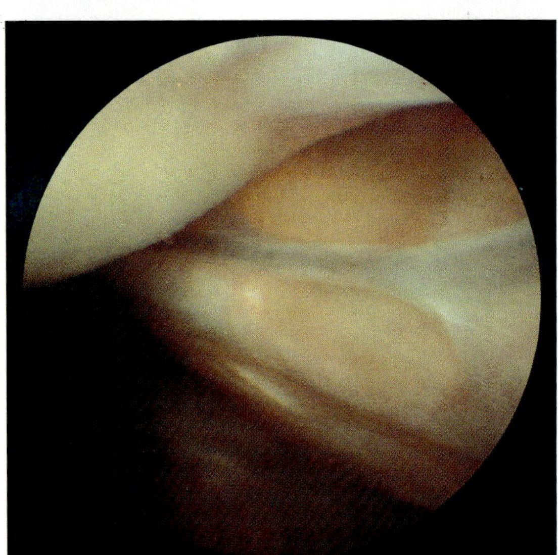

1.22

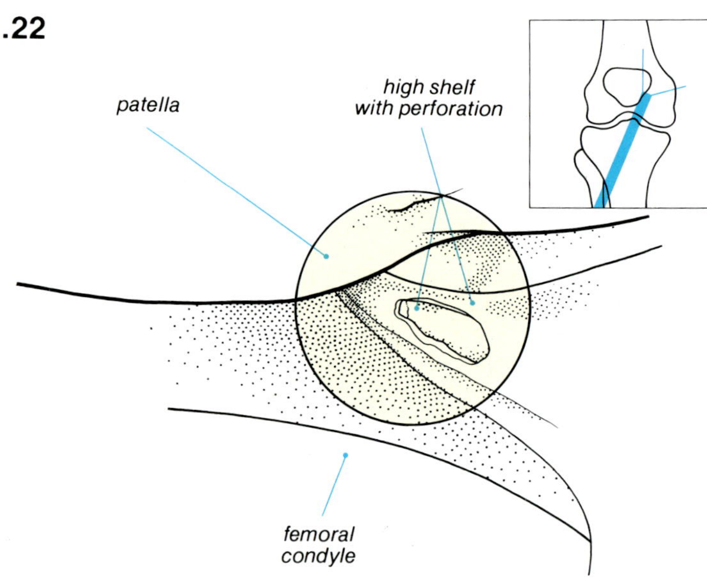

resemblance to the medial synovial shelf but in this patient were quite separate from the shelf and did not have the typical shelf-like appearance of Fig. 1.23.

The synovium in the suprapatellar pouch (Fig. 1.25) normally has a vertical and horizontal distribution of blood vessels rather like a gridiron. Fig. 1.25 was taken, like most of the others in this volume, with the leg elevated and a tourniquet applied and inflated but without exsanguination of the limb. The latter diminishes the vascular markings and gives the synovium a blanched appearance which elevation alone does not.

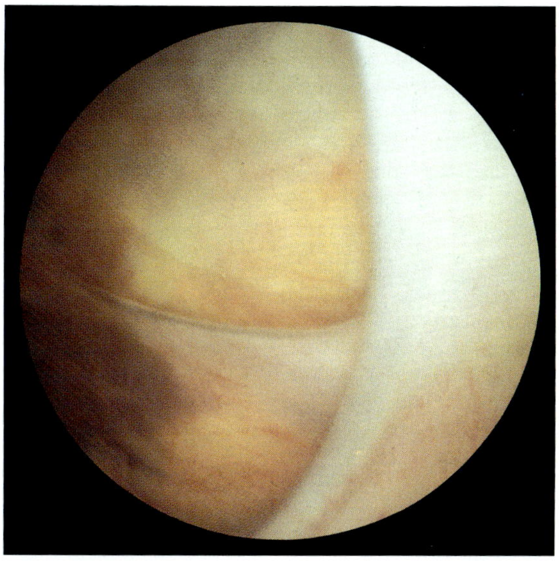

1.23

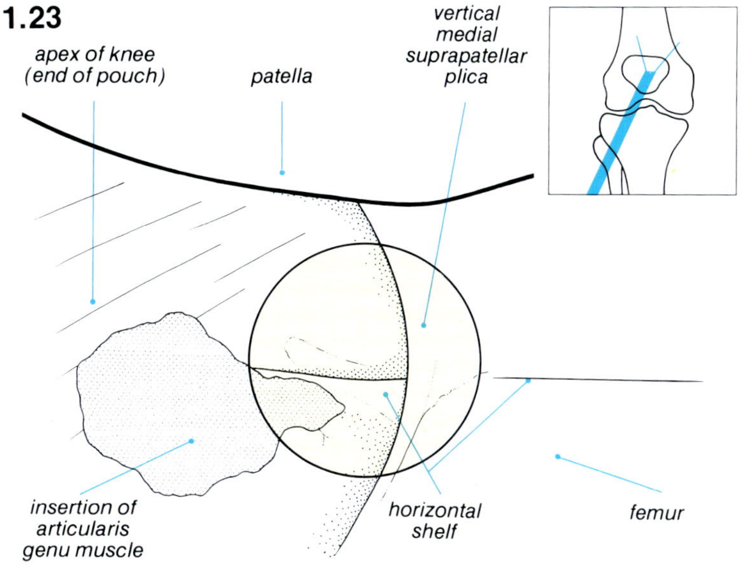

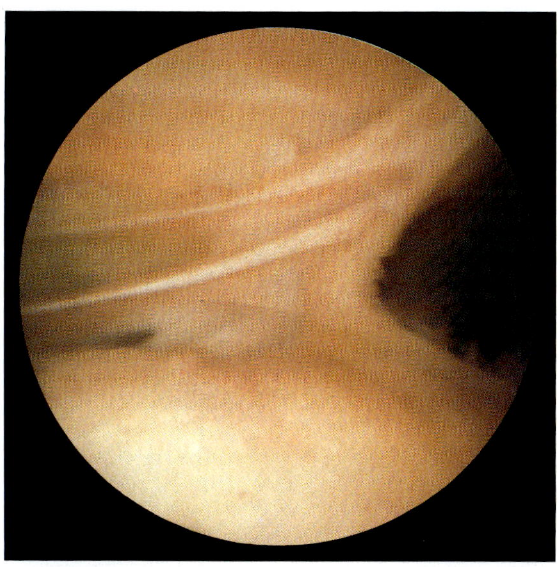

1.24

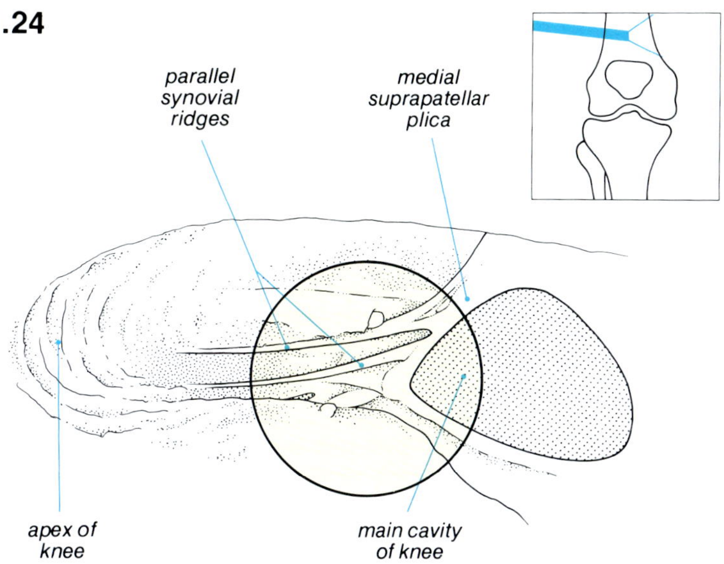

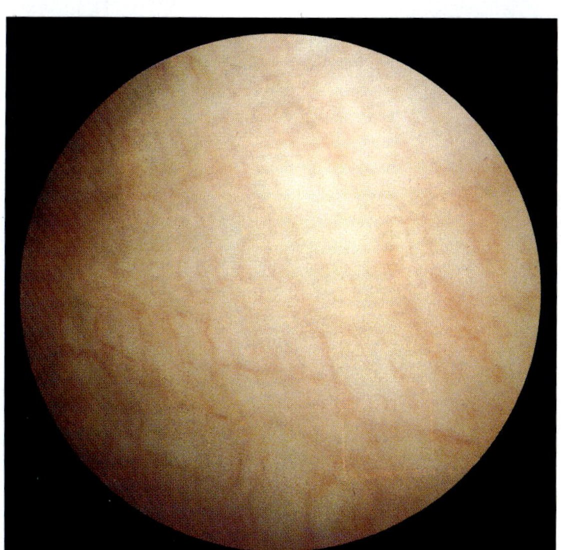

1.25

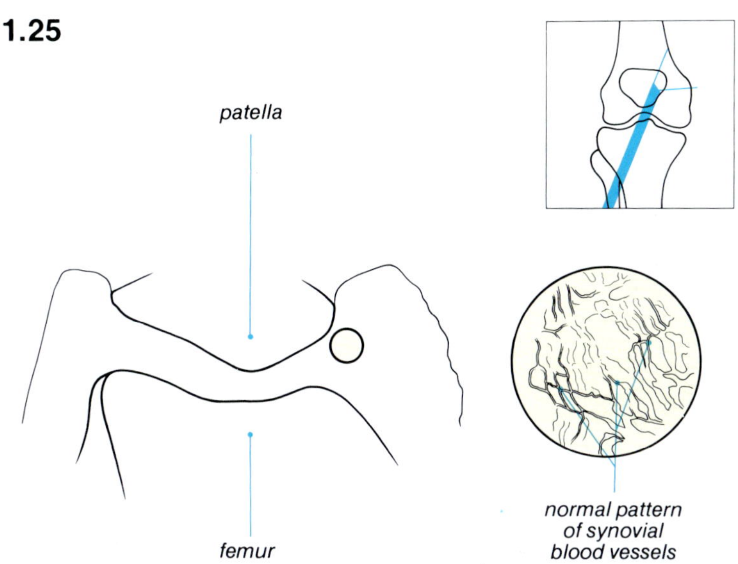

PATELLOFEMORAL JOINT

The patellofemoral joint is a difficult structure to examine with an arthroscope because its surface lies so close to the lens of the instrument and because the presence of the arthroscope and distension of the joint distorts the normal relationships of the structures.

The patellar surface is most easily assessed by moving the patella from side to side over the tip of the arthroscope so that the joint surface is 'swept'. Although this technique allows the entire surface to be inspected, it is still not possible to include the entire width of the patellofemoral joint in a single arthroscopic view.

When the patellofemoral joint is examined from below, it can be seen that the lateral facet is closely applied to the femur and lies slightly lateral to the centre of the intercondylar groove while the medial facet rises more steeply than the lateral (Fig.1.26). The medial facet is in contact with the femur in flexion, but this relationship cannot be seen with the arthroscope.

The patellofemoral joint can also be examined from above to demonstrate the relationship of the patella to the femur and the infrapatellar fat pad. In Fig.1.27 the lateral placement of the patella on the femur can be clearly seen as the median ridge of the patella lies well lateral to the centre of the intercondylar groove. The infrapatellar fat pad lies like a tongue between the patella and the femur, moving in and out of the patellofemoral joint as the knee is flexed and extended.

MEDIAL GUTTER

In systematic examination of the knee, the suprapatellar pouch is usually followed by the medial gutter. After thorough inspection of the suprapatellar pouch, including the medial synovial shelf, the tip of the arthroscope can be rolled round the medial femoral condyle as the knee is flexed.

On leaving the suprapatellar pouch the arthroscope will come to lie in the medial gutter where a fold of synovium may be seen passing from the medial femoral condyle to the capsule of the knee. This fold (Fig.1.28) is not one of the synovial 'plicae' normally described but is nevertheless a constant finding and has a counterpart in the lateral gutter (see Fig.1.71). The fold marks the boundary between the suprapatellar pouch above, the medial gutter below and the posteromedial compartment posteriorly. It has a spiral appearance, necessary because of its movement which can be felt against the bone on the medial side of the knee during flexion and extension.

When the arthroscope is moved downwards from the synovial fold (Fig.1.28), the superior meniscosynovial junction is seen. The appearance of the junction changes according to the stresses applied to the knee, the degree of ligamentous laxity and the state of the synovium. In Fig.1.29 the knee is lying in a neutral position with no valgus strain. The meniscosynovial junction therefore appears to be closed, without any obvious defect

1.26

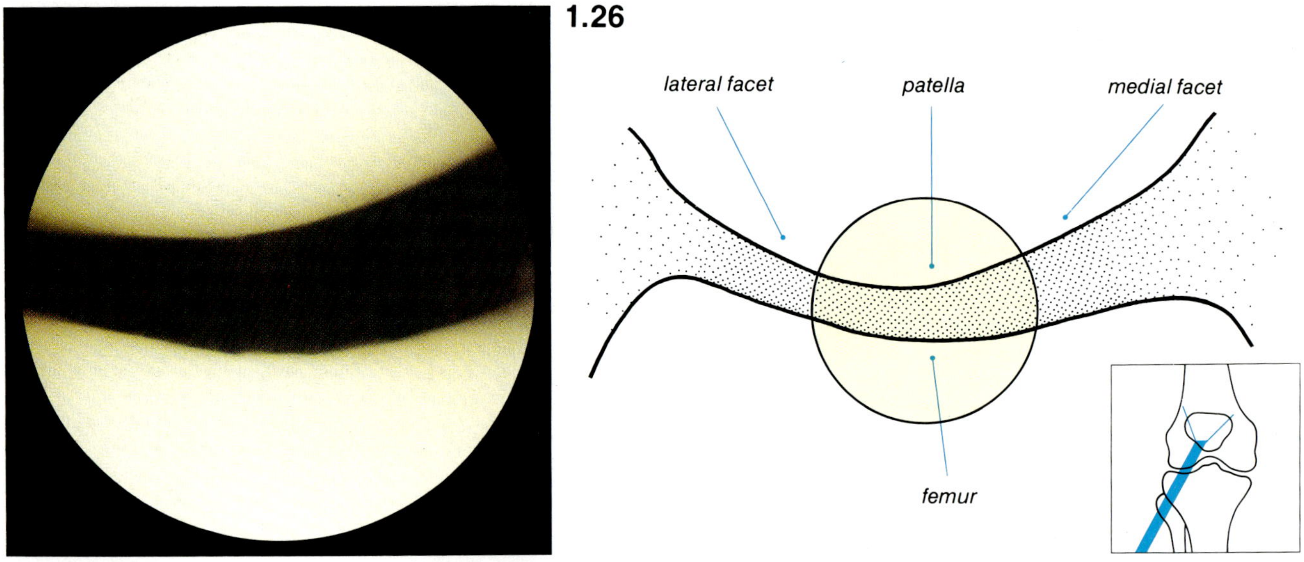

1.27

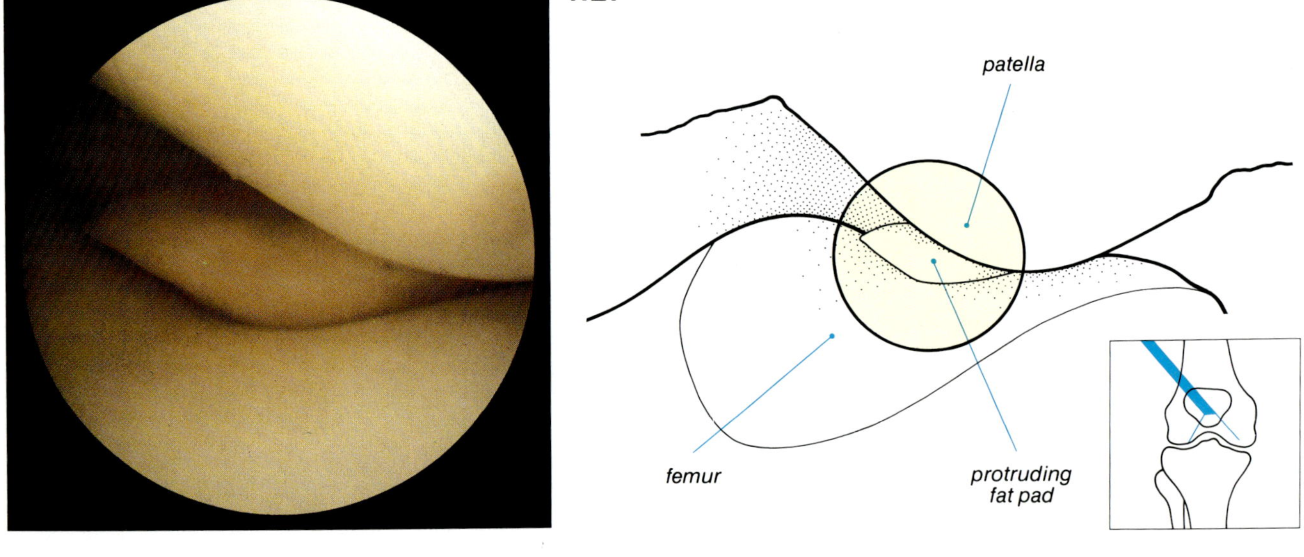

between the meniscus and the synovium. When a valgus strain is applied to the same knee, a deep groove appears between the meniscus and the synovium overlying the medial capsule. This groove (Fig. 1.30) is sometimes mistaken for a peripheral detachment of the meniscus during arthrography when the contrast medium may pool in the groove and give the appearance of a meniscal tear.

In Figs. 1.29 and 1.30 the synovium does not show inflammatory change but appears as a smooth even surface. If synovitis is present, the synovium becomes thickened and swollen, overlapping the meniscus and making it difficult to assess the integrity of the meniscosynovial junction without the use of a probing needle or a hook inserted through a second incision.

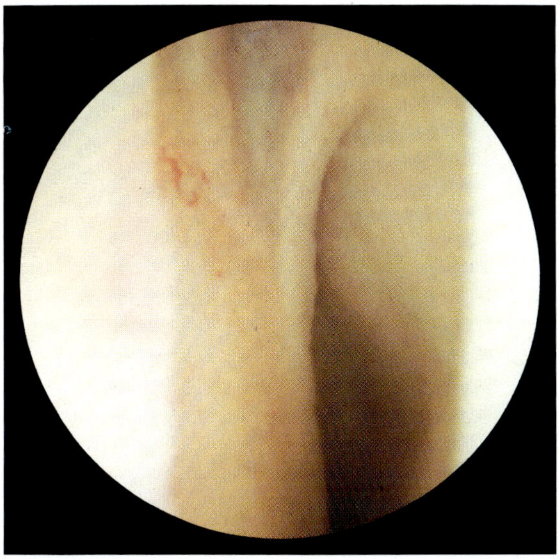

1.28

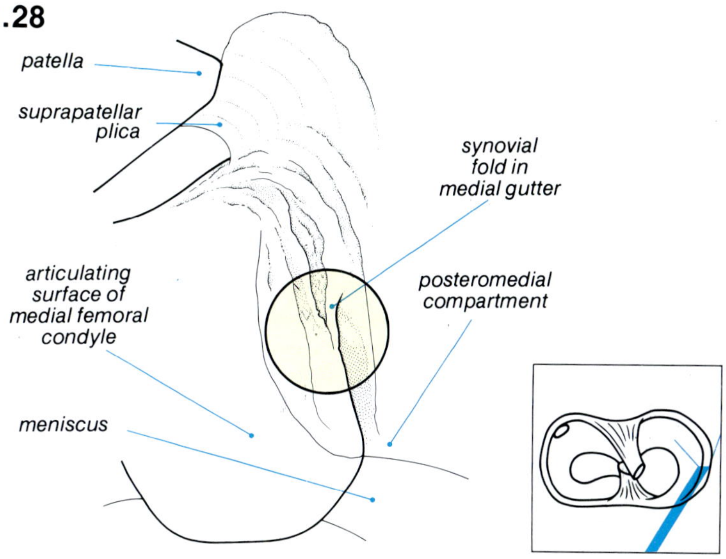

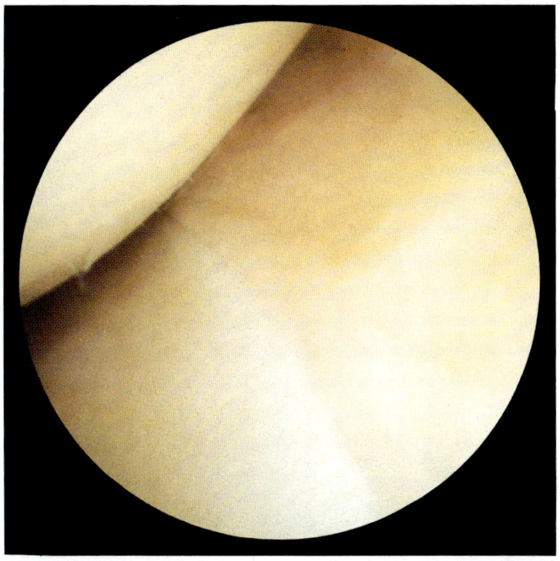

1.29

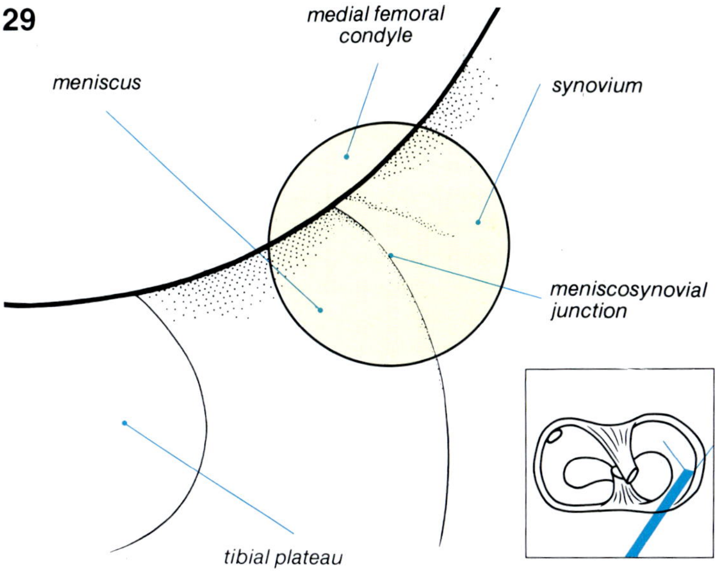

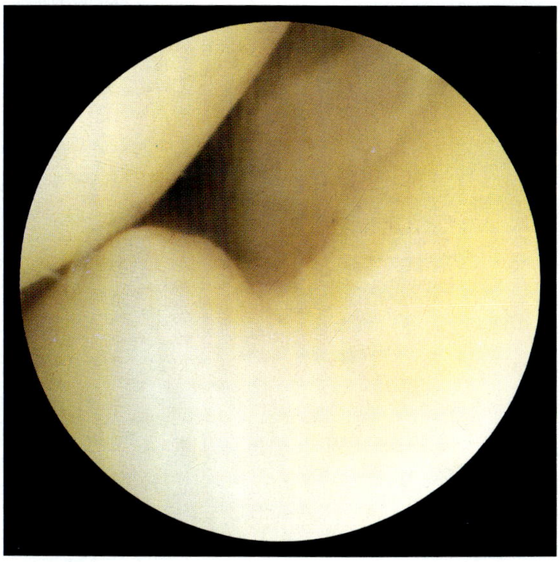

1.30

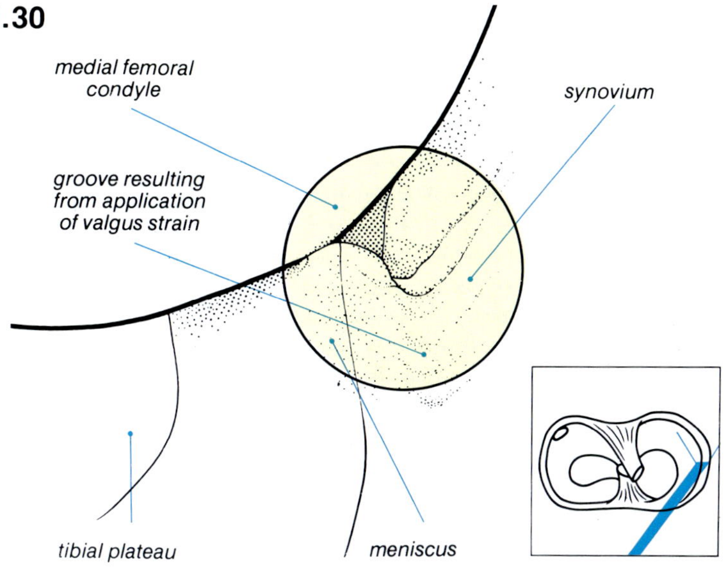

If the arthroscope is passed further back into the medial gutter, the meniscus will be seen sweeping behind the condyle and away from the capsule that forms the medial wall of the knee. At this point the firm fibrous consistency of the capsule and the medial ligament gives way to the softer tissues that form the medial wall of the posteromedial compartment and may present the appearance in Fig. 1.31 in which the posterior third of the medial meniscus leaves its medial attachment to lie behind the medial femoral condyle. This change in attachment of the meniscus may well act as a stress raiser and influence the pattern of tears in the posterior third of the medial meniscus. In the lateral compartment the popliteus tendon lies in a similar position and influences the pattern of lateral meniscal tears, as will be demonstrated later.

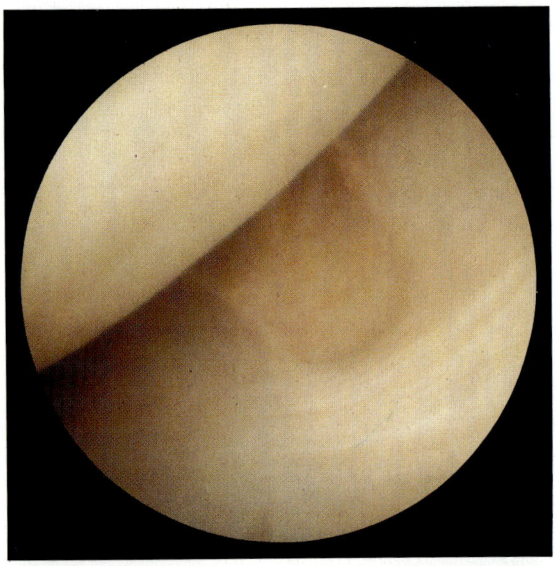

1.31

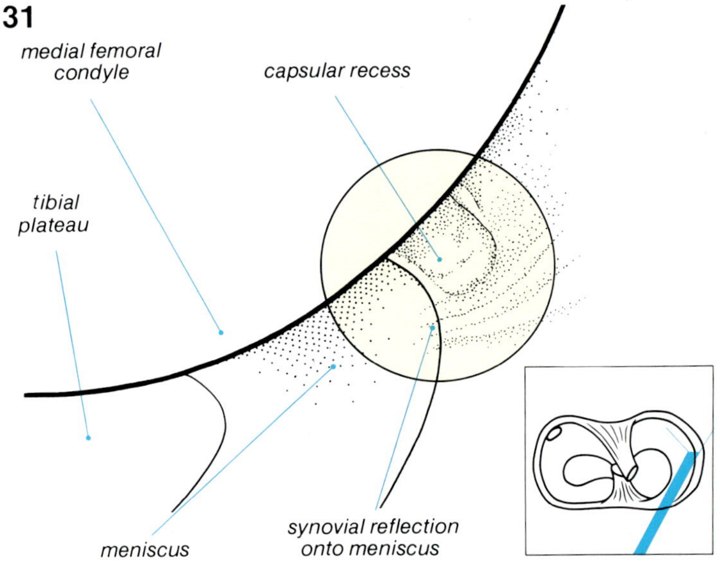

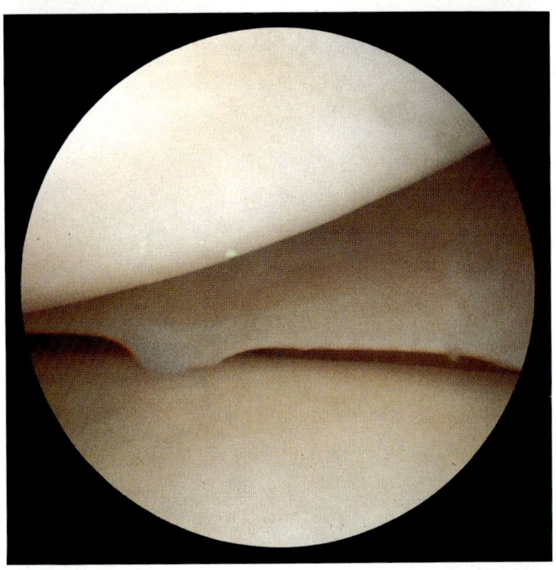

1.32

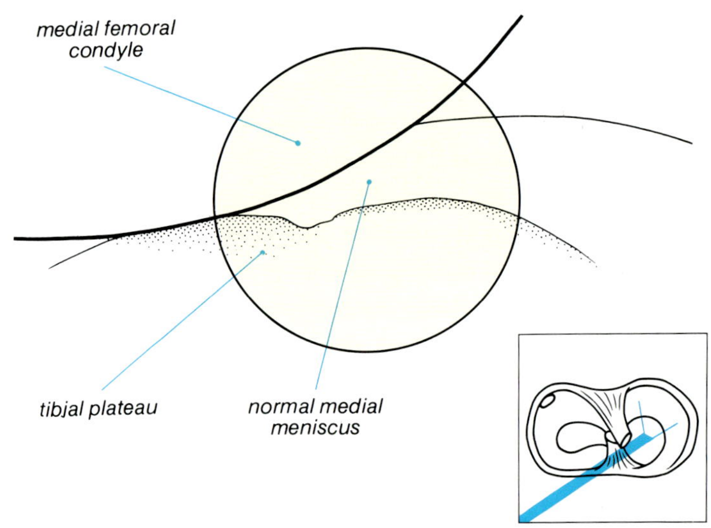

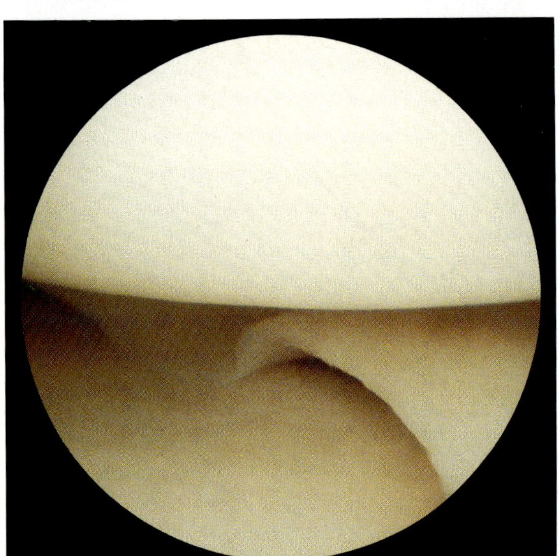

1.33

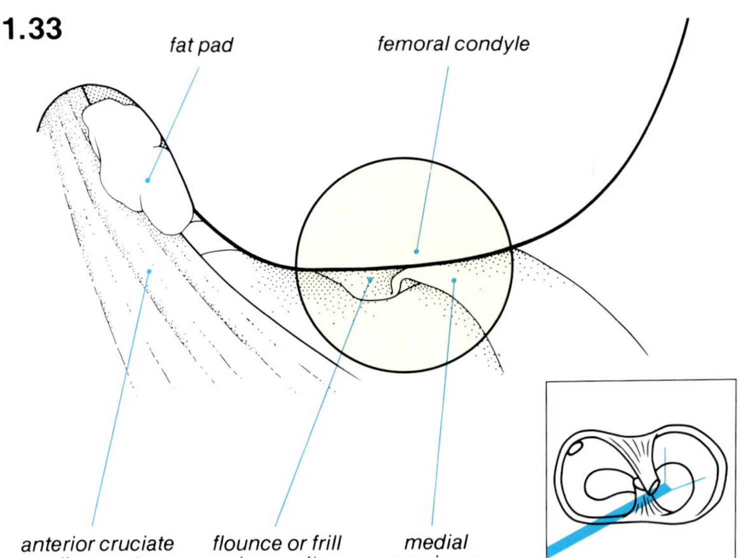

MEDIAL COMPARTMENT

After inspecting the medial gutter the tip of the arthroscope can be withdrawn to lie in the medial compartment, bringing the free margin of the medial meniscus into view. This is usually seen as a knife-like edge but will present slight irregularities in the older patient. The meniscus moves with the tibia during flexion and rotation of the knee but when relaxed will lie roughly parallel to the tibial plateau. In Fig. 1.32 the meniscus is lying slightly above the tibial plateau with a slight downward curve in the meniscal margin, but the meniscus is basically flat and relaxed.

Any sideways or rotational stress applied to the knee will, via the capsule and the medial ligament, influence the relative positions of the medial meniscus and the tibial plateau. In Fig. 1.33, a valgus and external rotational strain has been applied to the knee in thirty degrees of flexion. As a result, a frill or flounce occurs exactly opposite the point at which the meniscus sweeps away from the medial wall of the knee to lie behind the femoral condyle (Fig. 1.31). The flounce is not an indication of a meniscal tear but is a normal feature of variable size and is most marked in knees with lax ligaments. The flounce will also be unusually large and prominent if there is a tear in the posterior third of the meniscus, and evaluation of the integrity of the meniscus with a probing hook and needle is of particular importance if posterior horn tears are not to be missed.

Although the superior meniscosynovial junction is easily seen, the undersurface of the meniscus can only be examined with the help of a probing needle or hook. In Fig. 1.34 a needle has been passed beneath the meniscus to enter the knee at the inferior meniscosynovial junction which is clearly intact. Unlike the superior meniscosynovial junction, which varies greatly according to the strain upon the knee, the inferior meniscosynovial junction has a much more constant appearance and abnormal mobility usually indicates injury to the medial ligament rather than generalized ligamentous laxity.

The posterior attachment of the medial meniscus to the tibia can be difficult to see but will almost invariably come into view if a valgus and external rotational strain is applied to the knee in thirty degrees of flexion. The posterior horn is most easily seen in patients with small bones and generalized ligamentous laxity and is most difficult in patients with large bones, tight knees and a prominent tibial spine.

Fig. 1.35 shows the posterior attachment of the medial meniscus from the anterolateral approach. If the posterior horn cannot be identified from this approach for the reasons mentioned above, the anteromedial or central approach must be used.

Immediately above the posterior horn of the medial meniscus lies the entrance to the posteromedial compartment (Fig. 1.35) which is bounded by the

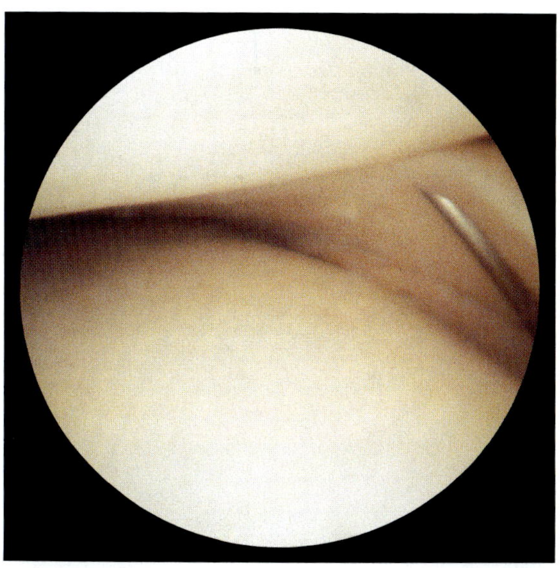

1.34

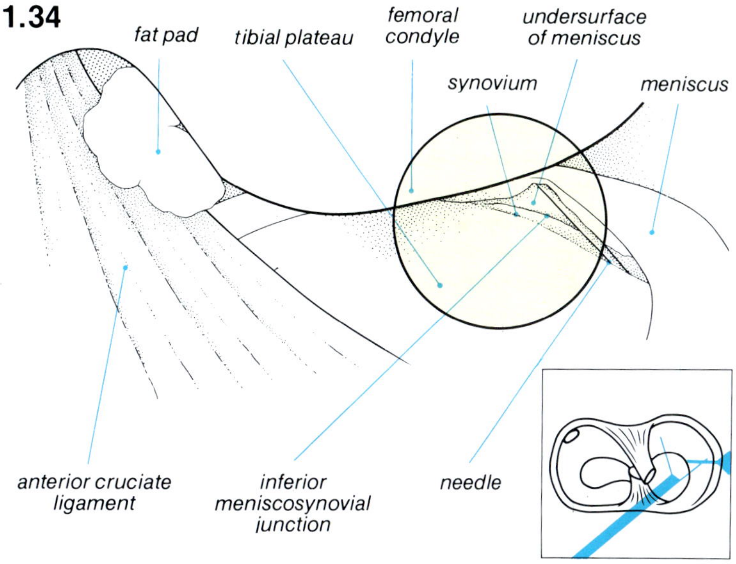

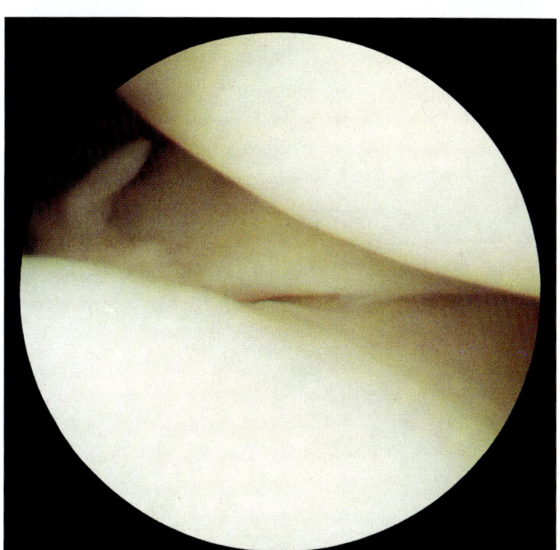

1.35

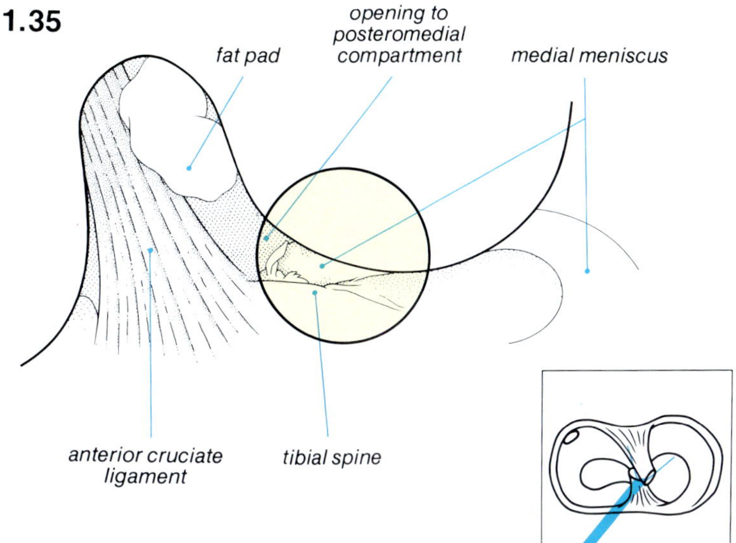

posterior cruciate ligament laterally, the femoral condyle above and medially, and the posterior horn of the medial meniscus below. The opening to the posteromedial compartment is large enough to accommodate a 5mm arthroscope if correctly inserted and aligned.

The medial femoral condyle presents a smooth appearance like a billiard ball (Figs.1.32-1.34) but an irregularity is often seen at the front of the medial compartment at the point where the medial femoral condyle comes into contact with the anterior horn of the medial meniscus in full extension. The lesion consists of a small ridge of heaped up synovium and articular cartilage that is firmly impacted against the anterior horn in full extension but lifts away in slight flexion. Fig.1.36 shows such an 'impingement' lesion in the position of full extension, with the small cushion of abnormal synovium resting against the anterior horn of the medial meniscus. In Fig.1.37, which shows the same knee as in Fig.1.36, the knee has been flexed slightly and the ridge lifted slightly away from its previous position to reveal a small depression behind it. The patient illustrated in Figs.1.36 and 1.37 was a nineteen-year-old girl; there was no sign of degenerative or other articular cartilage change in the knee.

The significance of the impingement lesion is unclear, but it is almost certainly involved as a cause of symptoms in the synovial shelf syndrome when the lesion comes into contact with the synovial shelf as the knee is flexed. The contact between a tight synovial shelf (see Fig.1.16) with a lesion such as in Fig.1.37 is very likely to cause clicking, catching and pain as the shelf moves over the irregularity of the articular cartilage. Some authors have reported a lesion of the articular cartilage in patients with the synovial shelf syndrome which is probably an impingement lesion seen with the knee flexed. Fig.1.38 shows the lesion with the knee flexed to approximately twenty degrees in a patient who had no synovial shef; if a shelf were present, the ease with which such a lesion would strike its free margin can be imagined.

Figs.1.36 and 1.37 showed the medial meniscus firmly attached to the anterior margin of the tibial plateau so that the femur strikes its anterior horn. In some patients the anterior horn is mobile and rides forward so that the femur comes into contact with the tibial plateau itself, without an intervening meniscus. Such an appearance is sometimes called a 'dislocating anterior horn' and operations have been devised for reattaching the meniscus to its correct position.

Fig.1.39 is of such a 'dislocating anterior horn' with the meniscus lying in front of the tibial plateau. The meniscus is seen using a seventy degree arthroscope inserted from the anterolateral approach. It is the author's opinion that this appearance is not pathological and that the presence of an intact but dislocating anterior horn of the medial meniscus is not invariably an indication for surgical intervention.

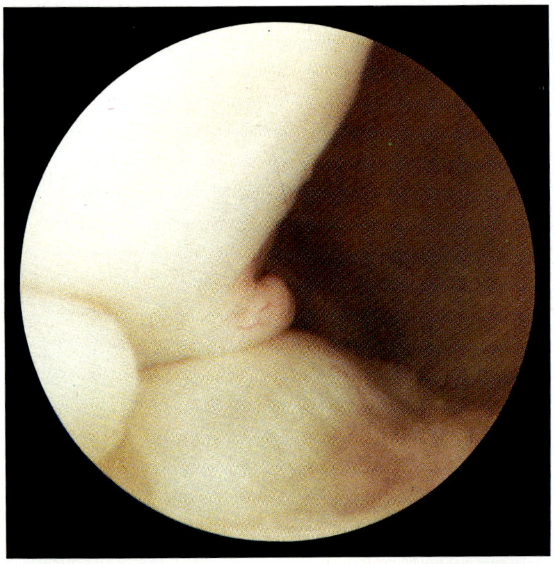

1.36

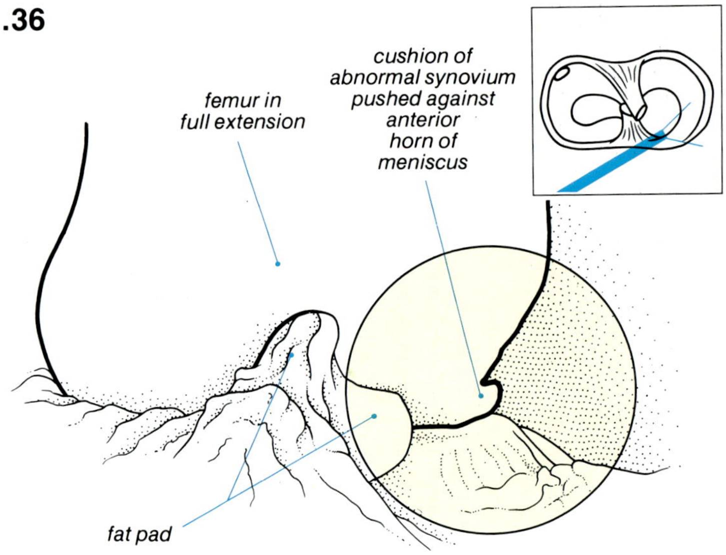

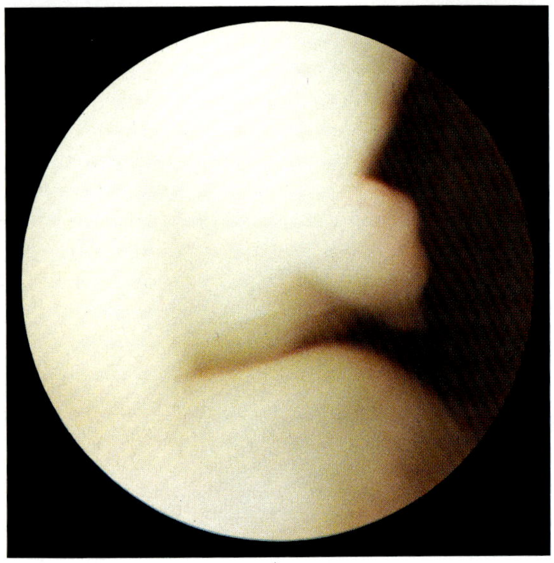

1.37

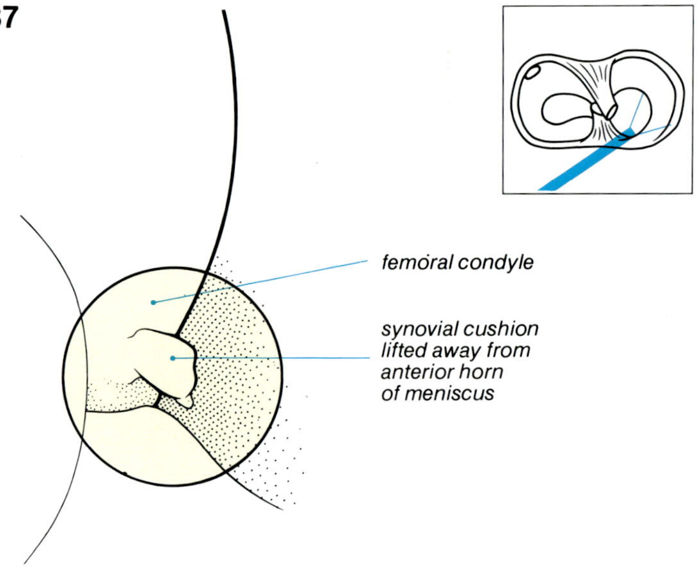

POSTEROMEDIAL COMPARTMENT

The posteromedial compartment can be entered with a 5mm arthroscope passed through the triangle shown in Fig. 1.35 if the knee is flexed to thirty degrees and a valgus and an external rotational strain applied. If osteophytes or a prominent tibial spine prevent entry from this approach, the anteromedial or central approaches must be used. With the tip of the arthroscope lying in the posteromedial compartment and the lens directed medially, the posterior horn of the medial meniscus will be seen attached to the tibia with the synovium sloping downwards and backwards away from the posterior meniscosynovial junction to the floor of the posteromedial compartment (Fig. 1.40).

1.38

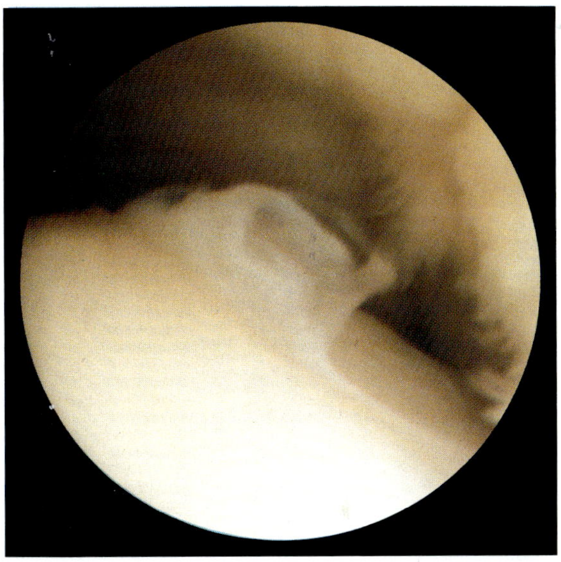

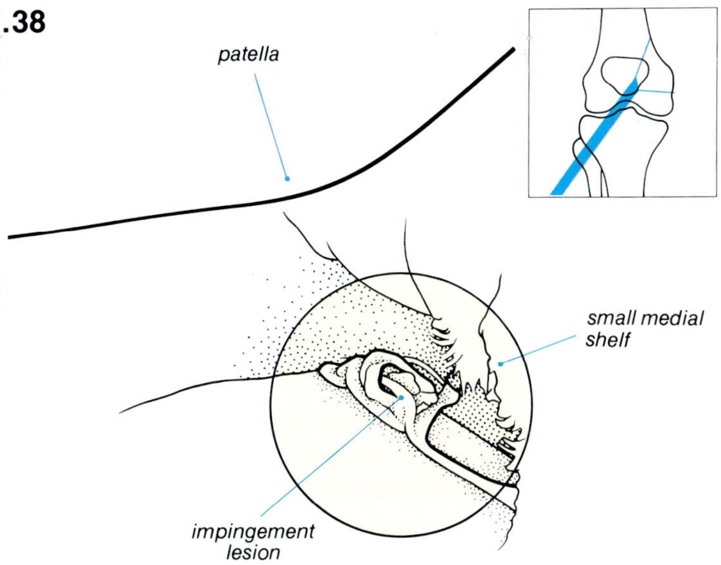

1.39

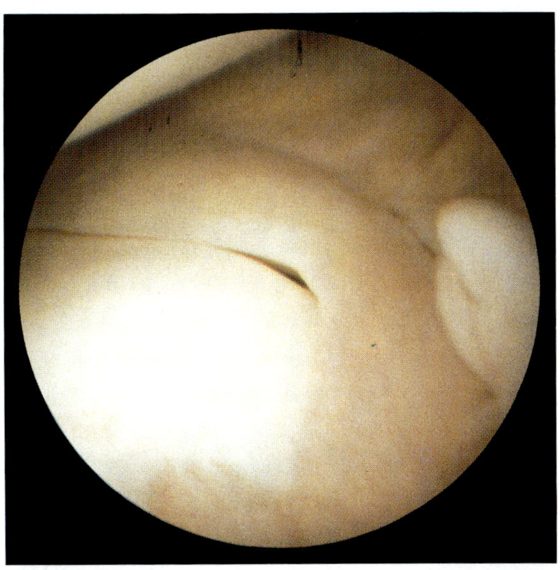

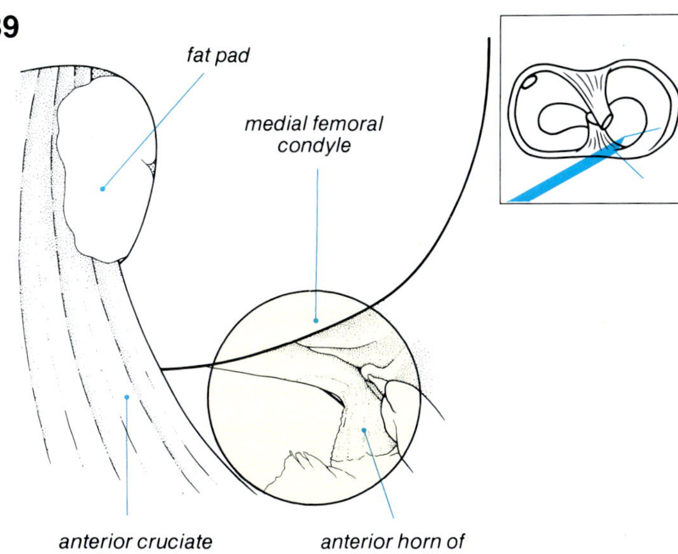

1.40

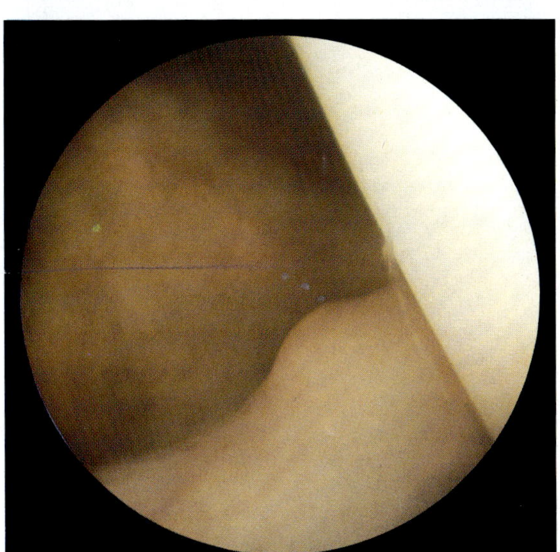

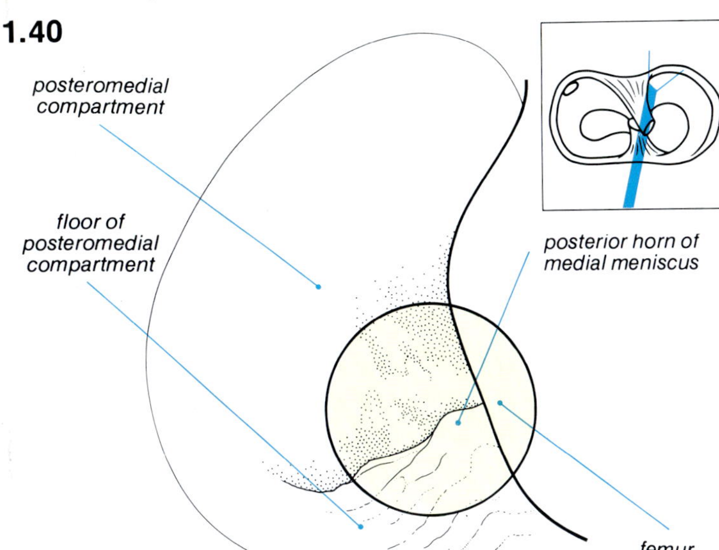

With the arthroscope inserted a little further, the floor of the posteromedial compartment can be seen, sometimes with a small ridge of synovium looking a little like a cockscomb arising from the synovial floor (Fig.1.41). This ridge, although a common finding, is not present in every knee and does not appear to be associated with symptoms. Fig.1.41 also shows the posterior third of the meniscal width lying behind the medial femoral condyle in its normal position.

In Fig.1.42, which shows the posteromedial compartment of a patient with an inflamed synovial fat pad whose symptoms were relieved by excision of the fat

1.41

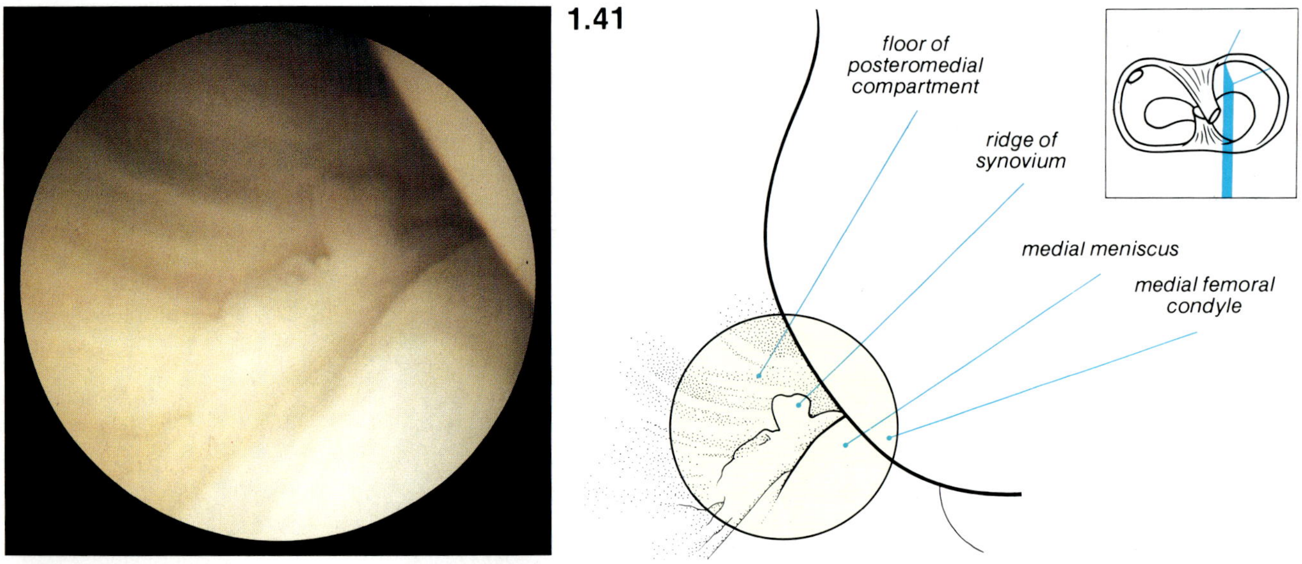

1.42

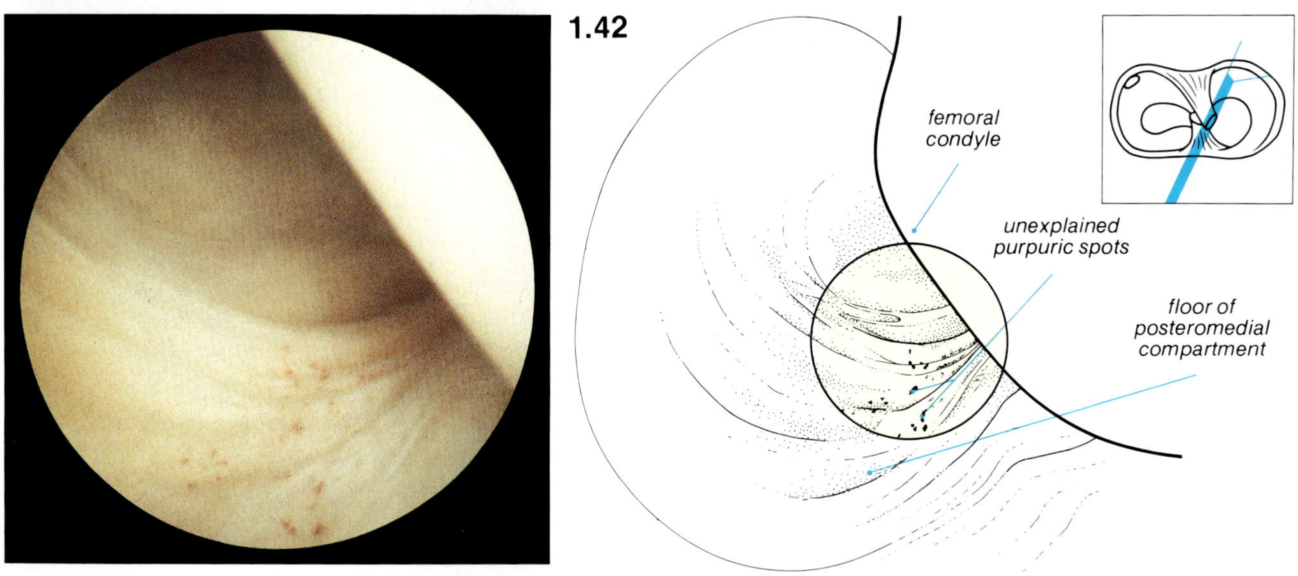

1.43

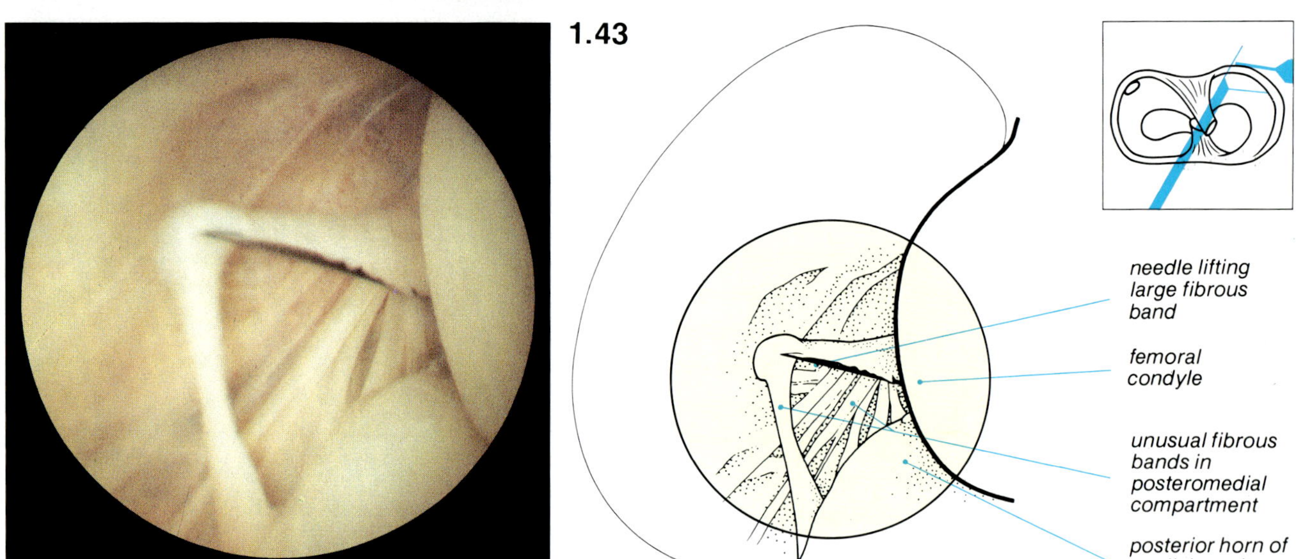

pad, the posteromedial compartment has no cockscomb but its floor bears a line of purpuric spots. These spots are an unusual finding and their significance is not known. Punctate haemorrhages of this type may also be seen around the sites of previous injury, as they are on other serous surfaces such as the peritoneum and pleura. The patient in Fig.1.42 had no history of injury and no explanation is offered for this appearance.

Many unusual appearances can be seen in the posteromedial compartment and one of these is shown in Fig.1.43. In this patient there was a collection of parallel fibrous bands running from the medial wall of the capsule to the back of the meniscus. One of these bands, which is particularly large, lies free, stretching across the compartment and has been lifted with a needle to demonstrate its position. No explanation is offered for these bands, but it is possible that they are due to hypertrophy of the capsule or posterior oblique ligament of the knee.

The posteromedial compartment can also be entered directly from the posteromedial approach. Insertion of the arthroscope directly through the posteromedial corner of the knee is safe provided that the knee is first distended with saline and the correct position of insertion confirmed by probing with a hypodermic needle; if saline runs back through the needle, the tip must be lying in the posteromedial compartment. When this approach is used the instruments should always be inserted with the knee flexed to ninety degrees.

From the posteromedial approach the back of the medial femoral condyle, the posterior surface of the meniscus, the meniscosynovial junction and the posterior cruciate ligament can be seen. These features are shown in Fig.1.44 in which the knee is flexed to approximately ninety degrees. The synovium at the back of the medial meniscus is clearly seen sloping down to the floor of the compartment, and the posterior cruciate ligament is in the background lying in its synovial sleeve.

The posterior cruciate ligament blocks entry into the posterolateral compartment from the posteromedial approach. If the posterolateral compartment can be entered from this side, there must be a deficiency of the posterior cruciate ligament. The ligament is normally covered with synovium, but on close inspection its fibres can be seen lying beneath the synovium. In Fig.1.45 the arthroscope has been passed as far as the posterior cruciate and its lens directed forwards so that it looks into the intercondylar notch from behind. A probing hook has been passed through the intercondylar notch from the anteromedial approach and its tip can be seen lying at the posterior edge of the posterior cruciate ligament, indenting its synovial sheath.

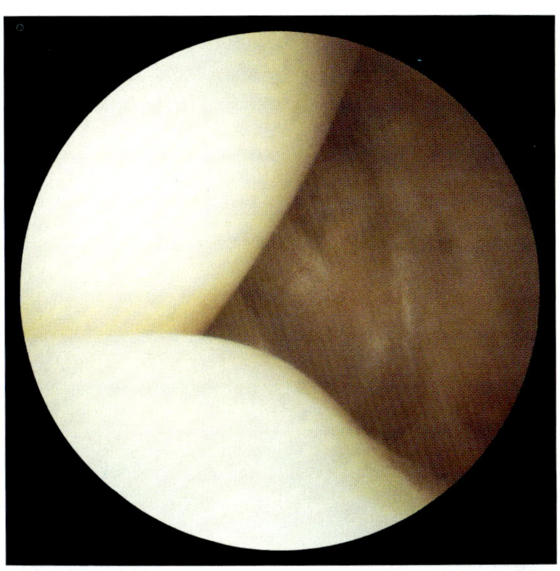

1.44

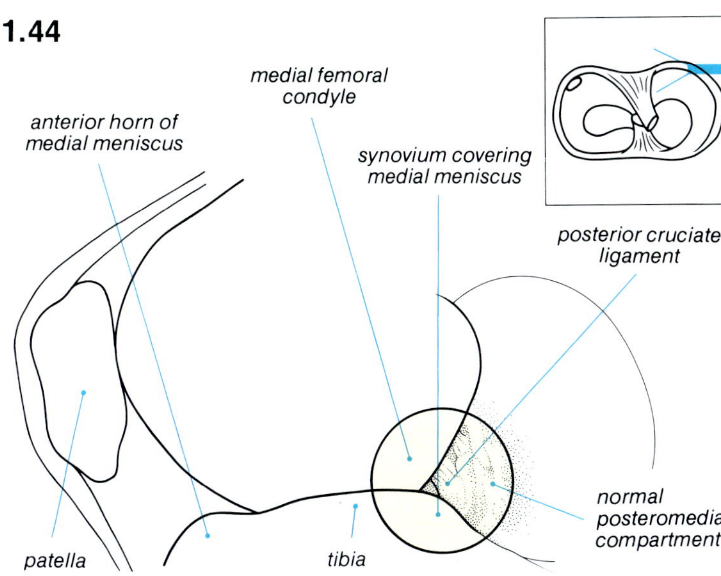

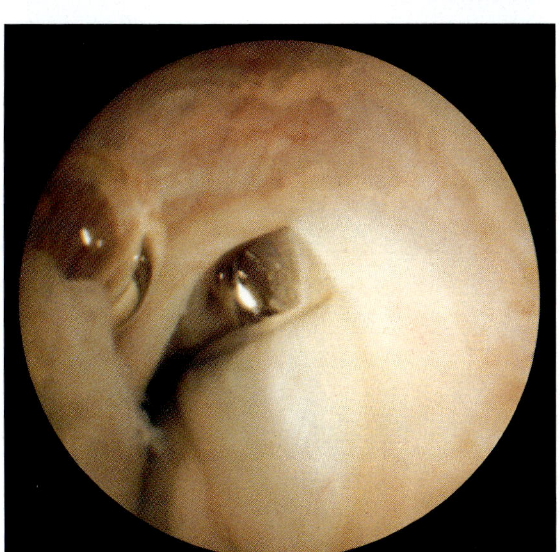

1.45

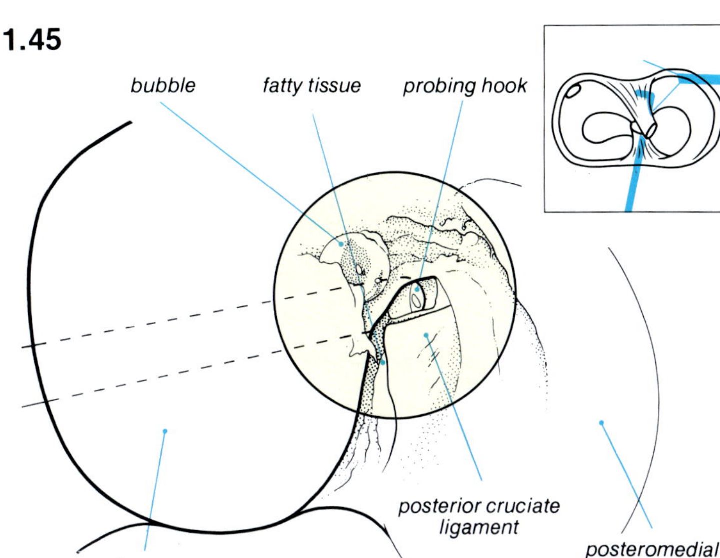

The posteromedial compartment is a comparatively small space and can be distended if the knee is filled with saline in the extended position and then flexed so that the synovium is placed under tension. The result is that the synovium which runs from the reflection of the posterior capsule onto the periosteum at the back of the femur is seen as an arched roof lying proximally. Fig.1.46 was made from the posteromedial approach using a seventy degree telescope looking directly proximally, or upwards, at the reflection of the synovium from the capsule onto the femur. There is a slight alteration in the vascularity of the synovium along the line of the reflection. The synovium appears a little swollen because of a generalized synovitis in the knee.

Fig.1.47 shows the synovial reflection when the knee has not been flexed as fully as in Fig.1.46. The reflection does not run as smoothly from the capsule to the femur and is indented by a short fibrous ridge.

INTERCONDYLAR NOTCH

The intercondylar notch can be a difficult area to examine with an arthroscope. If the arthroscope is inserted from the anterolateral, central or anteromedial approaches, its tip will lie in the intercondylar notch, making it difficult to hold the arthroscope away from the structures to be examined. Because of this the structures in the notch tend to be seen in close-up and their size and appearance can be distorted.

To make the examination even more difficult, the intercondylar notch is not an empty space but contains the anterior and posterior cruciate ligaments, the infrapatellar fold (also known as the ligamentum mucosum and the plica synovialis infrapatellaris), the tibial spine and the fat pad. Fig.1.48 shows the ligamentum mucosum, or infrapatellar fold, at its attachment to the femur. The ligamentum mucosum can be easily distinguished from the anterior cruciate ligament by its flimsy consistency and its insertion into the apex of the intercondylar notch rather than into its posterolateral corner.

The infrapatellar fold is very variable in size and when absent altogether (Fig.1.49) results in the entire anterior cruciate ligament being seen clearly from its tibial to its femoral insertion, an unusual appearance. In other patients, the infrapatellar fold may occupy the entire intercondylar notch as a vertical wall without an opening through which the arthroscope can be passed. Fig.1.50 shows such an infrapatellar fold from the lateral suprapatellar approach. The crescentic fold runs from the femur to the fat pad, which appears as a three-lobed structure. In such patients, the infrapatellar fold can be negotiated by passing the arthroscope above it or directly through it. Alternatively, the arthroscope can be inserted from the anteromedial approach to be passed through the membrane so that the lateral compartment can be examined. Whichever of these techniques is

1.46

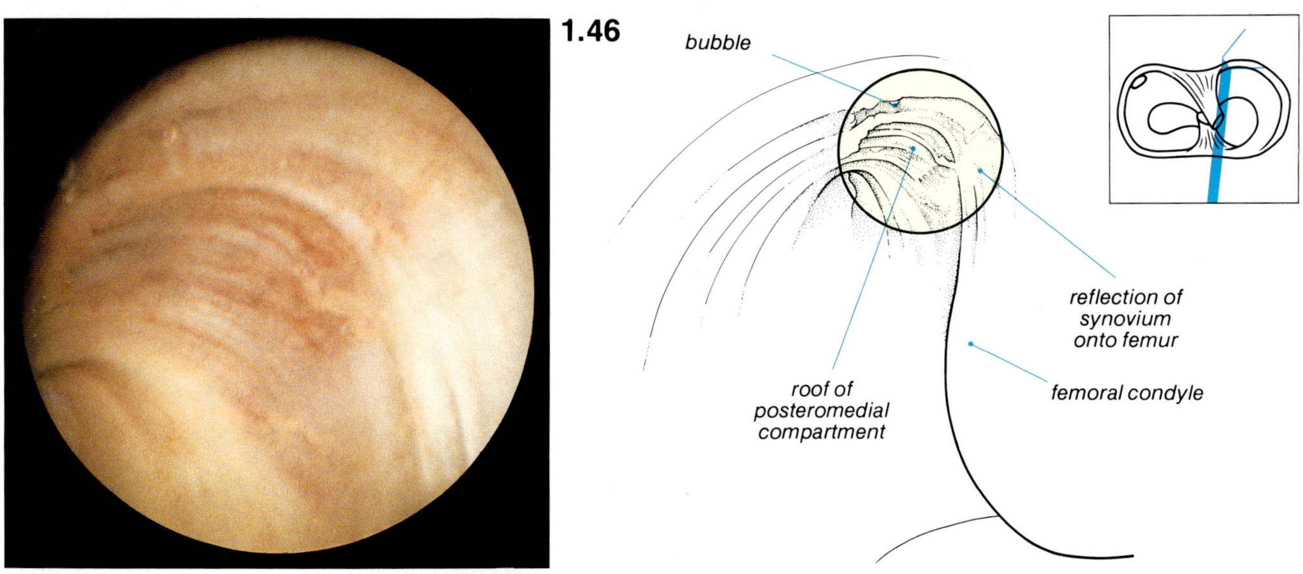

1.47

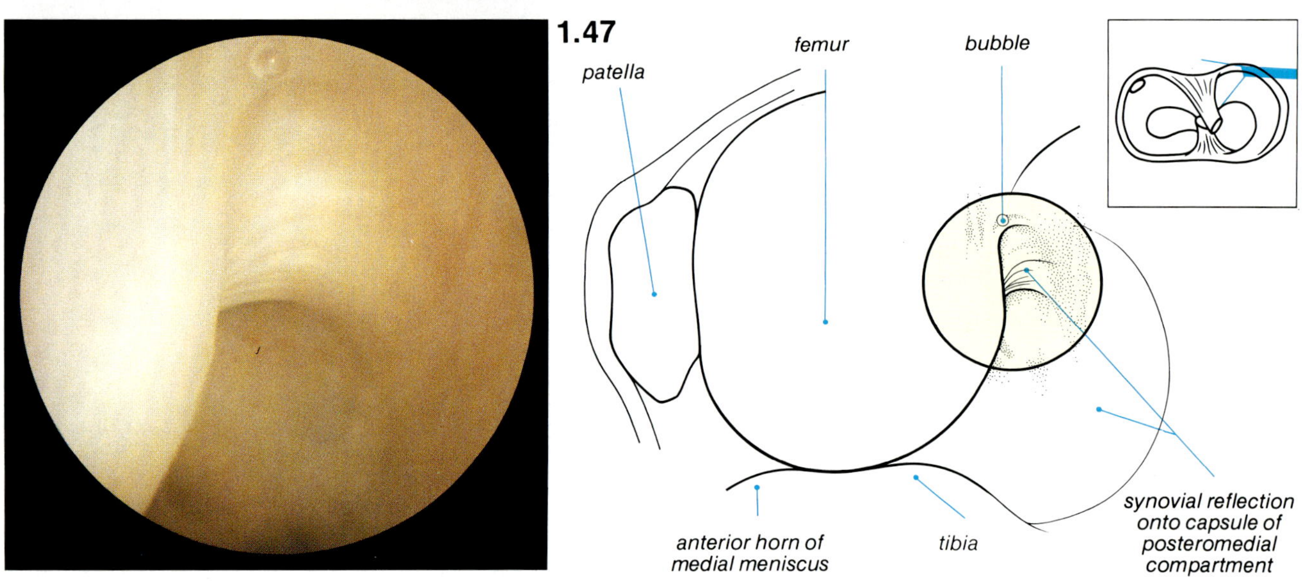

preferred, the complete infrapatellar fold is best seen from above.

The anterior and posterior cruciate ligaments lie in the same synovial sheath which is a prolongation of the synovium overlying the posterior capsule. The relationship of the synovium covering the posterior cruciate ligament to the posterior capsule is comparable with that of the mesentery in the abdomen and with other structures which invaginate a serous membrane, such as the lung. The area of synovium overlying the cruciate ligaments is considerable and may be affected by synovitis. In Fig. 1.49 the synovium overlying the anterior cruciate ligament is intensely inflamed, with a great increase in the vascular markings. The appearance is that of pannus spreading over the anterior cruciate ligament from the tibial insertion upwards. The patient

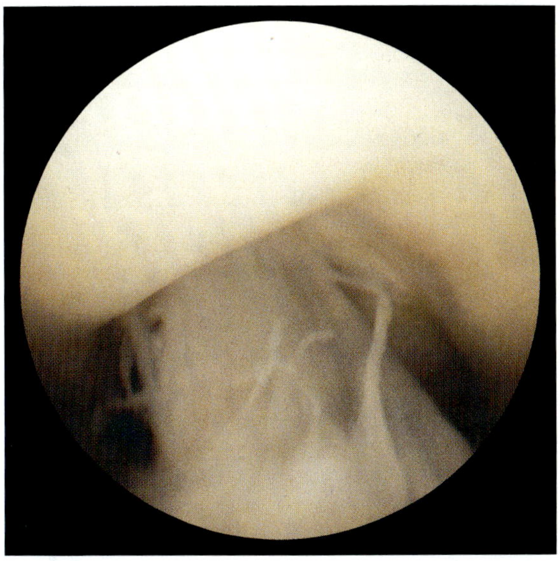

1.48

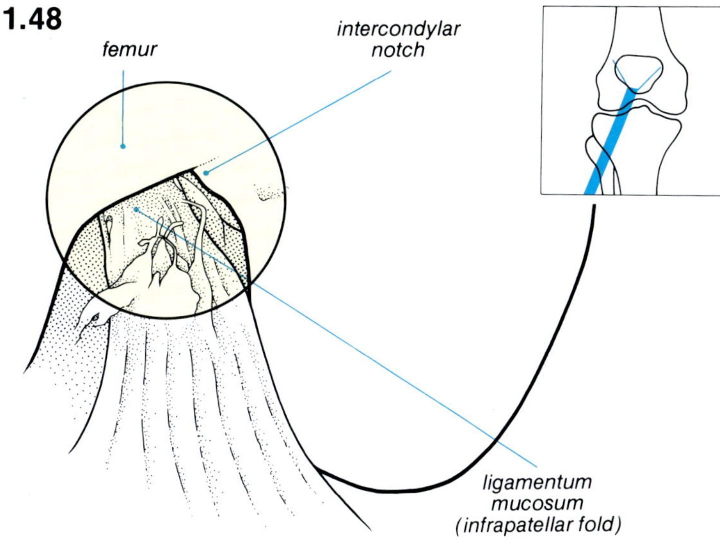

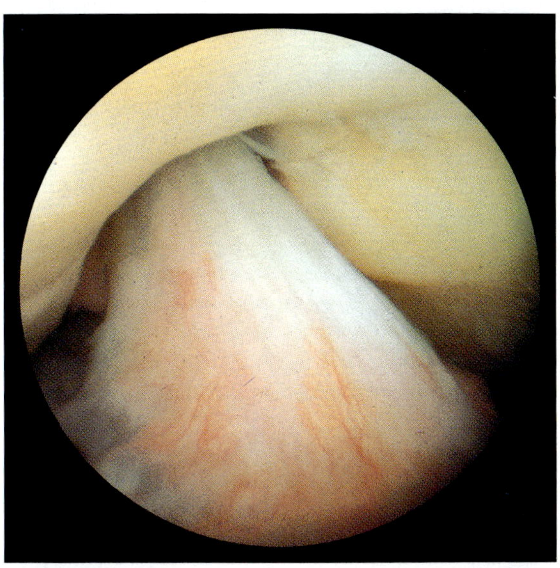

1.49

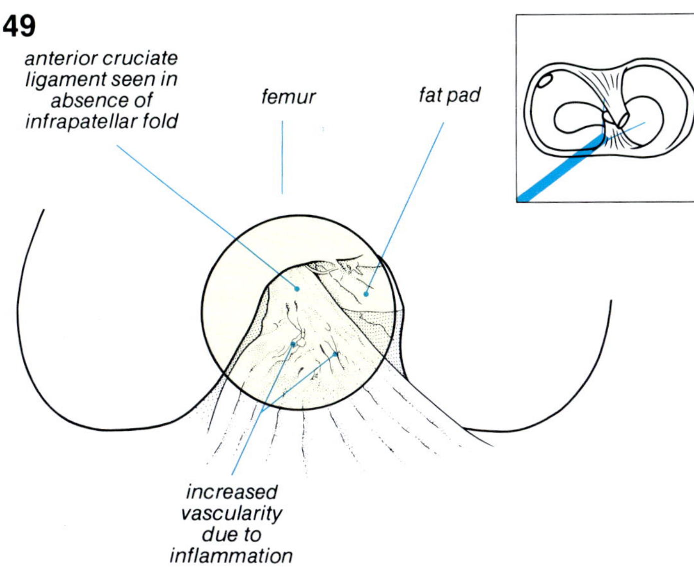

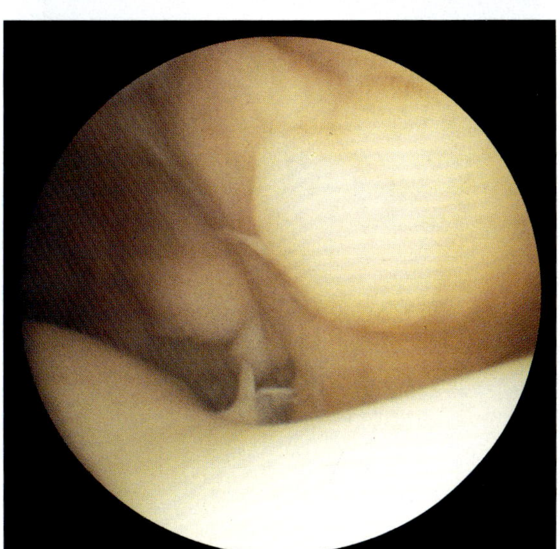

1.50

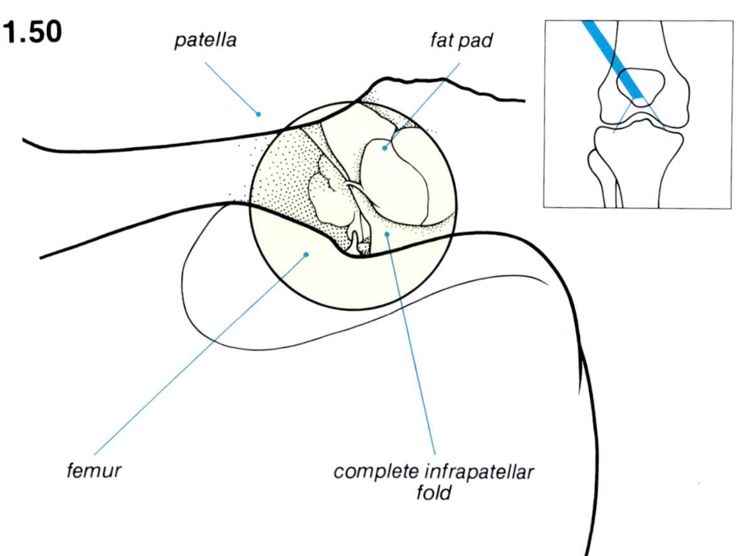

had a torn lateral meniscus and synovitis most marked in the lateral half of the knee.

Because the anterior and posterior cruciate ligaments are covered in the same sleeve of synovium and the anterior cruciate ligament lies in front of the posterior, it is unusual to see the posterior ligament in the intercondylar notch from the anterior approach. In Fig.1.51 the fat pad overlying the femoral insertion of the posterior cruciate ligament has been pulled forward with a blunt hook to reveal the ligament. Its fibres cannot be seen because of the synovial sheath.

In Fig.1.52, the synovium overlying the posterior cruciate ligament is torn and exposes fibres of the ligament itself as it crosses behind the anterior cruciate ligament. This appearance, though unusual, is not uncommon in older patients. The tear in the synovium does not appear to be associated with any history of injury and is probably of no pathological significance.

The femoral attachment of the posterior cruciate ligament is concealed by a small pad of fat which lies beneath the synovium covering the ligament and occupies the space between the anterior cruciate ligament and the anterior margin of the medial femoral condyle. This fat pad is variable in size and in Fig.1.53, which shows the knee in slight flexion, the fat pad is lifted slightly away from the anterior cruciate ligament. When the knee is extended fully, the posterior cruciate fat pad comes into close contact with the anterior cruciate, as in Fig.1.54 which shows an unusually large and succulent fat pad.

Although there is no definite evidence that abnormalities of the posterior cruciate fat pad can be the cause of symptoms, the structure is in such a vulnerable position that it seems very likely to give rise to pain on full extension and external rotation of the tibia on the femur if the fat pad is inflamed or abnormally sensitive for any reason. In some patients with posterior cruciate ruptures, haemorrhage in this fat pad may contribute to the patient's symptoms.

After running with the anterior cruciate ligament within the synovial sheath (Figs. 1.51 & 1.52), the posterior cruciate enters a short synovial tunnel to insert onto the back of the tibia. This synovial tunnel (Fig. 1.55) receives little mention in standard anatomical texts, but

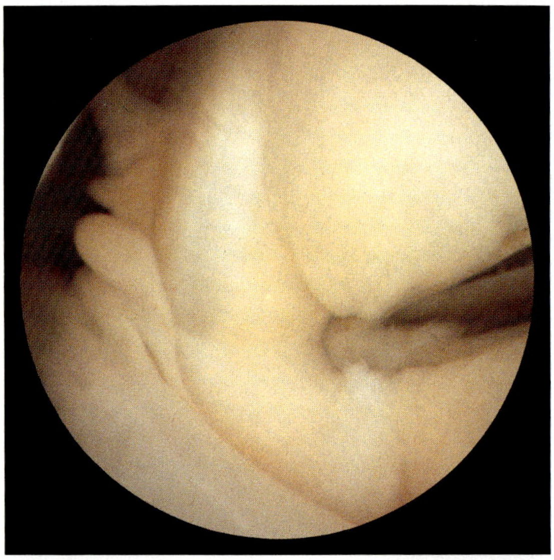

1.51

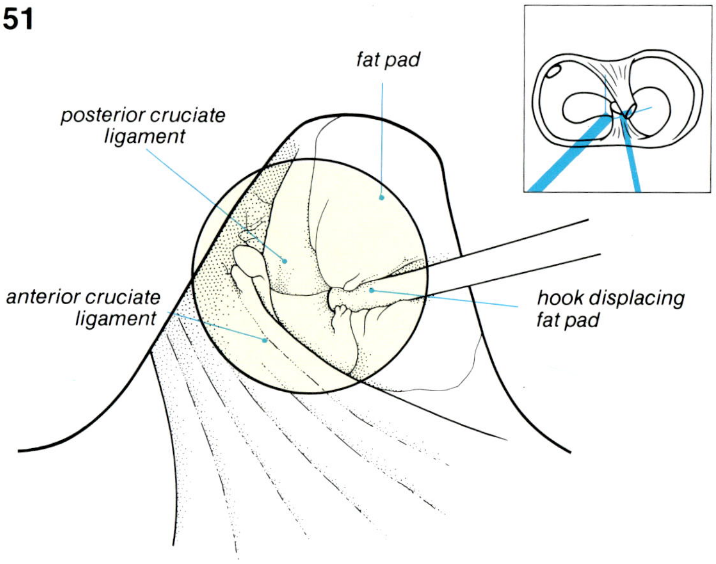

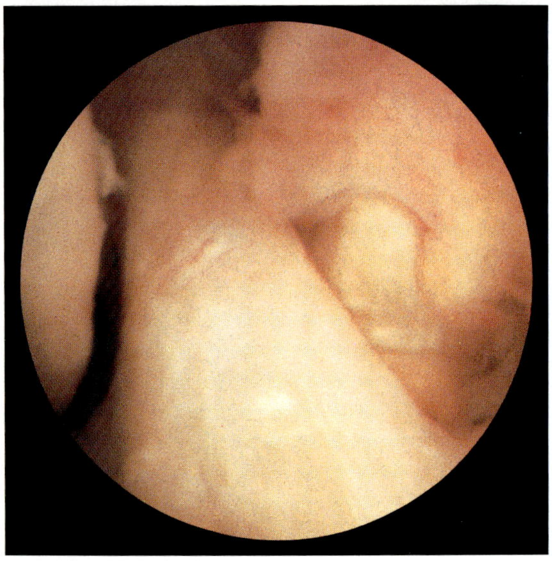

1.52

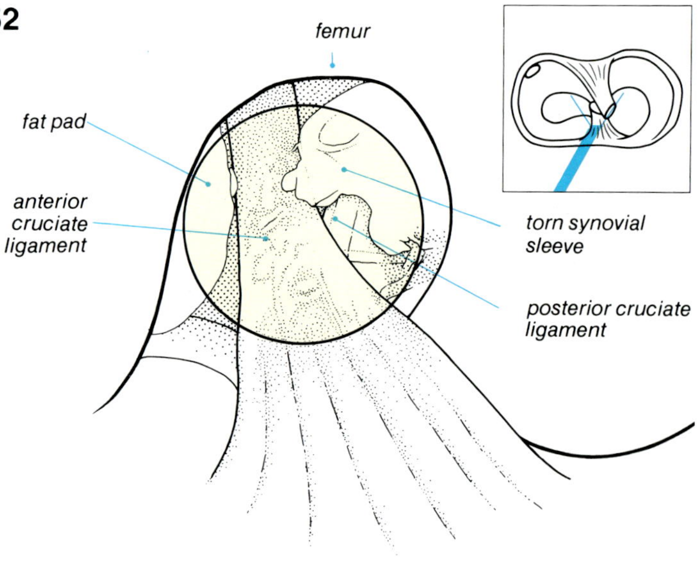

it is a constant feature of the knee and is bounded on its medial side by the posterior horn of the medial meniscus and on its lateral side by the synovium that runs forward to surround the anterior cruciate ligament. The posterior cruciate tunnel is particularly obvious in patients with ruptures of the posterior cruciate ligament. The tunnel is narrow but large enough to contain small loose bodies and even fragments of instruments fractured during arthroscopic surgery.

1.53

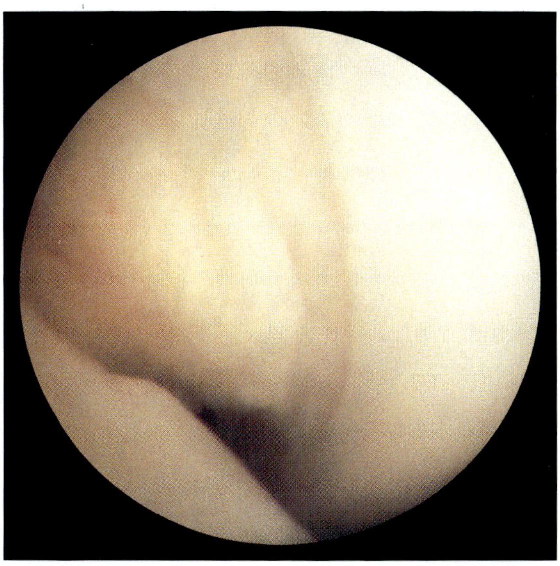

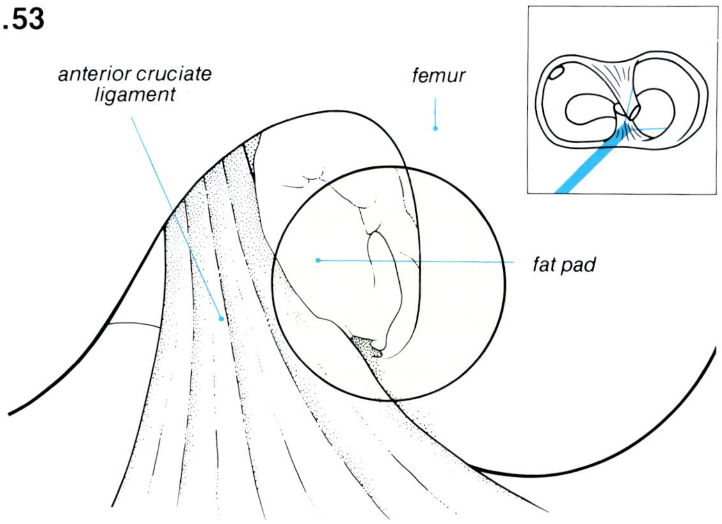

1.54

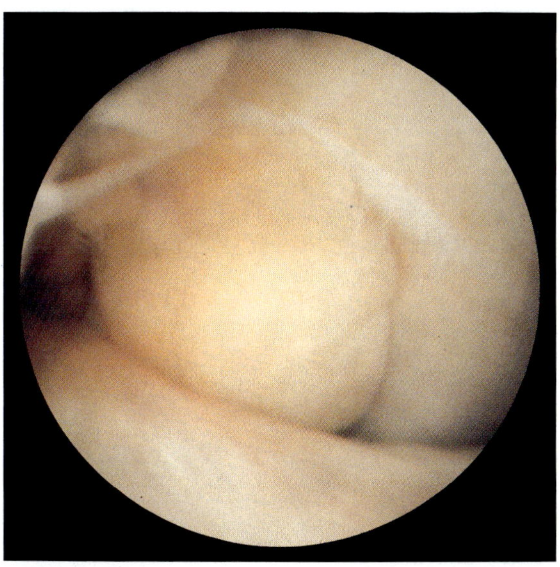

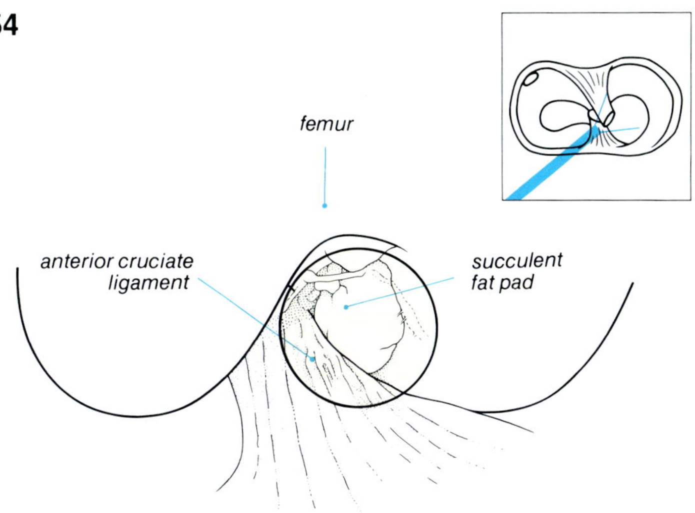

1.55

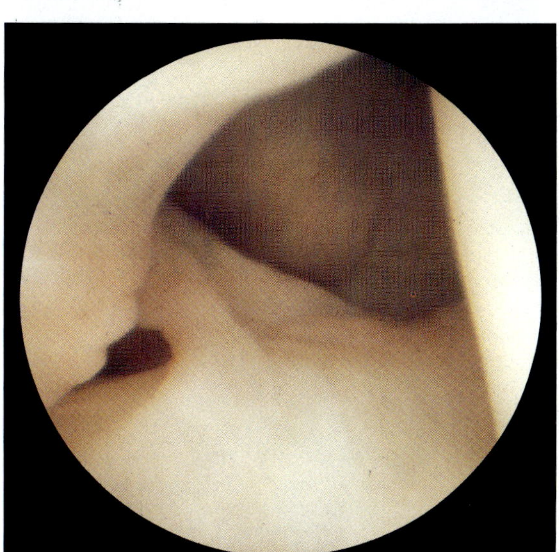

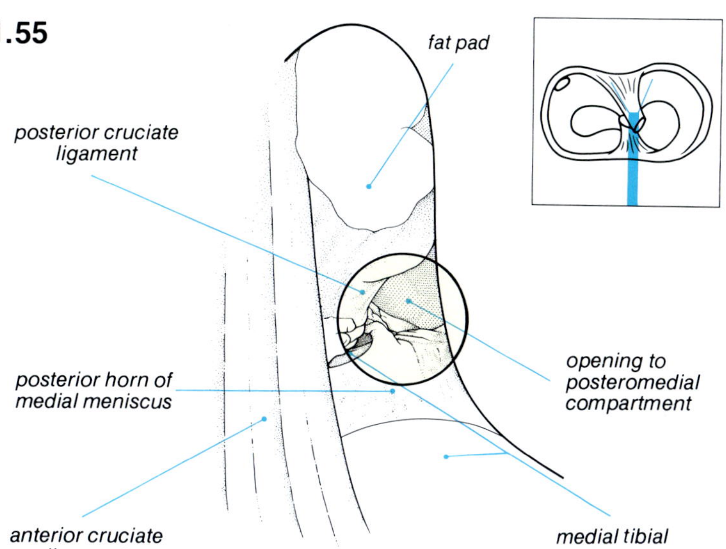

The cleft between the lateral femoral condyle and the cruciate ligaments is narrow but will accommodate a 5mm arthroscope and provide access to the posterolateral compartment. The anterior cruciate ligament is attached to the lateral condyle of the femur at the posterior margin of the intercondylar notch but the insertion is less conspicuous than that of the posterior cruciate. Although the synovium can be seen sweeping off the ligament onto the femoral condyle at its upper end (Fig.1.56), there is no fat pad to mark the attachment of the ligament to bone as there is on the medial femoral condyle where the posterior cruciate is inserted. The proximity of the ligament to the lens and the narrowness of the intercondylar notch at this point make

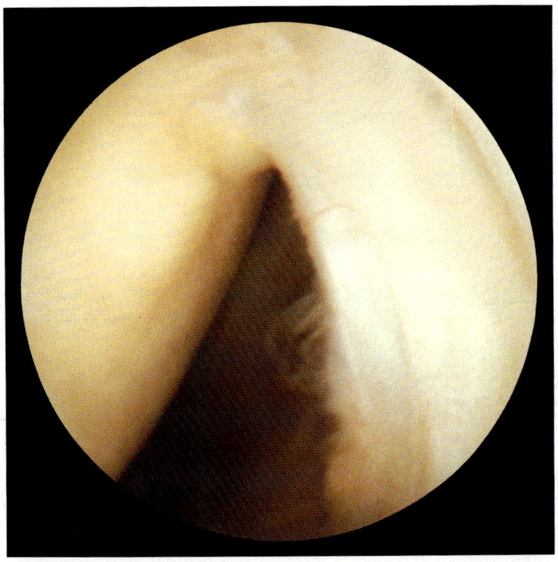

1.56

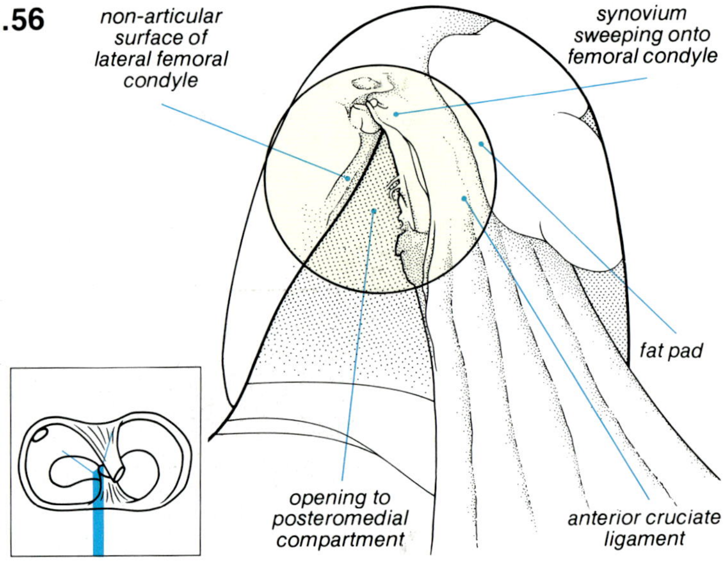

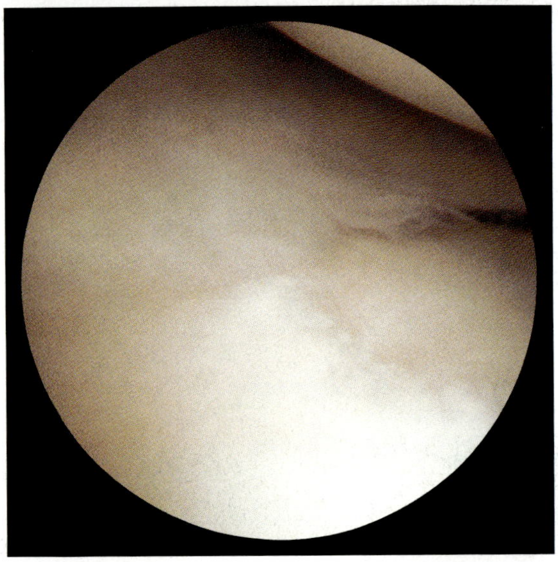

1.57

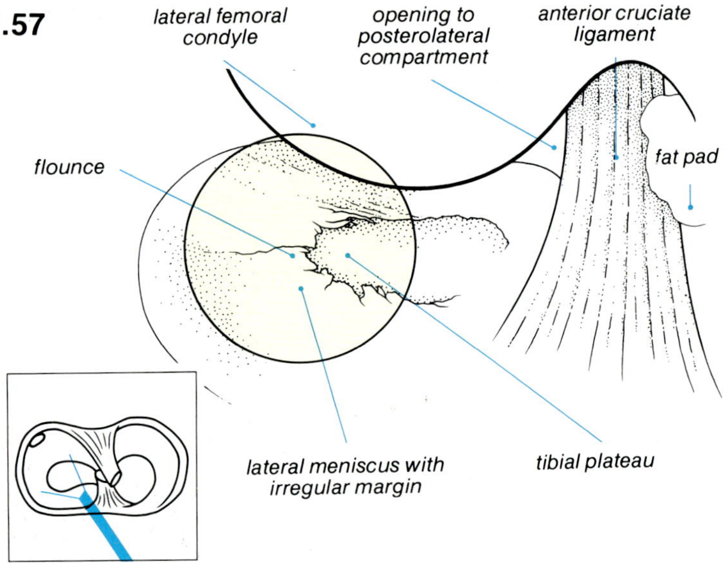

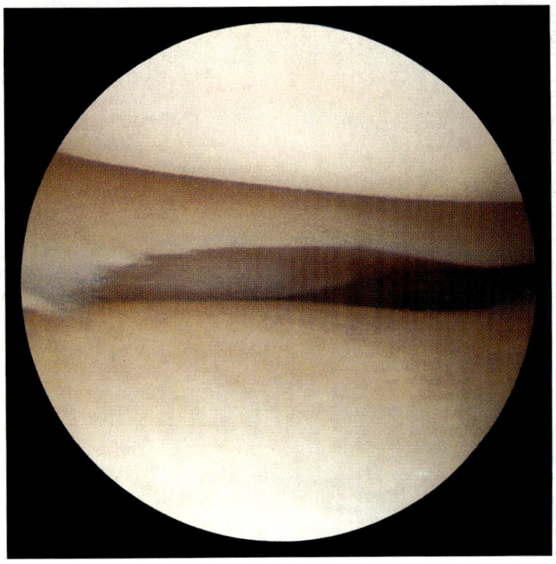

1.58

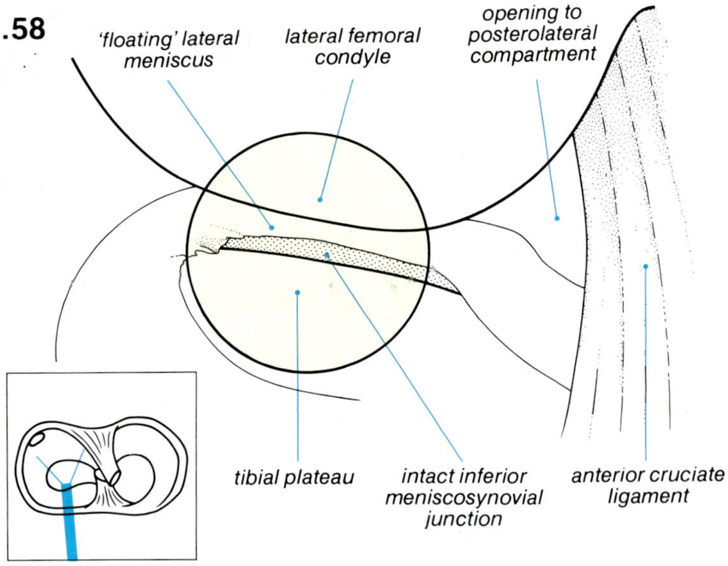

examination of this area very difficult, particularly if there is an abnormality to cause swelling or haemorrhage beneath the synovium (see Fig. 4.35).

LATERAL COMPARTMENT

From the intercondylar notch the arthroscope can be moved into the lateral compartment for inspection of the lateral meniscus. The lateral meniscus differs from the medial in that it is smaller and more circular in shape, its anterior and posterior attachments lying closer to each other than in its medial counterpart. However, like the medial, the lateral meniscus may also present a frill or flounce on its upper surface; but the flounce is more usually directed upwards rather than downwards as in the medial compartment. Although the margin of the meniscus is usually sharp and blade-like, a few fine irregularities are often seen but can be considered normal (Fig. 1.57).

Whereas the medial meniscus hugs the tibial plateau closely when varus or valgus strains are applied, the lateral meniscus will ride above the plateau when a varus strain is applied to the joint. In Fig. 1.58, in which a varus strain is applied to the knee, the meniscus is floating slightly above the tibial plateau. Beneath it can be seen the intact inferior meniscosynovial junction overlying the popliteus tendon which is not visible.

In Fig. 1.59, again showing a lateral meniscus with a varus strain applied to the joint, the entire length of the meniscus can be seen including both the anterior and posterior horns. The posterior horn rises above the tibial plateau, but this is a normal appearance that foes not indicate pathological laxity of the lateral ligament complex. The margin of the meniscus shows a slight irregularity in its posterior third. Irregularities of this type are often seen in older patients and are probably of no significance. Their size and position do not suggest that they are likely to become a larger lesion as, for example, do radial tears in the midportion of the meniscus.

The space beneath the lateral meniscus is considerable, quite large enough to accommodate a loose or foreign body (see Fig. 4.36). In Fig. 1.60 the lateral meniscus has been lifted off the tibial plateau with a hypodermic needle passed directly through the skin and used as a probe. The space beneath the meniscus is clearly seen and the popliteus tendon is just visible through the synovium.

The anatomy of the posterior horn of the lateral meniscus is very variable and differs markedly from that of the medial meniscus. The ligaments of Humphry and Wrisberg are well described in standard anatomical texts, but several variations of these two ligaments are

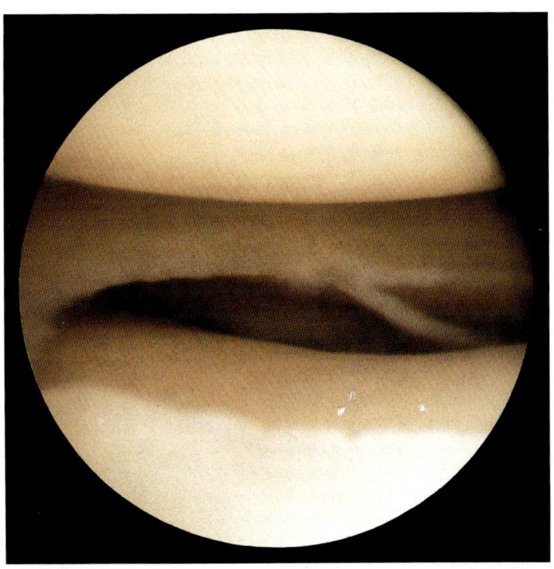

1.59

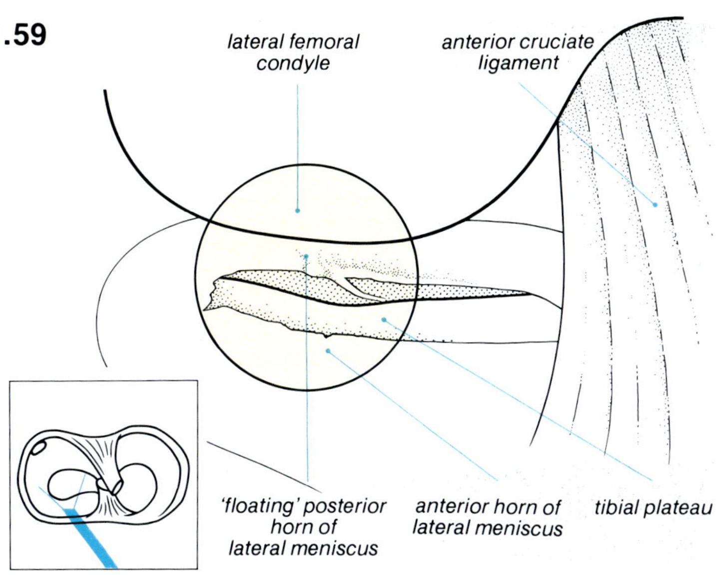

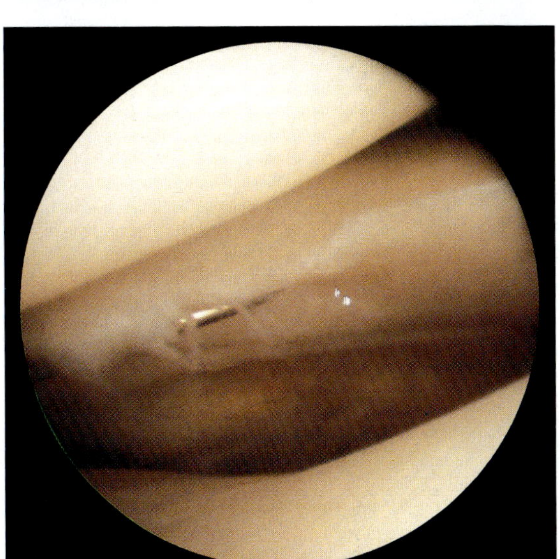

1.60

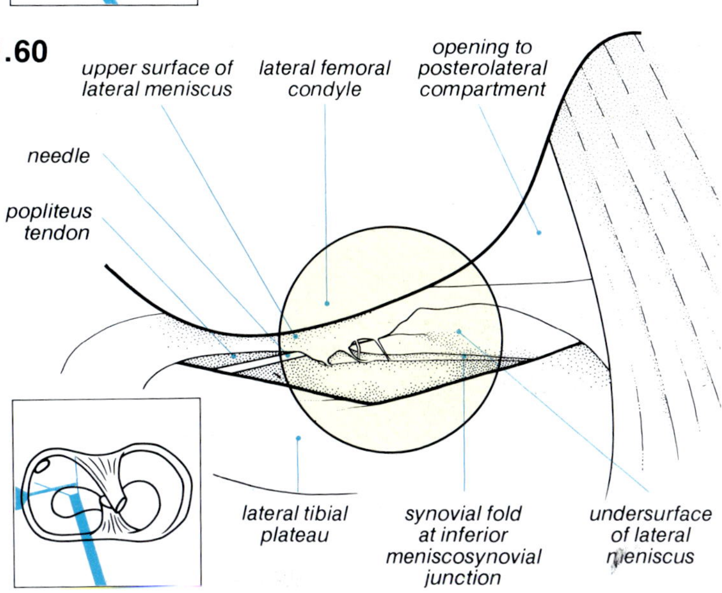

sometimes seen. Fig. 1.61 shows one variant; a triangular ligament arises from the apex of the intercondylar notch immediately in front of the insertion of the anterior cruciate ligament and passes downwards rather like a sail, with one corner tethered posteriorly to the posterior capsule of the knee and another to the insertion of the lateral meniscus onto the tibia.

In addition to the smaller size, mobility and circular appearance of the lateral meniscus, the anatomy of the lateral compartment differs from the medial in several other respects. The lateral tibial plateau is smaller than the medial and is arched so that the tibial plateau is higher at the centre than at either the anterior or posterior horn of the meniscus. In contrast, the medial tibial plateau is concave at its centre. The convexity of the lateral tibial plateau (Figs. 1.58-1.60) probably contributes to the 'floating' appearance of the lateral meniscus.

To accommodate the arching of the lateral tibial plateau, the femoral condyle is often concave. The curvature of the two joint surfaces is best appreciated at arthroscopy when the slight shadow cast by the arthroscope reveals the high ground at the centre of the plateau and the slight concavity on the femoral condyle. Fig. 1.62 shows the concavity of the femoral condyle, which appears as a darker area in the centre of the condyle. The convexity of the tibial plateau may also be seen with the meniscus lying level with the tibial plateau when the knee is in a neutral position with no varus strain.

POPLITEUS TUNNEL

The popliteus muscle runs from the lateral femoral condyle proximally to the back of the tibia distally and rotates the femur externally in relation to the tibia or, conversely, rotates the tibia internally on the femur. The tendon of the popliteus courses through the lateral side of the knee by way of a tunnel that lies between the lateral edge of the lateral meniscus and the joint capsule. As the tendon enters the popliteus tunnel it lies completely free of the meniscus on its medial side, the meniscus arching over it. On the lateral side, the tendon is free of the synovium above the meniscus, but below this level it blends into the synovial wall to leave the synovial cavity. The space between the meniscus and the capsule is variable but is usually large enough to accommodate a 5mm arthroscope as well as the popliteus tendon if the knee is held in neutral abduction with approximately fifteen degrees of flexion. Fig. 1.63 shows the popliteus tendon sweeping lateral to the meniscal margin towards its insertion at the back of the tibia.

The popliteus tunnel lies at the junction of the middle and posterior thirds of the lateral meniscus, at the point where the meniscus leaves the capsule of the knee and sweeps centrally to insert into the tibia. The tunnel

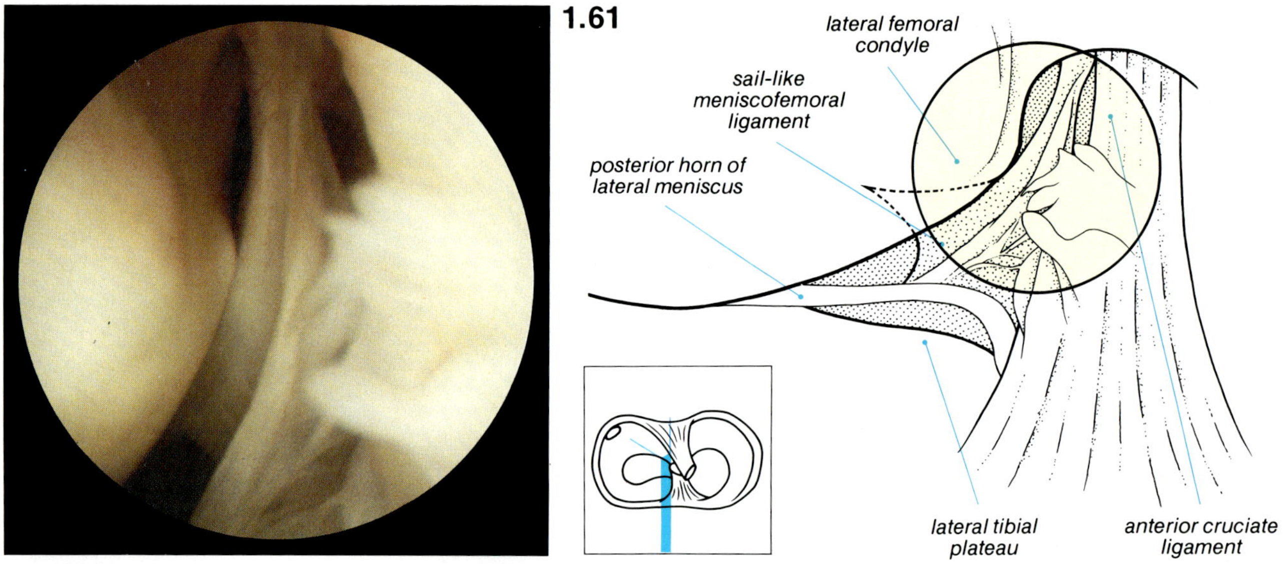

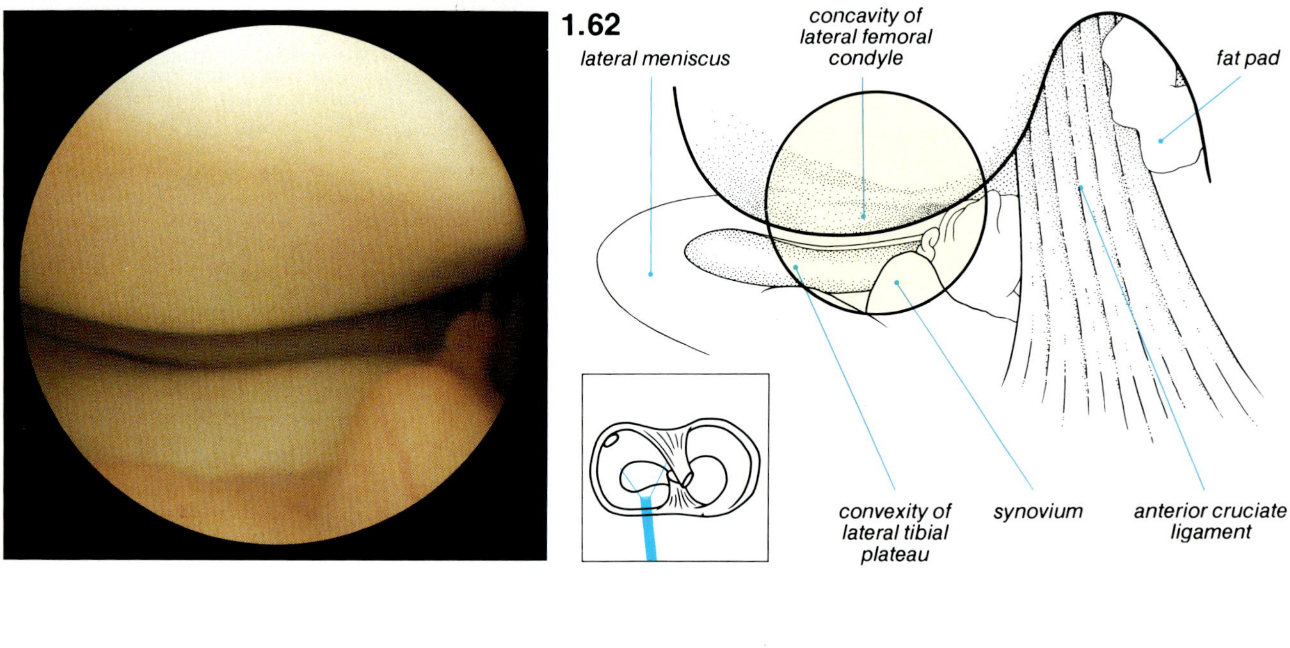

therefore acts as a 'stress raiser' in the lateral meniscus and has a great influence on the pattern of tears by creating a point of weakness at which the tear may begin. The relationship of the tendon to the meniscus can be seen in Fig. 1.63 which was taken from the anterolateral approach, but is perhaps more clearly seen in Fig. 1.64 which was taken from the lateral suprapatellar approach and shows how the popliteus tendon occupies a tunnel between the meniscus medially and the capsule of the joint laterally.

When the knee is fully extended, the insertion of the popliteus tendon comes to lie close to the upper surface of the meniscus and may well be forced firmly against it in hyperextension. In Fig. 1.65, taken with the knee almost fully extended, the attachment of the popliteus tendon to the femoral condyle is lying close to the lateral meniscus

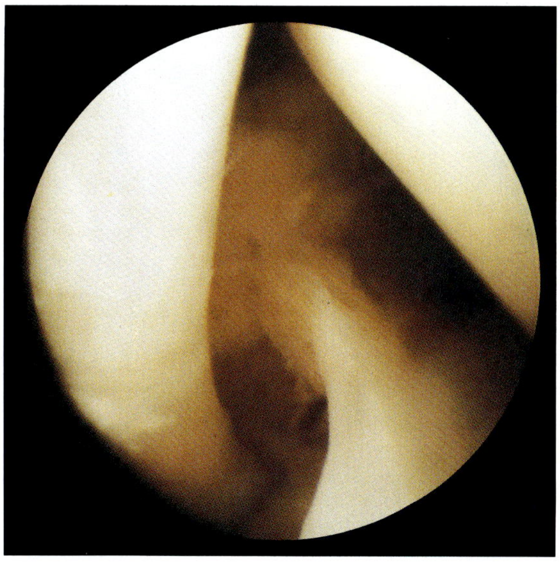

1.63

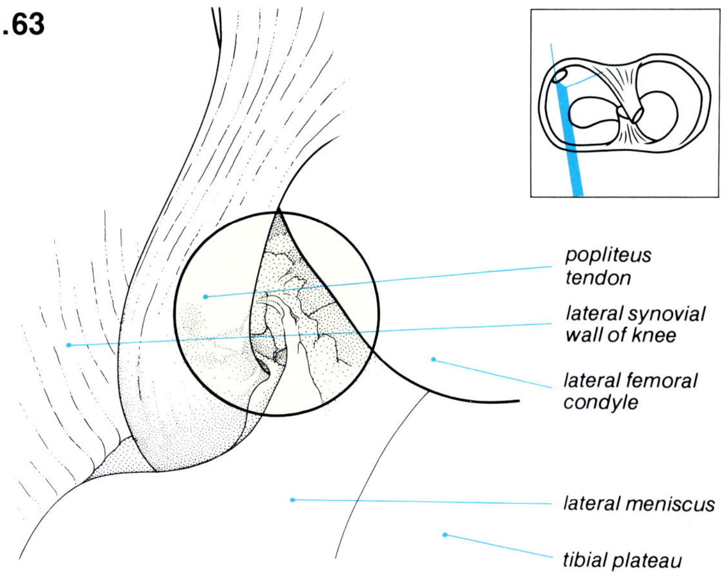

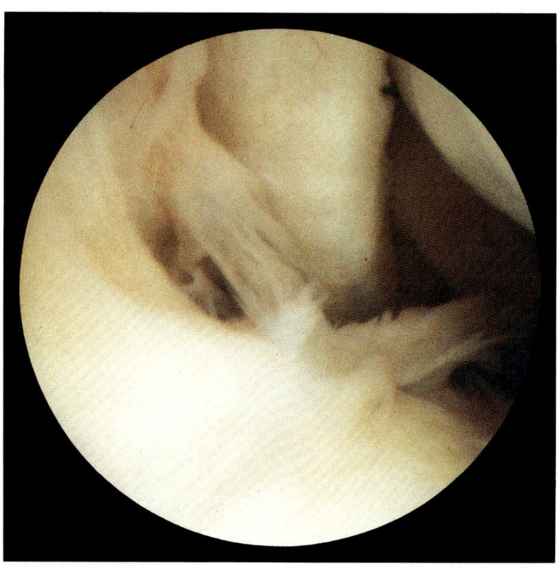

1.64

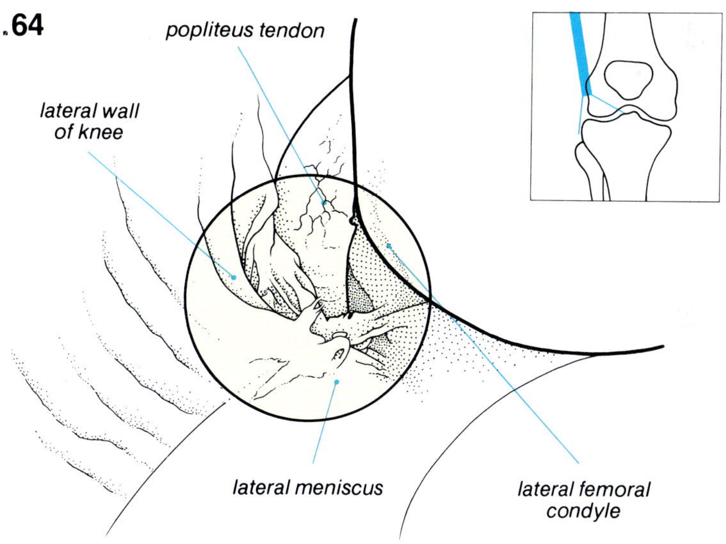

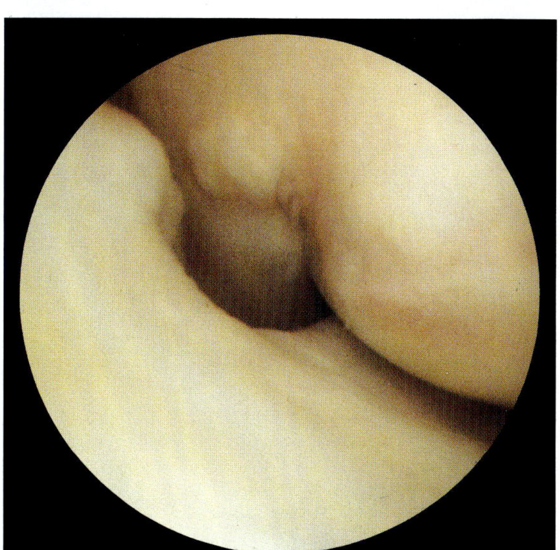

1.65

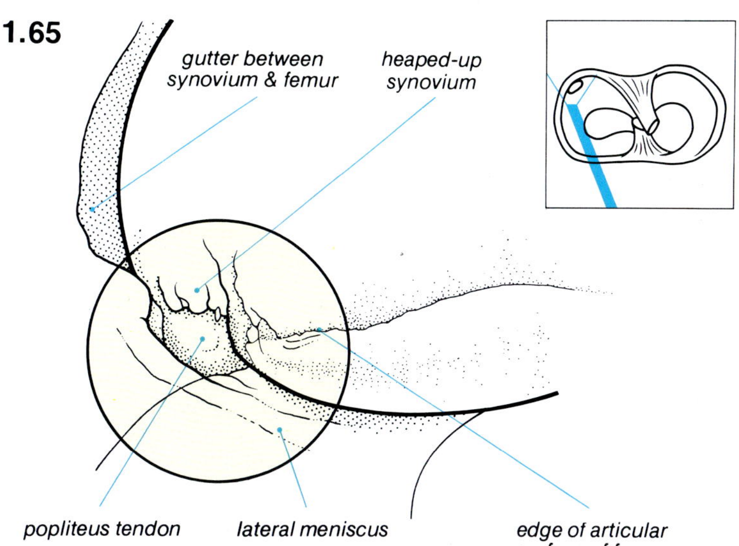

and there is a heaped up area of synovium on the otherwise smooth surface of the tendon. This appearance is comparable to the impingement lesion seen on the medial femoral condyle in full extension and may perhaps be an indication of the force with which the popliteus insertion is applied to the lateral meniscus in full extension.

When the popliteus tendon is passing lateral to the meniscus and the lateral femoral condyle is pressing it firmly against the tibia, the tendon and its insertion act as a clamp to secure the meniscus to the tibial plateau. It is easy to imagine how a sharp twisting force applied to the knee in this position could lead to a tear at this site and this may well be the cause of most complex oblique, or 'parrot-beak', tears of the lateral meniscus. Fig.1.66 shows the popliteus tendon lying between the lateral

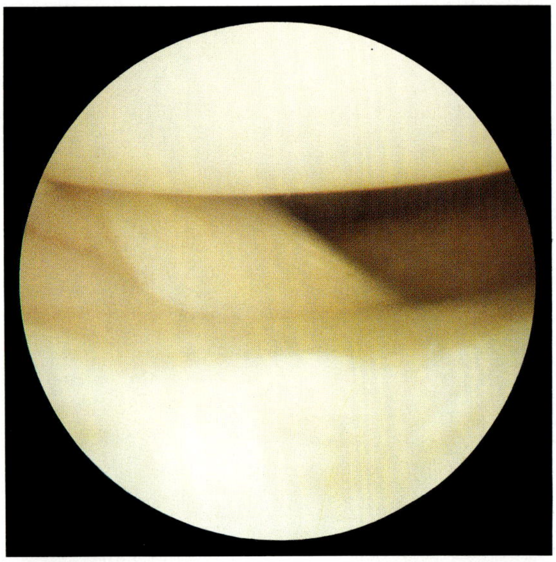

1.66

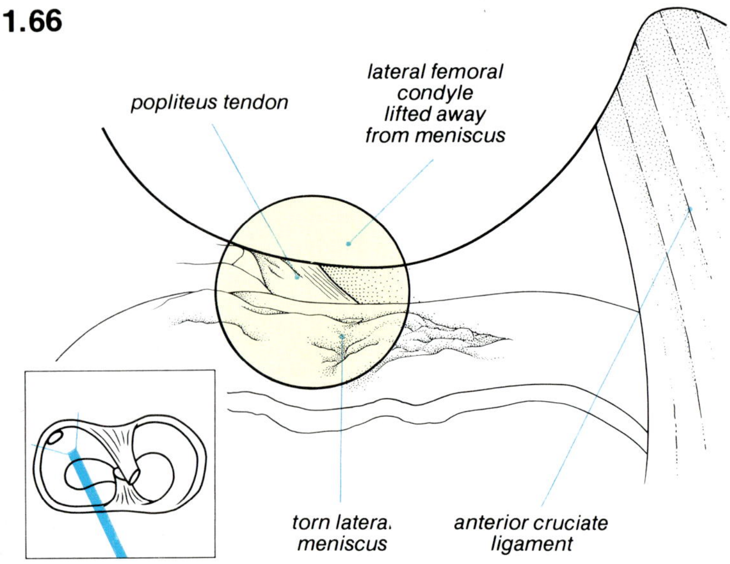

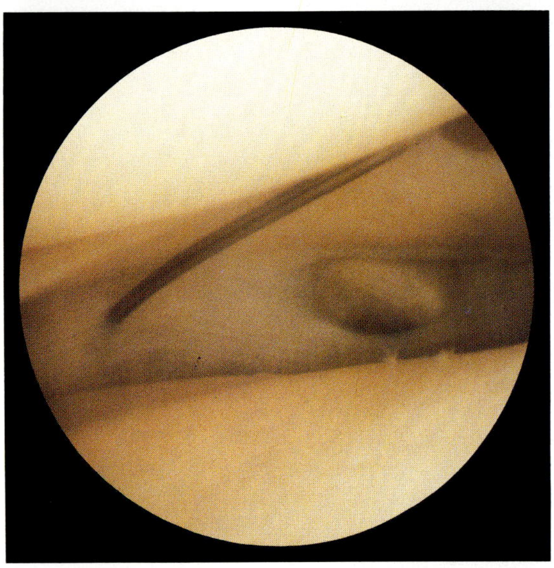

1.67

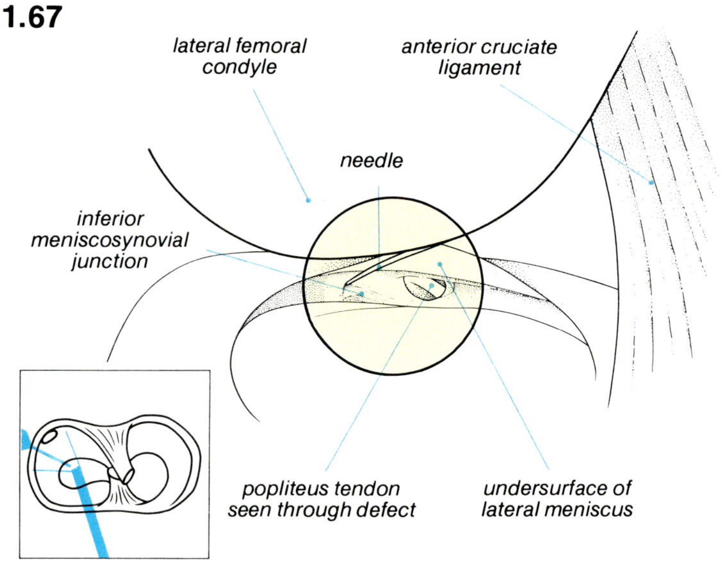

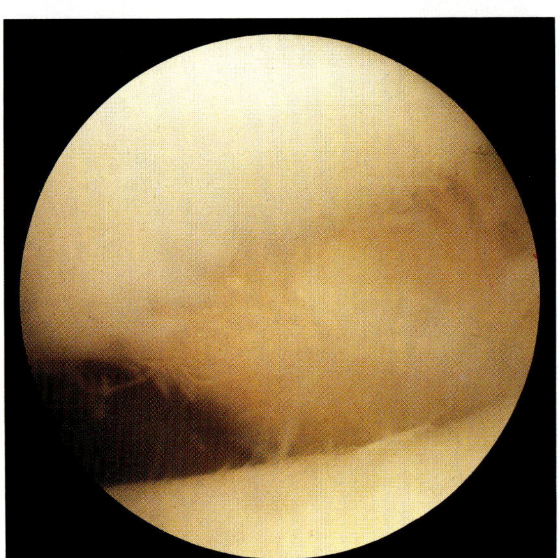

1.68

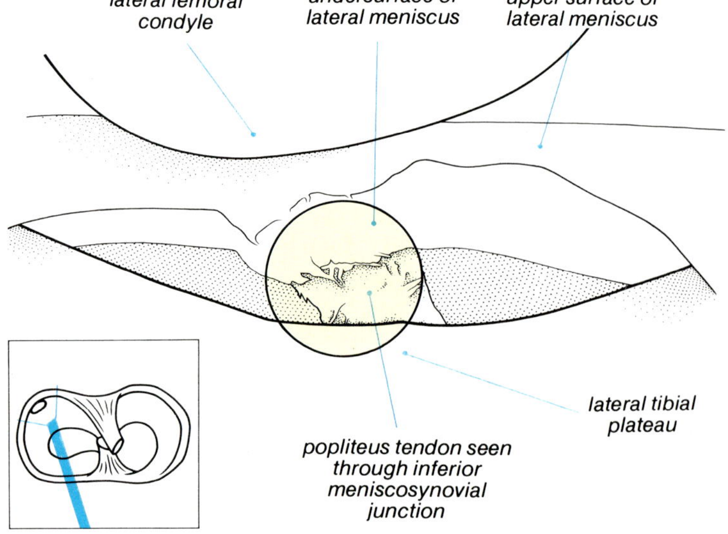

femoral condyle and the lateral meniscus of a patient who had a complex oblique tear opposite the popliteus tunnel. It is not always possible to see the popliteus tendon in this space, but in patients with unusual joint laxity, as was the case here, the tendon can be clearly seen.

In Fig.1.58 the popliteus tendon could not be seen beneath the meniscus because of an intact inferior meniscosynovial junction. In Fig.1.67, however, the meniscus has been lifted with a needle and the popliteus tendon is clearly visible through a defect in the inferior meniscosynovial junction. The defect has smooth edges and does not have the appearance of a recent injury. The patient had no symptoms referrable to the lateral side of the knee and the defect was regarded as an incidental finding, but it may be that the knees with such a defect are more subject to tears of the lateral meniscus.

Although it is alarming to find a defect in the inferior meniscosynovial junction with exposed popliteus tendon (Fig.1.67), the normal inferior meniscosynovial junction appears to be insubstantial. In Fig.1.68 the arthroscope has been placed beneath the lateral meniscus and the inferior meniscosynovial junction is clearly seen. The popliteus tendon and its fibres shine through the thin synovial covering and it is difficult to see how such a structure could contribute usefully to the stability of the lateral meniscus.

Figs.1.69 and 1.70 show a recent tear of the inferior meniscosynovial junction from the lateral side. A 5mm arthroscope has been placed in the popliteus tunnel alongside the tendon and its lens directed medially. In Fig.1.69 the tendon has blended with the lateral wall of the tunnel so that only its medial surface is truly intra-articular. The tendon leaves the joint at the level of the tibial plateau. A tear can be seen in the inferior menisco-synovial junction with clean and sharp edges suggesting recent injury (compare with Fig.1.67).

In Fig.1.70, the same knee as in Fig.1.69, the lateral meniscus has been displaced medially with a percutaneous needle to demonstrate the mobility of the meniscus. The tibial plateau is visible through the tear in the inferior meniscosynovial junction. The significance of lesions of this type is not clear, but they may well be responsible for excessive mobility of the lateral meniscus and possibly for locking of the knee in full flexion. The posterior extent of the tear in the inferior meniscosynovial junction determines the mobility of the meniscus and assessment of such menisci can be extremely difficult.

If all abnormally mobile lateral menisci were removed, it is likely that many unnecessary meniscectomies would be performed, while leaving menisci that are a little loose may lead to continued symptoms but perhaps to a lower incidence of degenerative osteoarthritis. Repair of the inferior meniscosynovial junction and reattachment of the meniscus may be appropriate for some but the exact

1.69

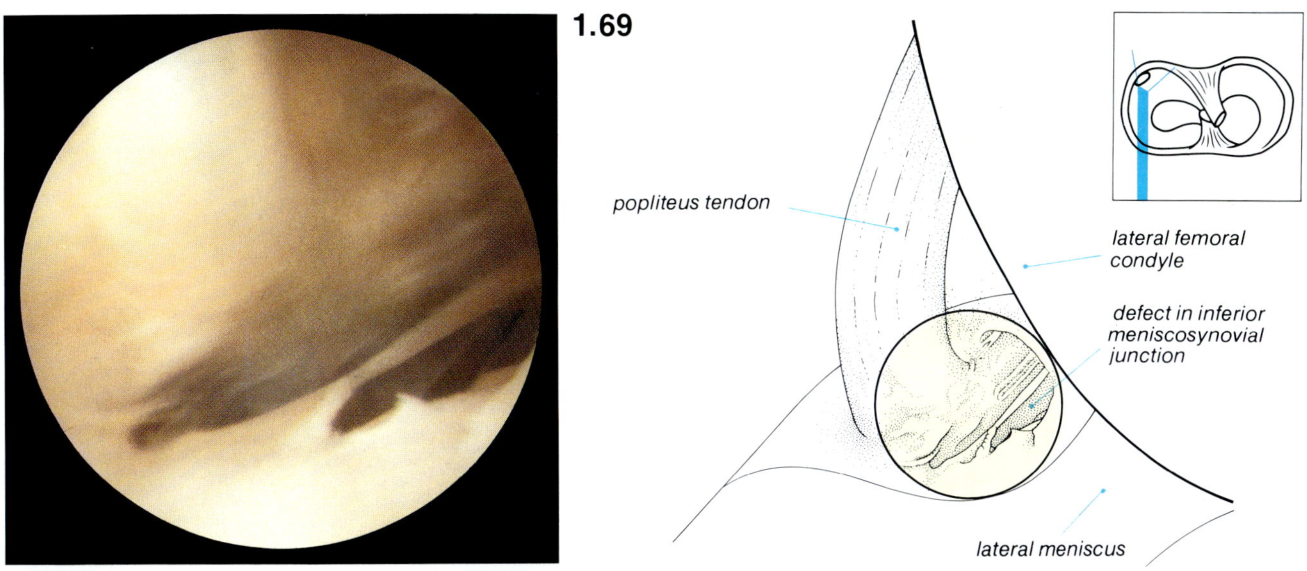

1.70

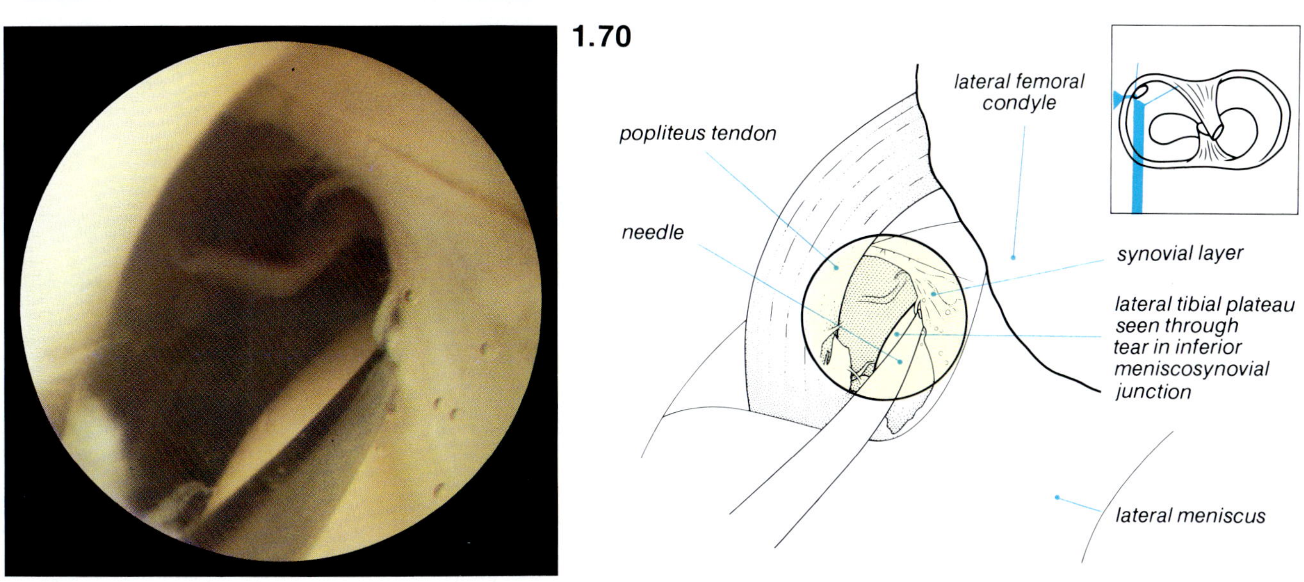

role of meniscal reattachment for this type of lesion has yet to be determined.

LATERAL GUTTER

After withdrawal of the arthroscope from the popliteus tunnel, it may be moved up the lateral gutter towards the suprapatellar pouch. On leaving the lateral gutter, a spiral fold of synovium is encountered (Fig.1.71). This synovial fold is comparable to that in the medial gutter (see Fig.1.28) and is not of pathological significance. The fold is easily felt through the skin, particularly if the synovium is inflamed when it may be palpated as a tender ridge. The recess behind the fold is a frequent refuge for loose bodies and can best be seen from the lateral suprapatellar approach. The spiral nature of the fold is dictated by its position near the axis of rotation of the knee and by the need of the synovium to move during flexion.

POSTEROLATERAL COMPARTMENT

Like the posteromedial compartment, the posterolateral compartment can be entered either by passing the arthroscope through the intercondylar notch beside the cruciate ligament or by making a separate incision into the compartment directly. The posterolateral compartment is smaller than the posteromedial and does not have such a deep recess behind the posterior horn of the meniscus. Fig.1.72 shows the posterolateral compartment with the knee in approximately ninety degrees of flexion. The arthroscope has been passed through the intercondylar notch and its lens directed laterally. The synovial slope from the back of the meniscus to the floor of the compartment is not as steep as in the posteromedial compartment, but a ridge of fat is present on the floor as it is on the medial side.

With a thirty degree telescope, the popliteus tendon can only just be seen with the arthroscope placed in the intercondylar notch and then only if the arthroscope is placed well to the back of the posterolateral compartment and if the tibia is held in external rotation so that the popliteus tunnel is drawn posterolaterally. Although the tendon cannot be seen clearly, the synovium overlying it can usually be seen as a low ridge. Fig.1.73 shows the popliteus tendon in the background, beyond the femoral condyle and above the lateral meniscus. A sharp knife-like fold of synovium passes forwards from the posterior capsule to the upper limit of the articular surface. This sharp crescent of synovium is easily identified from the posterolateral approach at arthrotomy, when it can be felt with the gloved finger.

Fig.1.74 shows the posterolateral compartment of a patient with a damaged posterior cruciate ligament which has allowed the tibia to fall backwards in relation to the femur, bringing with it the popliteus tendon. If, as here, the popliteus tendon can be seen clearly, abnormal laxity of the posterior cruciate ligament or of the

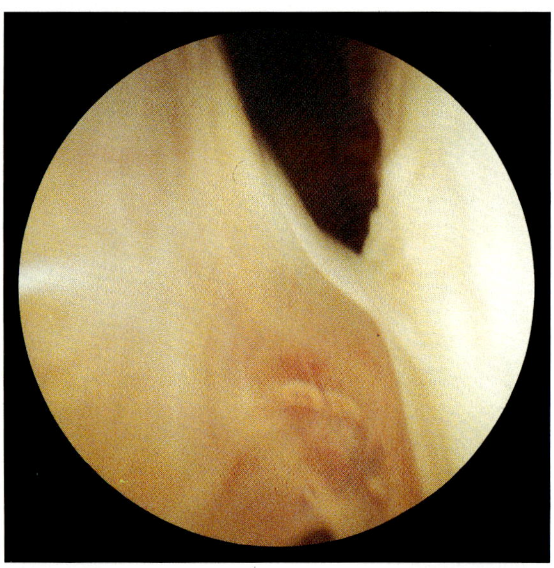

1.71

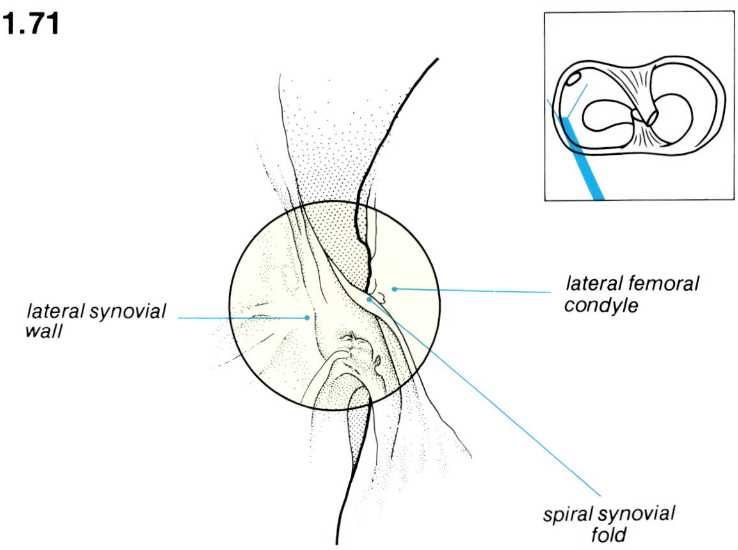

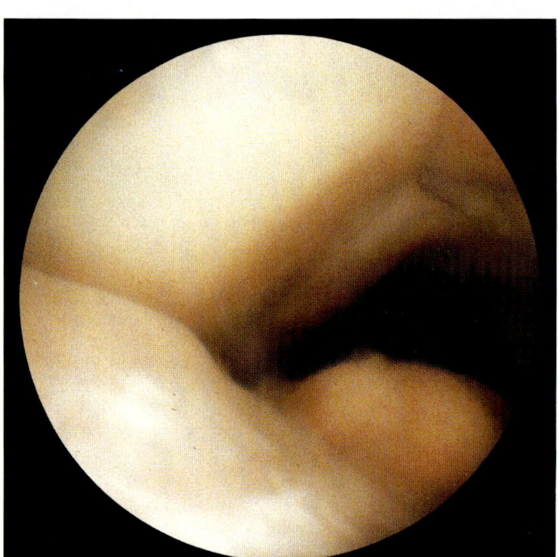

1.72

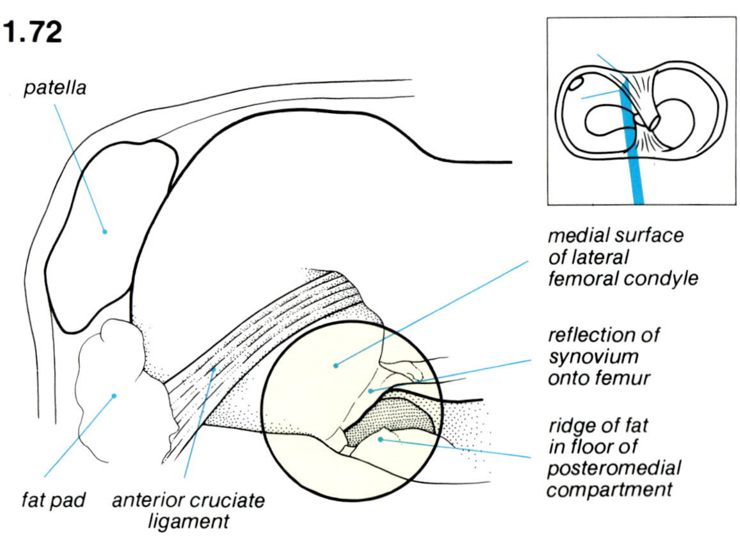

posterolateral corner of the knee must be suspected. The synovium is slightly pigmented and inflamed, the result of repeated haemorrhage into the joint due to the posterior cruciate laxity. Although Fig.1.74 indicates a pathological appearance, it is included in this section on normal appearances because it demonstrates the relationship of the popliteus tendon, the meniscus and the femoral condyle.

If the arthroscope is placed in the posterolateral compartment through a separate posterolateral incision rather than through the intercondylar notch, the centre of the joint can be seen with the synovium sweeping forwards from the posterior capsule to leave the posterior oblique ligament as it does in the posteromedial compartment, but with the difference that it may appear as a tight crescentic fold. Fig.1.75 shows such an

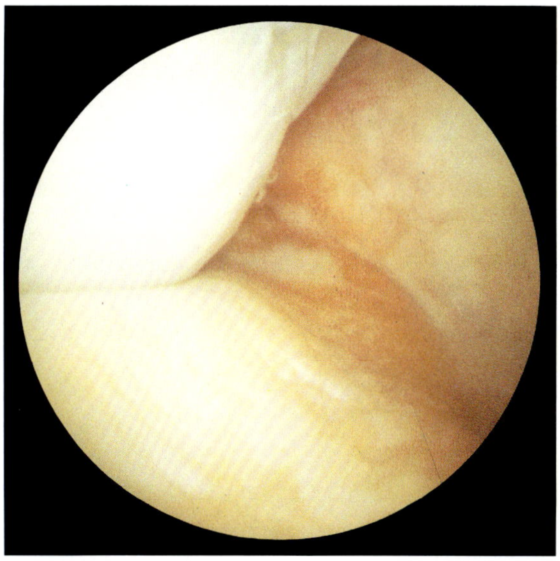

1.73

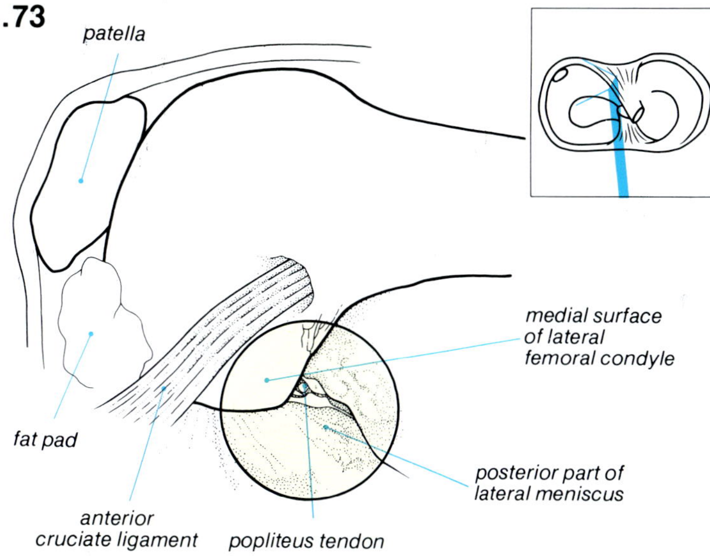

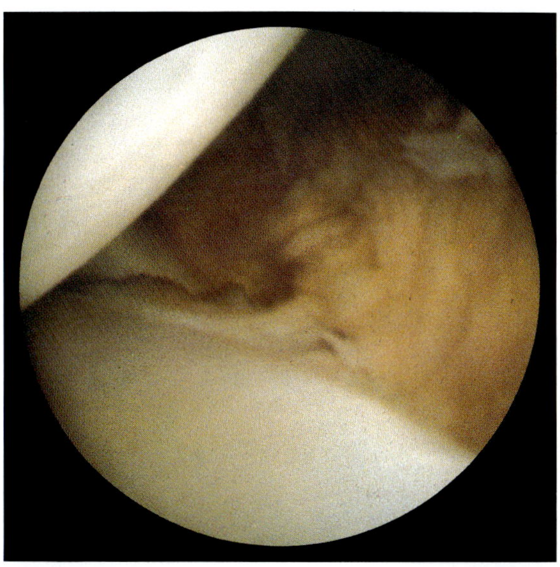

1.74

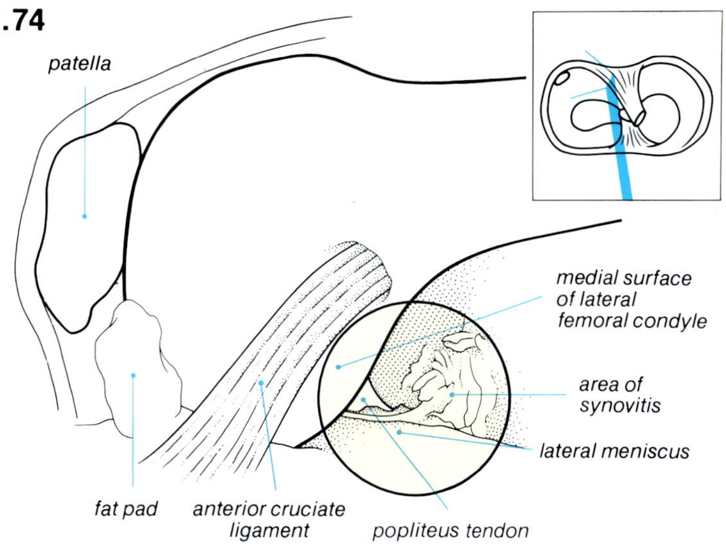

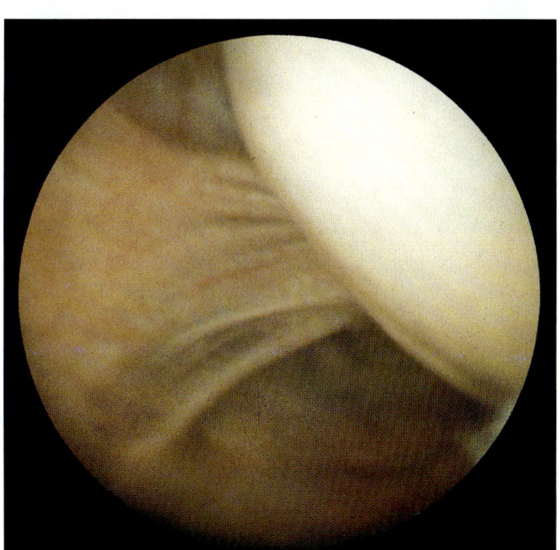

1.75

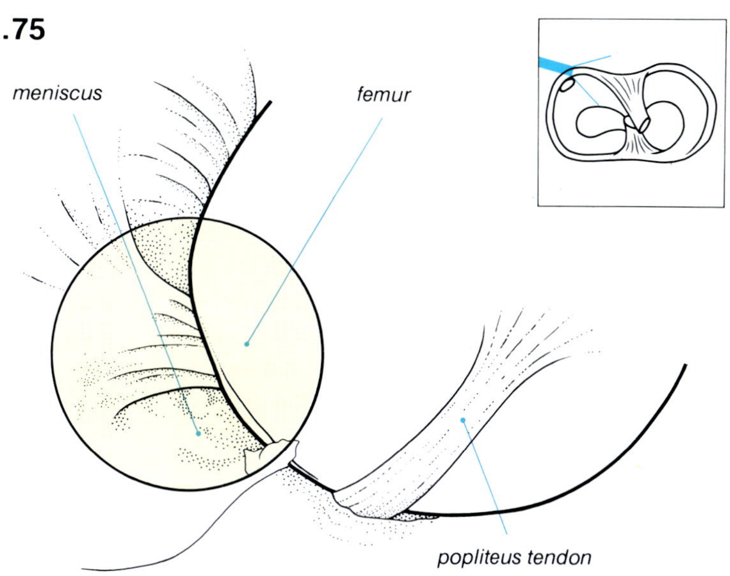

abnormal fold moving forwards lateral to the posterior cruciate ligament to be joined onto the back of the intercondylar notch. Fig.1.61 demonstrated another pattern of abnormal fold in this part of the joint. Neither of these folds corresponds to any of the commonly described constituents of the oblique posterior ligament.

Fig.1.76, a view from the posterolateral approach, shows pit-like depressions in the synovium lying in a line parallel to the upper surface of the lateral meniscus. These pits are rarely seen but are a curious feature and do not appear to be associated with any symptoms. No explanation is offered for their presence.

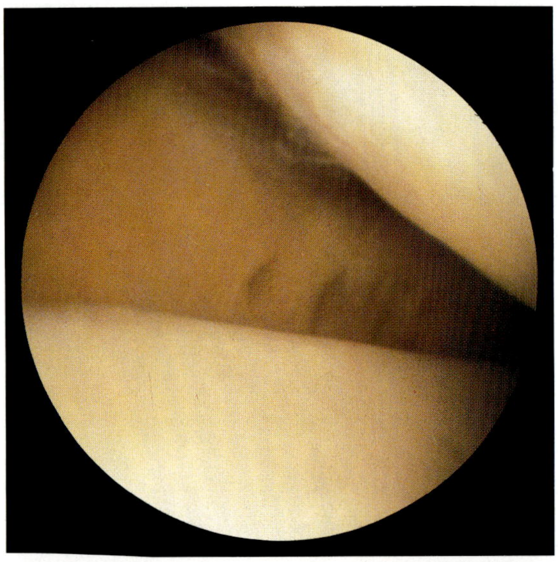

1.76

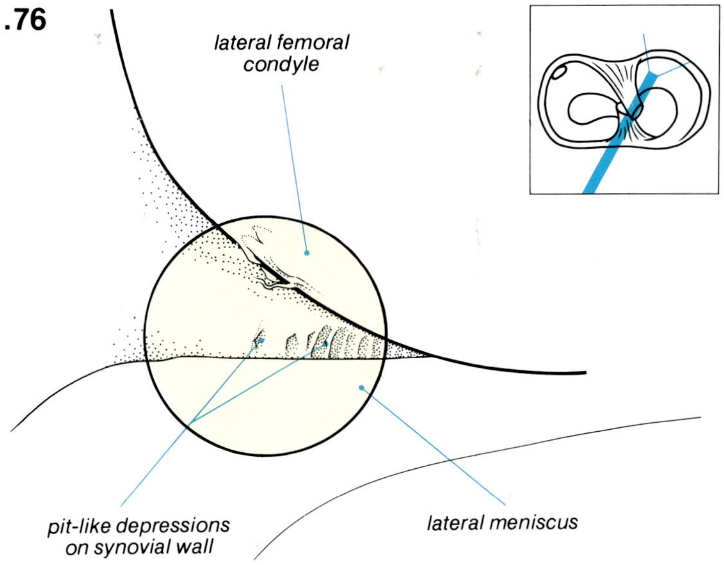

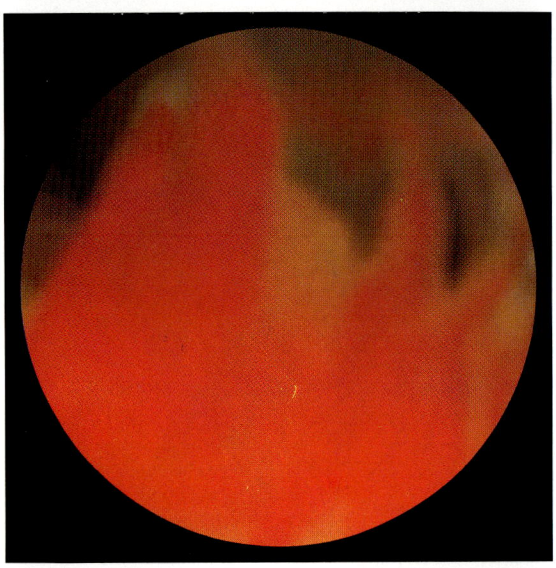

1.77

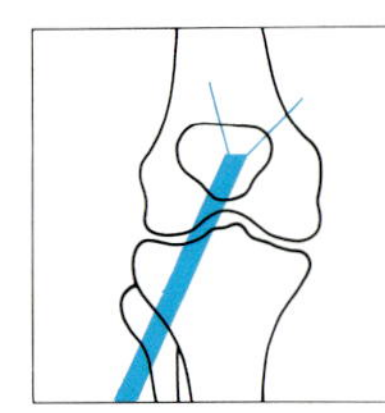

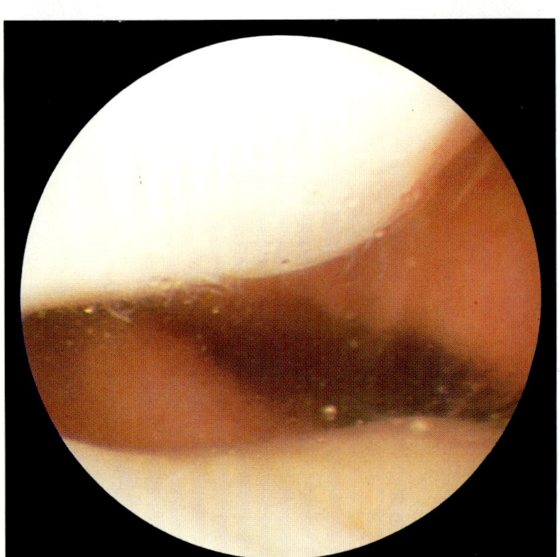

1.78

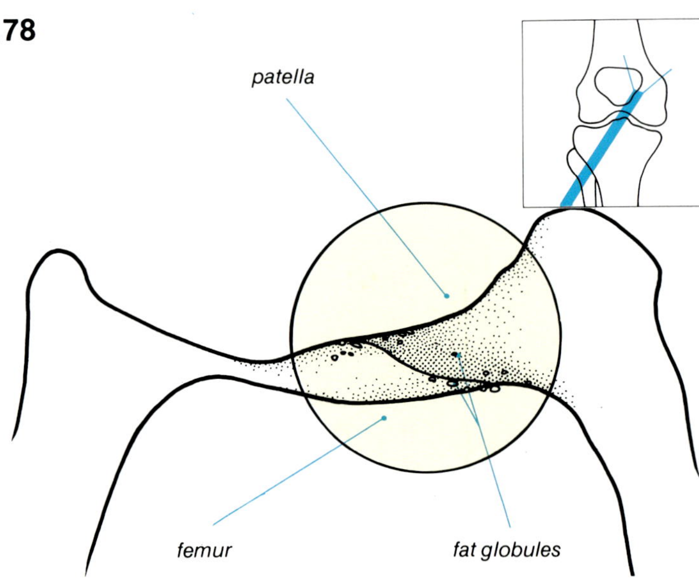

ARTEFACTS

Although arthroscopy should involve little damage to the joint, the operation itself can give rise to unusual appearances which may be puzzling. Difficulties in examination, sometimes due to deficiencies in surgical technique or in handling of the instruments, can also contribute to diagnostic difficulty.

Fig.1.77 shows bleeding into the joint. The flow of saline from the tip of the arthroscope to wash the blood away from the tip of the instrument has produced a flame-like appearance. If the irrigation fluid is run into the knee through a separate needle or channel but leaves the knee via the arthroscopic sheath, blood will be washed towards the tip of the arthroscope, creating problems of visibility. If haemorrhage is present in the knee, the tourniquet should be inflated and the joint irrigated with adequate quantities of irrigation fluid.

In Fig.1.78, floating between the femoral condyle and patella are small pearl-like globules of fat. These globules may be present in the knee if there is a recent fracture or if a bony defect has been drilled, but in Fig.1.78 they are the result of damage to the extrasynovial fat during insertion of the arthroscope. In general, floating fat globules are more likely to be seen in the obese patient during operations requiring repeated insertion of the arthroscope and if instruments have been handled vigorously, excessively or clumsily. Fat globules cause no problems apart from interfering with vision.

Bubbles of air rise to the uppermost part of the knee and if fat globules are present, they too will float upwards and come to lie trapped between the saline below and the undersurface of the air bubble above. Fig.1.79 shows the solid patella above and the air bubble below it with the arthroscope tip reflected as an incomplete ellipse. Lenticulate globules of fat are caught between the bubble and the saline. The air may be removed by perforation of the bubble with a needle and the fat by thorough irrigation.

Blood, fat and air in the synovial cavity can easily be removed but saline in the subsynovial tissue presents a more difficult problem because such a situation may cause the synovial cavity to be obliterated by a boggy mass of swollen tissue. Fig.1.80 shows a knee in which this mishap occurred as the result of inadvertent injection of saline between the front of the femur and the synovium. The resulting mass of swollen and soggy tissue is almost effervescent in appearance.

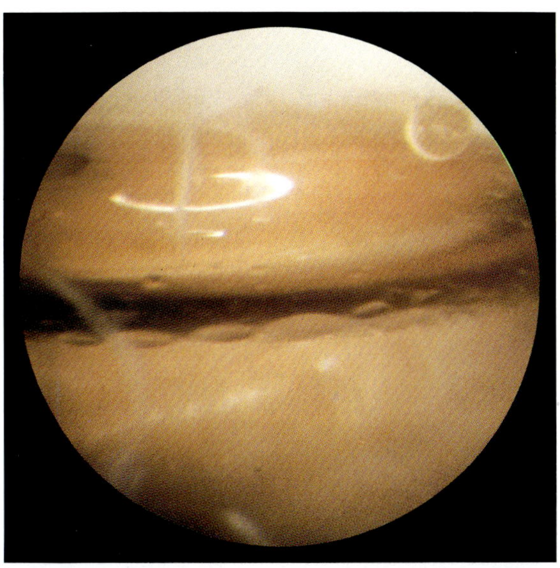

1.79

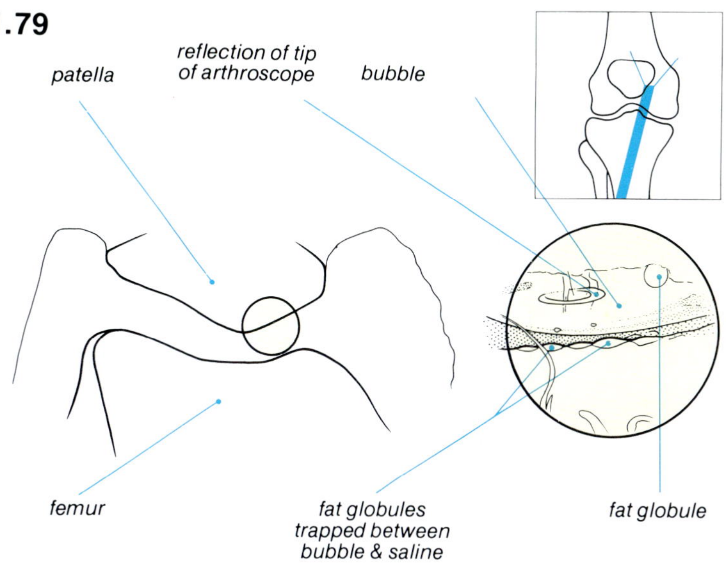

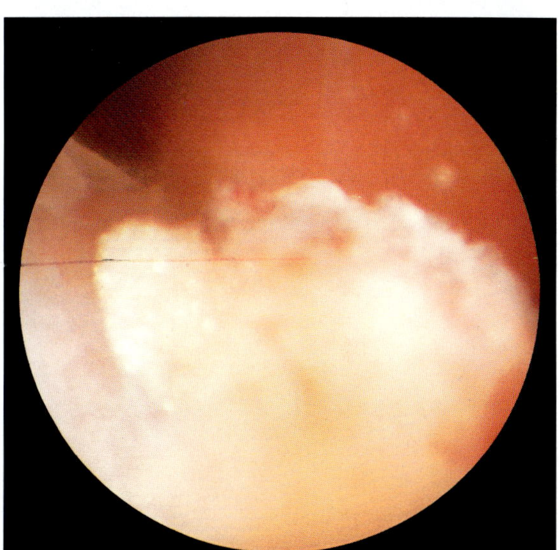

1.80

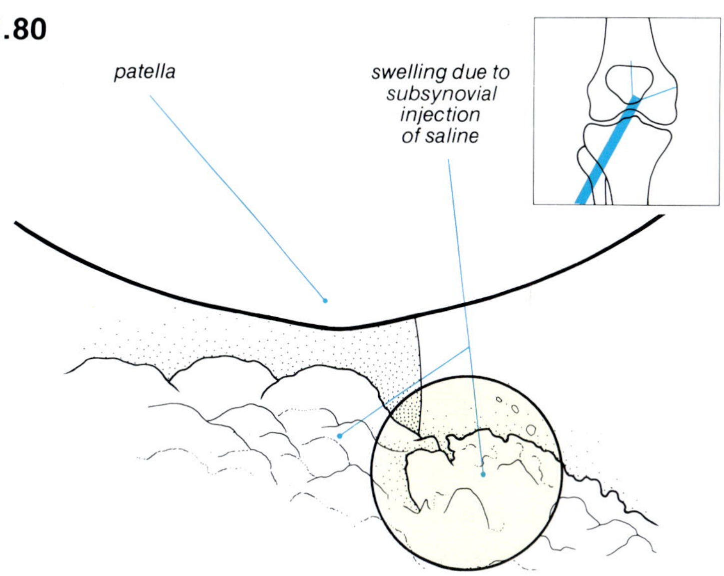

As the arthroscope is inserted and withdrawn from the knee, it must pass through the subsynovial tissues, most commonly in the area of the infrapatellar fat pad, an area particularly susceptible to distension by saline. Fig.1.81 shows the arthroscopic view of the interior of the fat pad, with an opening into the joint at the far end of a fatty tunnel. The saline was flowing from the tip of the arthroscope as this photograph was taken and resulted in considerable distension of the fat pad. If such an appearance is observed, the flow of saline should be stopped at once.

Synovium heals well after injury, but a scar can usually be identified at the site of a previous arthrotomy or wound. Fig.1.82 shows the site of an earlier arthrotomy and is marked by a festoon of fibrous arches. Blood vessels are also seen in the subsynovial tissues and are often noted at the site of scars. Although these vessels are well marked and run parallel to each other, suggesting that they are normal structures, it is curious that they should be so closely related to the wound and run so exactly parallel to it. Scars running along the line of arthrotomy incisions are an unusual observation but nevertheless are occasionally seen.

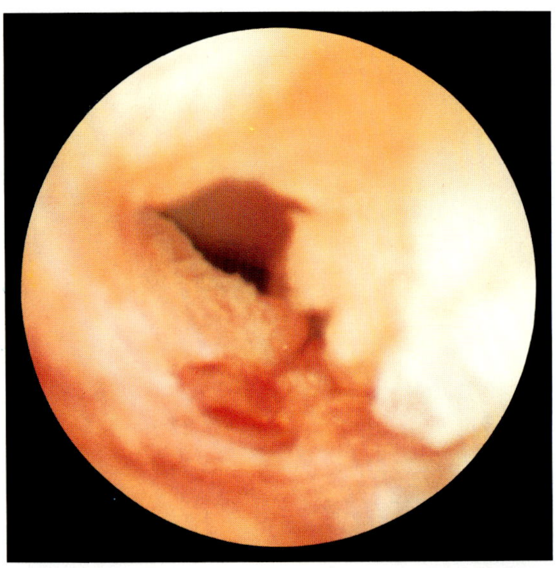

1.81

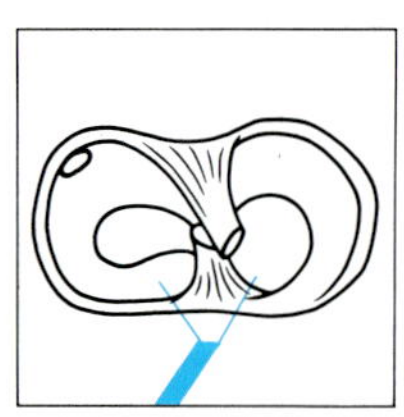

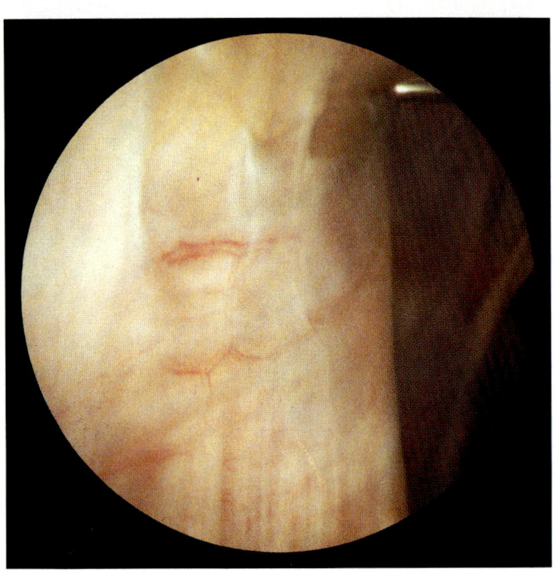

1.82

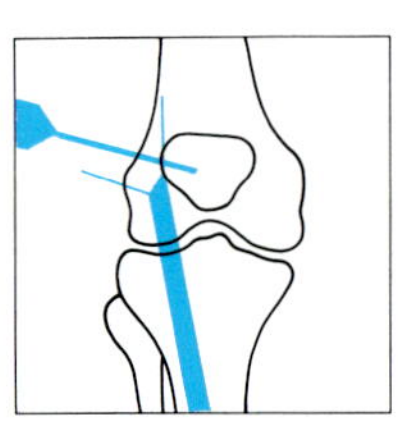

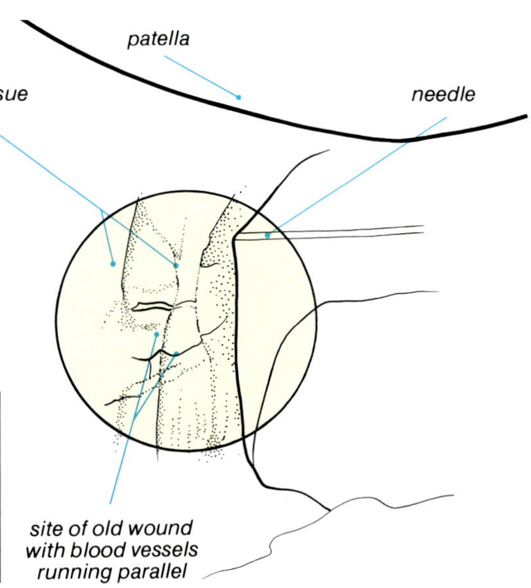

2
Synovial Disorders

Trauma

Direct trauma to the synovium results in bruising and haemorrhage. Fig.2.1 shows bruising of the infrapatellar fold after an injury to the knee that also disrupted the anterior cruciate ligament. The patient had a small effusion and was unable to straighten the leg. On clinical examination the knee appeared to be fixed in thirty degrees of flexion and the features were those of a locked medial meniscal fragment. At arthroscopy with the patient anaesthetized and the knee extended fully, the notch was found to contain much haemorrhagic and swollen tissue. Fig.2.1 shows an area of haemorrhage in the infrapatellar fold immediately below the apex of the intercondylar notch where it would have been compressed during full extension of the knee.

A late effect of injury to the synovium is adhesion formation. Fig.2.2 shows a blood-stained adhesion crossing the joint from the undersurface of the quadriceps mechanism to the anterior surface of the femur. On flexing the knee the adhesion became tense and could be seen pulling on the synovial lining of the joint. Isolated solitary adhesions of this type are not an uncommon finding at arthroscopy and are probably of no significance even though they are well placed to cause pain by traction of the synovium. The adhesion in Fig.2.2 was approximately 1mm in diameter and was divided arthroscopically; the knee was otherwise normal. The patient was suffering from anterior knee pain and the symptoms were not improved by the operation.

Fig.2.3 shows a stouter adhesion crossing the suprapatellar pouch transversely near its upper limit. Scarring of the suprapatellar pouch followed a previous operation, but movement in the knee was complete although accompanied by a dull pain on full flexion. The adhesions were divided arthroscopically and the patient reported that the pain on flexion had been relieved.

Adhesions in the suprapatellar pouch are sometimes so dense that the pouch is almost completely obliterated. These appearances are often seen after patellectomy or other trauma to the suprapatellar pouch. Fig.2.4 shows a dense bridge of fibrous material crossing the suprapatellar pouch transversely at the former site of the patella which had been removed because of persistent pain following a fracture one year earlier. The knee had been immobilized in extension after operation and would flex only to sixty degrees. Release of adhesions under arthroscopic control improved the range of flexion to one hundred and thirty degrees, but movement was

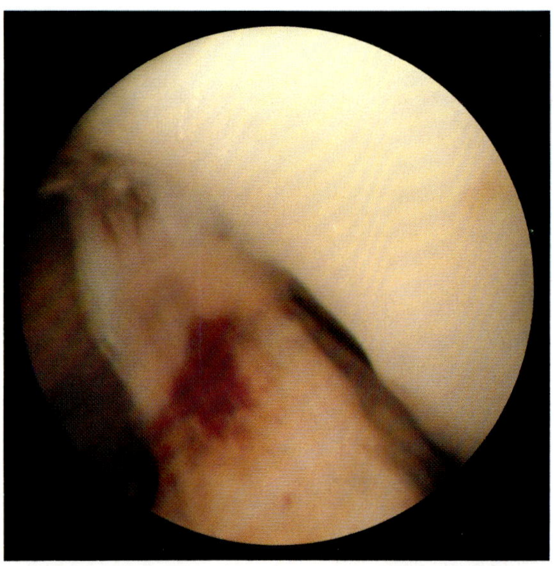

2.1

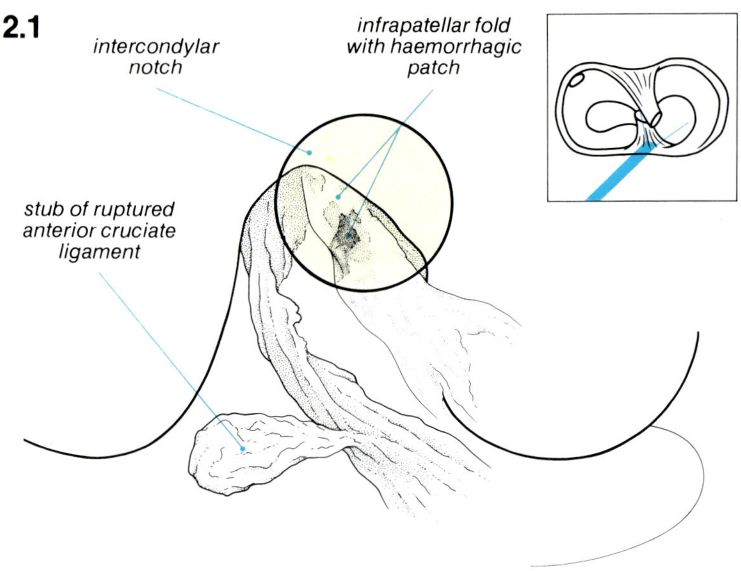

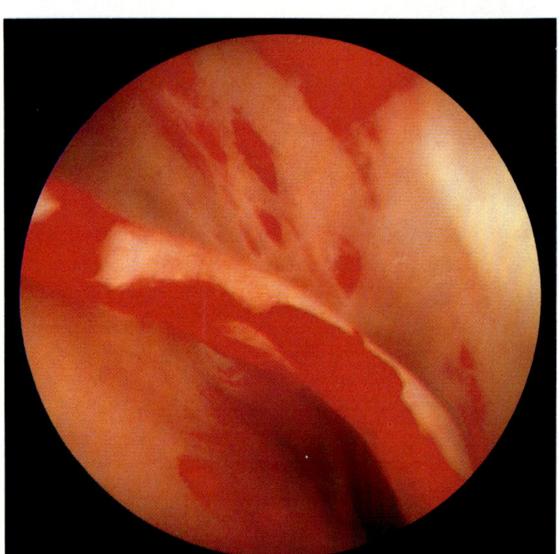

2.2

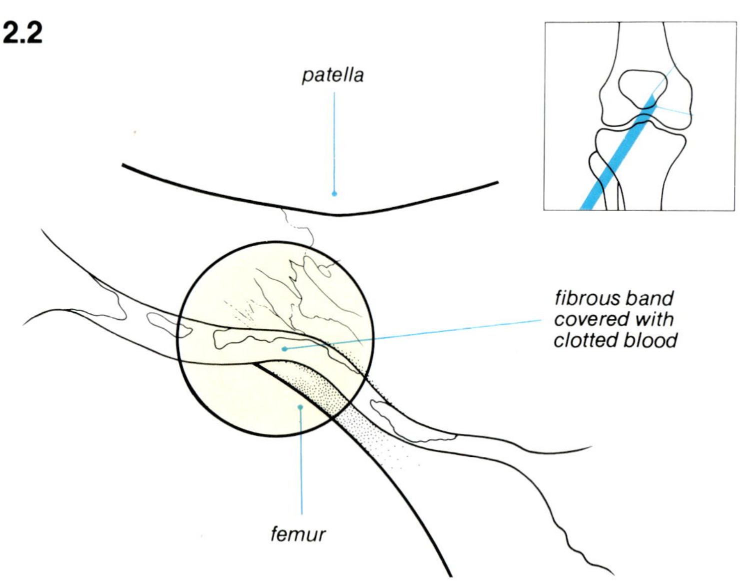

painful. It took many months to achieve a pain-free range of movement.

The suprapatellar pouch is the most common site for adhesions but they do occur elsewhere in the knee. Fig.2.5 shows an unusually dense adhesion in the posteromedial compartment, running from the back of the femoral condyle to the posterior capsule. The adhesion was divided arthroscopically. The patient had suffered a haemarthrosis following a fracture of the femur, and adhesions were present throughout the knee.

2.3

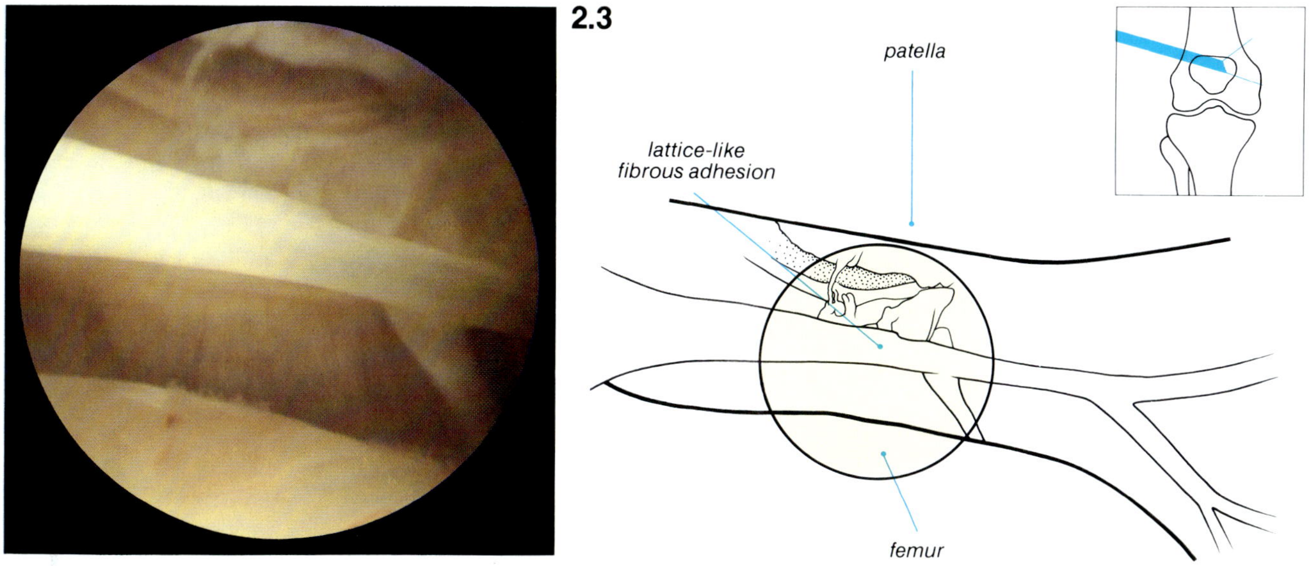

2.4

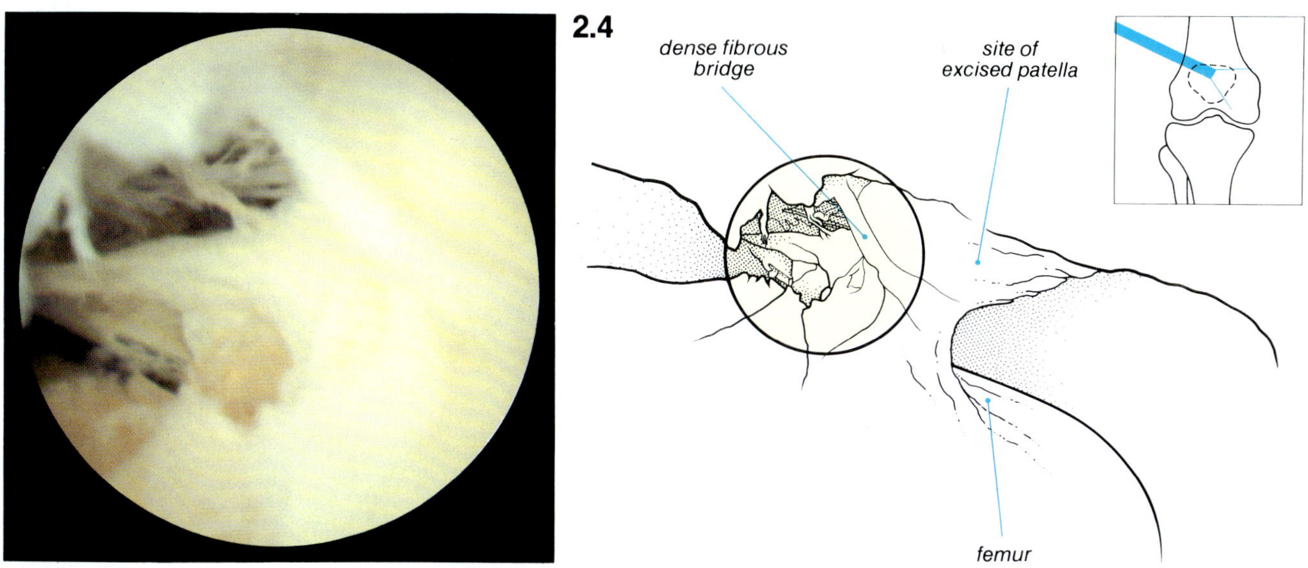

2.5

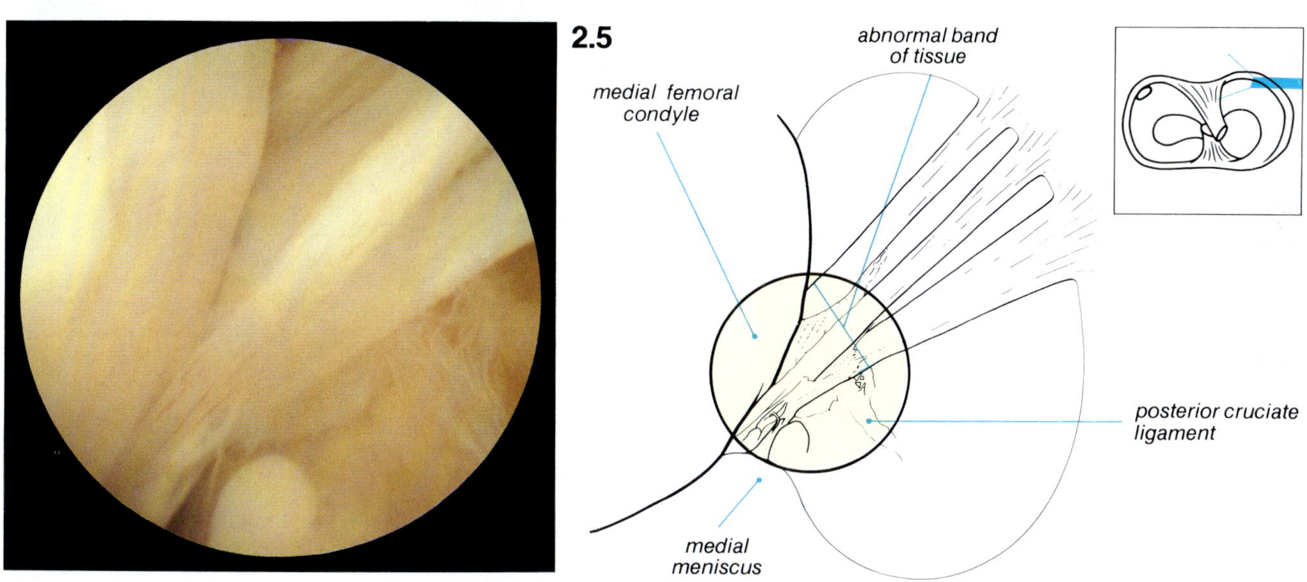

Scarring of the synovium can also occur after excision of the medial synovial shelf (Fig.2.6). Because the medial synovial shelf runs in a crescentic manner, excision of the shelf is likely to cause contracture across the base of the excised area as one might expect after, for example, excision of the skin web between the thumb and index finger. The resultant scarring may be denser and tighter than the original shelf and in this patient there was no relief of symptoms. A fibrous band slightly thicker than the original shelf can be seen at the site of excision. If the shelf is completely excised, taking the excision into the surrounding synovium, the scarring may be even more marked than in Fig.2.6.

Synovitis

The causes of inflammation of the synovium are many, and include trauma, infection, diseases such as rheumatoid arthritis, chemical irritation from blood, and irritation from fragments of articular cartilage.

Chronic localized irritation produces an increase in vascularity of the synovium and an overgrowth of pannus so intense that it can resemble granulation tissue. The knee in Fig.2.7 had a loose body jammed in the intercondylar notch for six months before operation. The patient was a busy man who could not afford time away from his work to undergo operation and had walked with a slightly flexed knee throughout this period, practicing knee extension exercises diligently and vigorously in the hope that operation could be avoided. Fig.2.7 shows the result of constant irritation of the synovium overlying the anterior cruciate ligament. After removal of the loose body, the range of movement was improved but pain on extension persisted for over three months.

Small purpuric spots are usually seen as an incidental finding (see Fig.1.42). But in Fig.2.8 they are found in a knee with a large effusion, no history of injury and no sign of joint disorder elsewhere. All serological tests were negative. Histological examination (Fig.2.9) showed increased vascularity and an infiltration of chronic inflammatory cells.

Septic arthritis leads to a variety of arthroscopic

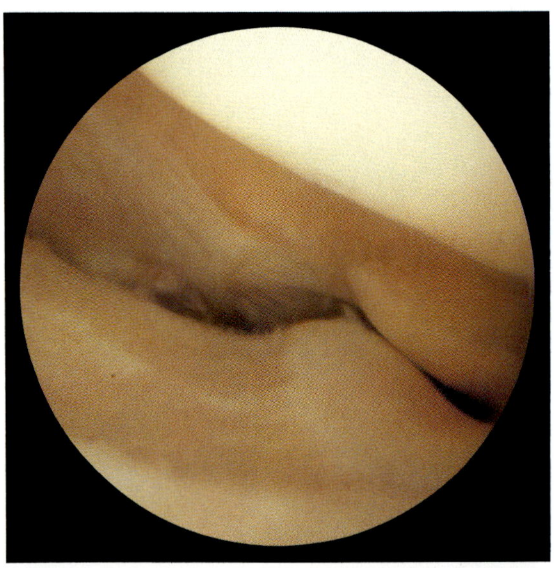

2.6

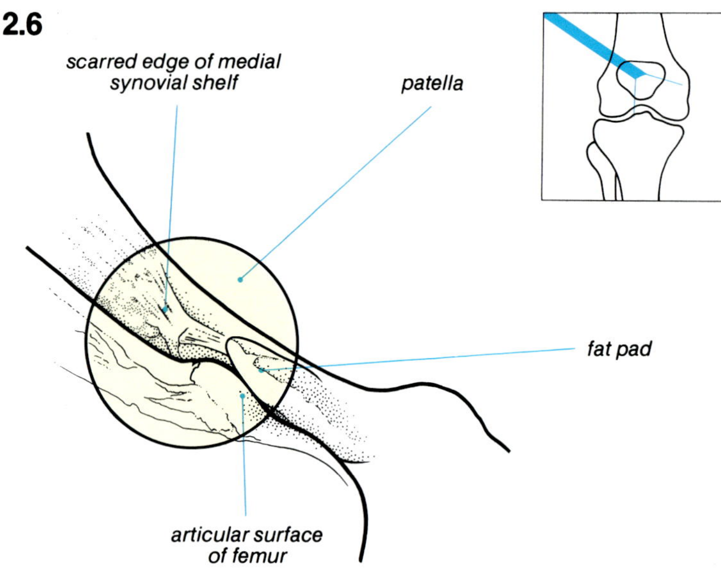

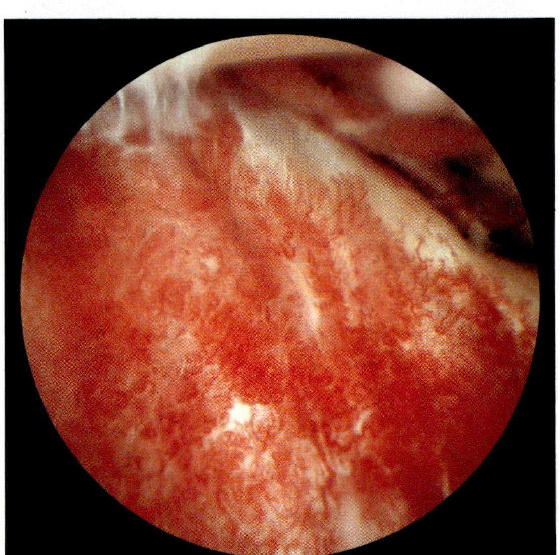

2.7

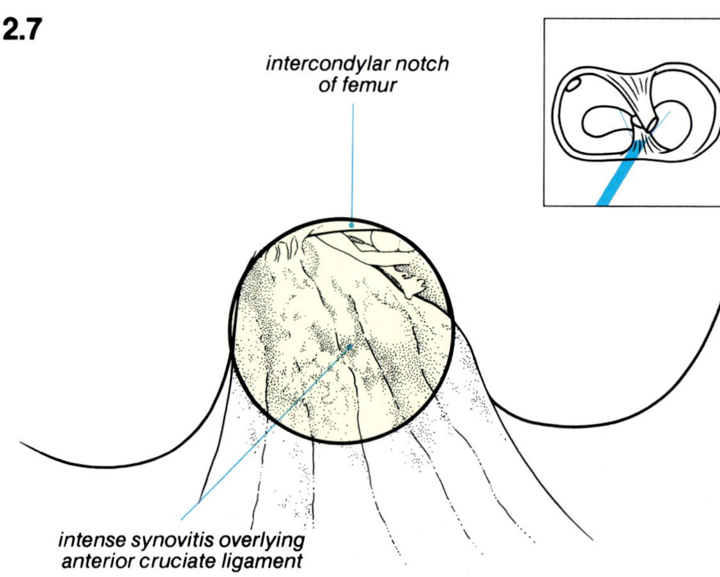

appearances, perhaps depending on the organism involved. Fig.2.10 shows the synovium of a 12-year-old boy who knelt on a rusty needle that broke and left a fragment of metal in the joint. The synovium was thrown into thickened folds with many small punctate haemorrhages on its surface. The haemorrhages are slightly larger than those in Fig.2.8 and more diffuse. The joint swelled, haemolytic streptococci were isolated, and the patient made a good recovery following thorough arthroscopic irrigation of the joint and adequate

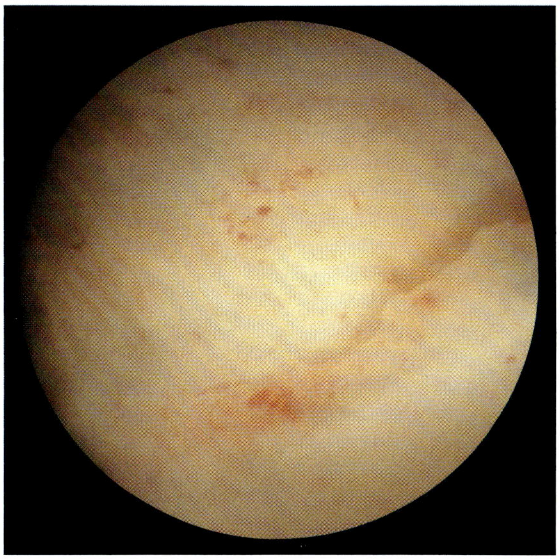

2.8

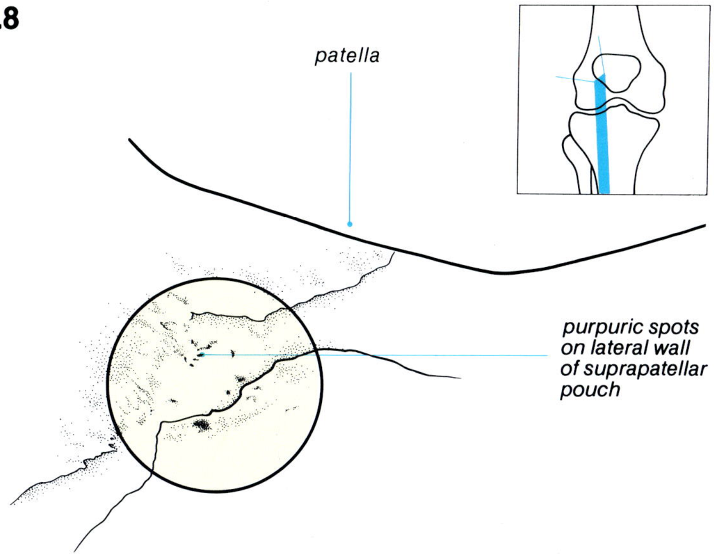

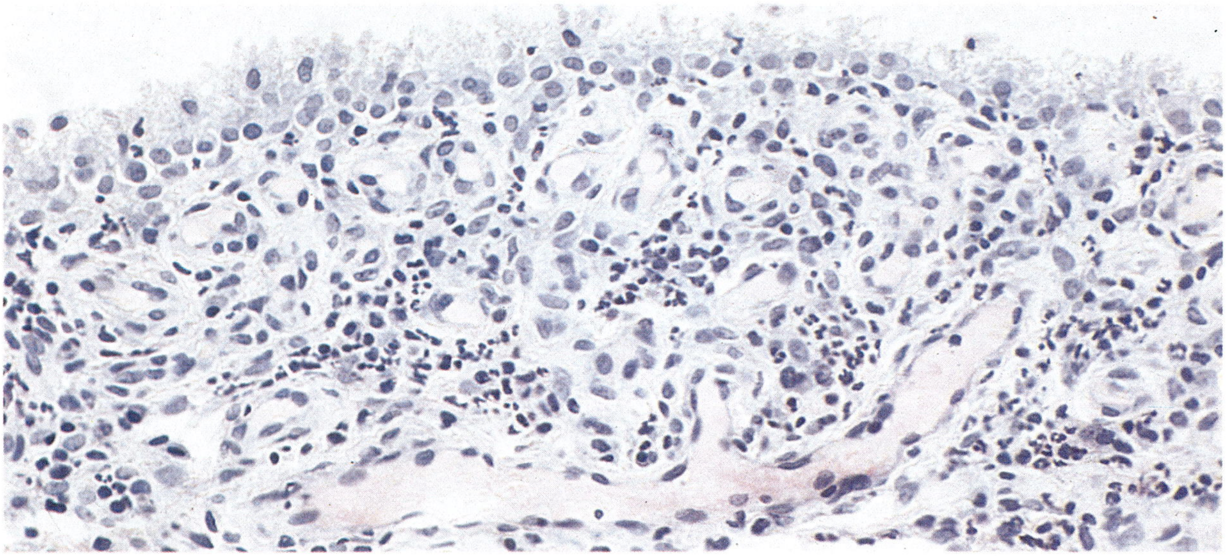

2.9

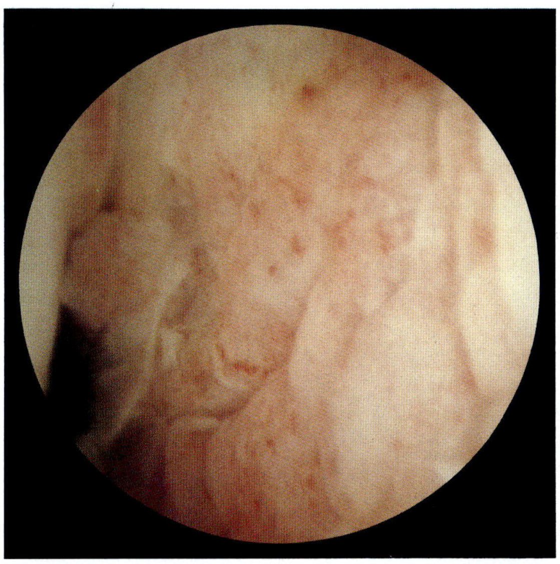

2.10

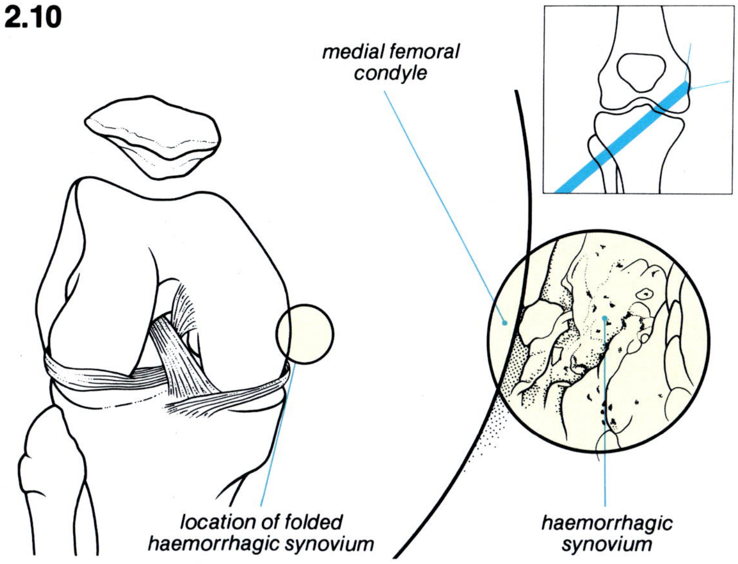

antibiotic treatment. Fig.2.11 shows the meniscosynovial junction of the same knee as in Fig.2.10. The meniscal and articular surfaces appear entirely normal but the synovium is grossly thickened and the normal depression at the meniscosynovial junction is lost.

Fig.2.12 is of a knee that had been infected five years previously. The patient did not receive medical treatment until the infection was well established and the joint became stiff with only thirty degrees of flexion. At arthroscopy the suprapatellar pouch was found to be obliterated by fibrous tissue. The undersurface of the patella consisted of subchondral bone without a covering of articular cartilage and with haemorrhagic fibrous tissue below it.

Acute synovitis of the knee from any cause can lead to the appearance in Fig.2.13. This knee was affected by pyrophosphate arthropathy and became acutely swollen without trauma. The synovium showed many thickened polyps with dilated vessels. Histological examination (Fig.2.14) showed intense plasma cell infiltration with some neutrophils.

As the synovitis begins to resolve, the polyps 'deflate' slightly, leaving a pointed tip at the end of the villus as if the swelling had started to resolve at the top and was extending proximally (Fig.2.15). The villi also bear a fine glaze of fibrin and white fibrinous strands extend from the tips of several of the villi. Like the appearances of Fig.2.13, those of Fig.2.15 are non-specific but are most commonly seen in patients with acute rheumatoid arthritis.

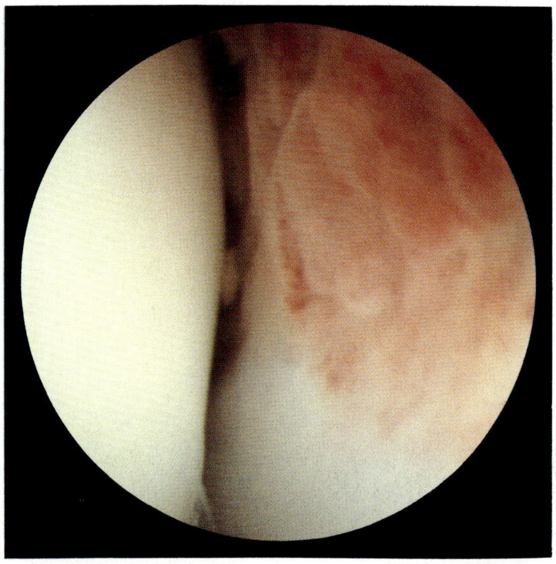

2.11

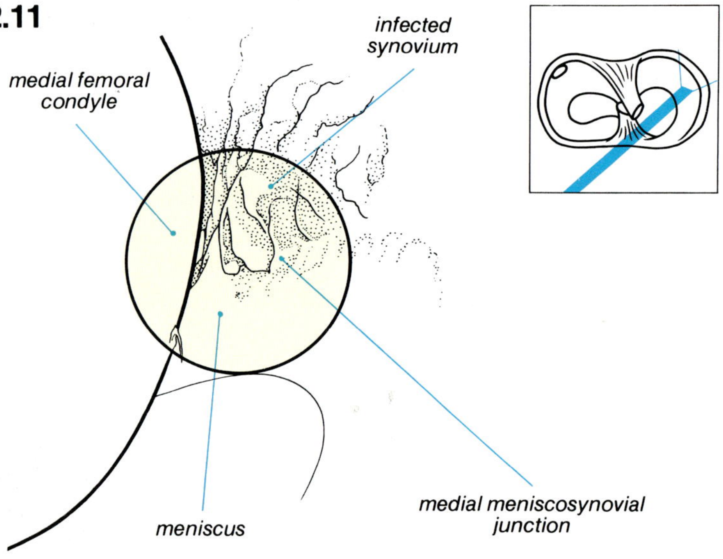

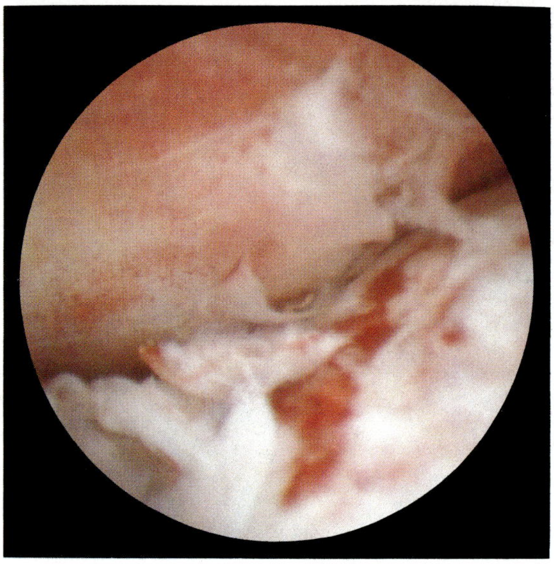

2.12

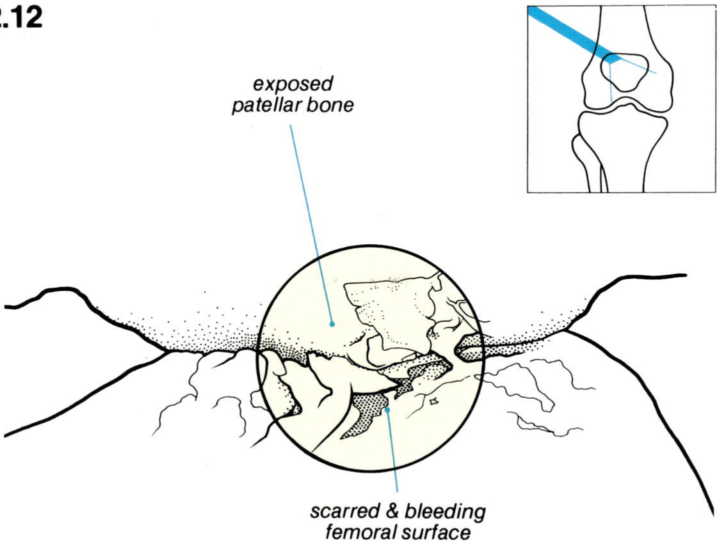

Rheumatoid arthritis

Chronic rheumatoid arthritis gives a slightly different appearance from those of Fig.2.13 and 2.15. Patients with rheumatoid arthritis may have superimposed degenerative change and areas of pigmentation due to repeated bleeding into the knee. For these reasons the synovial changes in these patients can vary widely and the changes due to rheumatoid arthritis alone may be

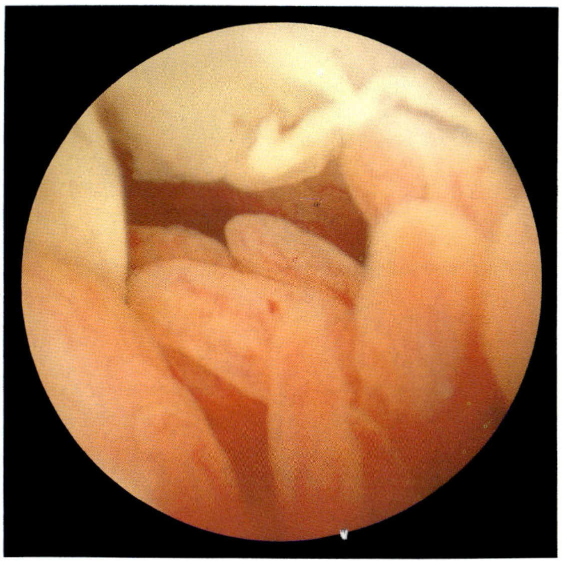

2.13

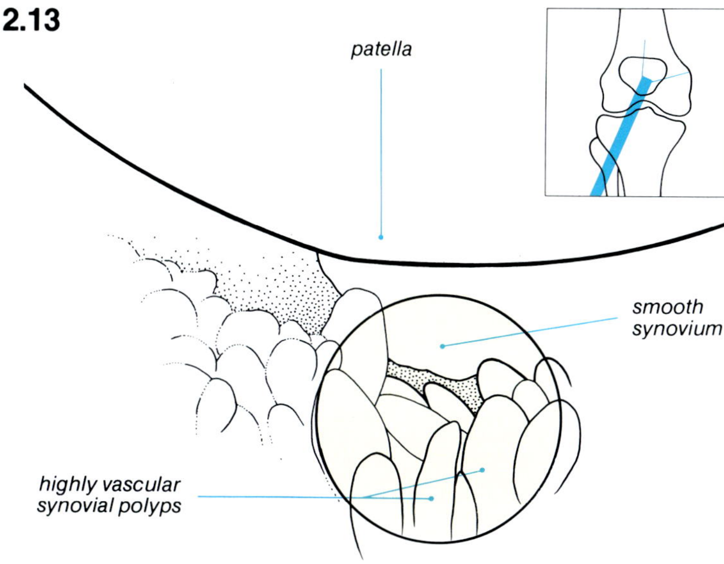

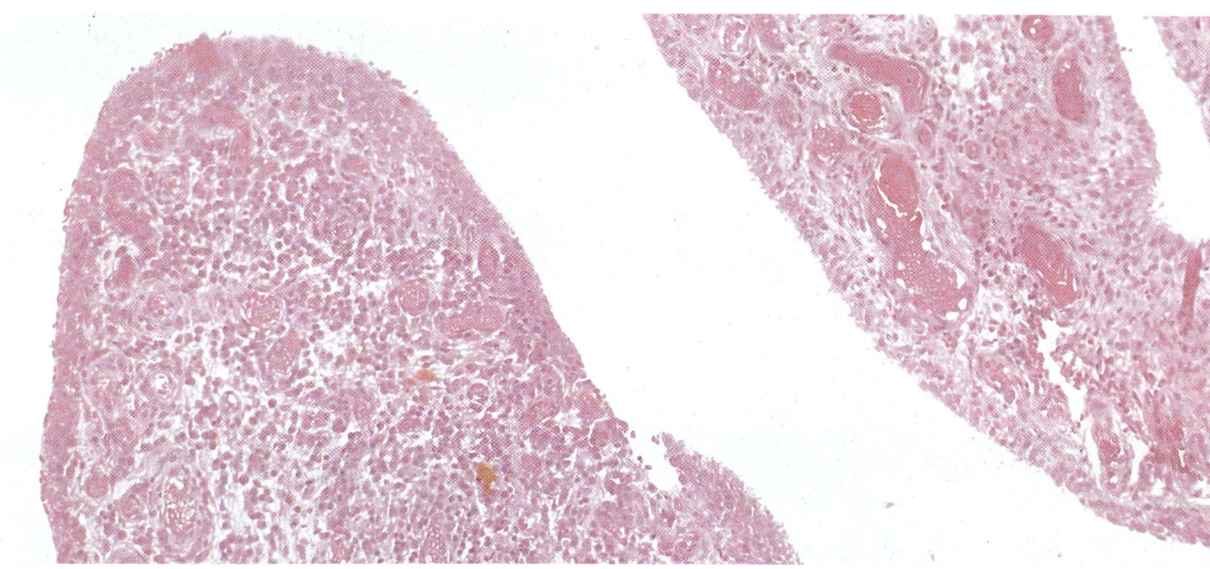

2.14

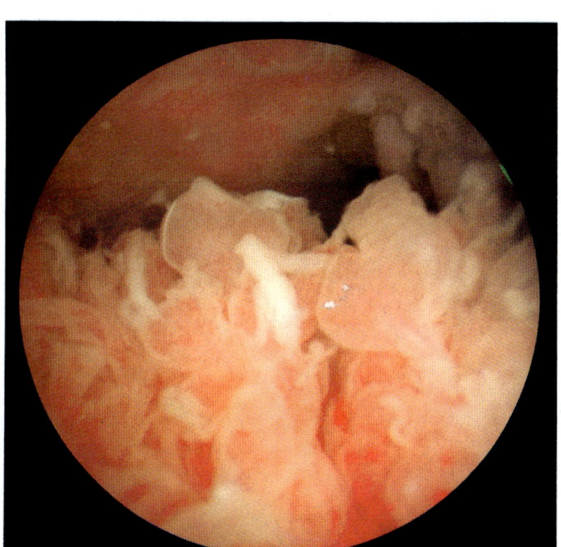

2.15

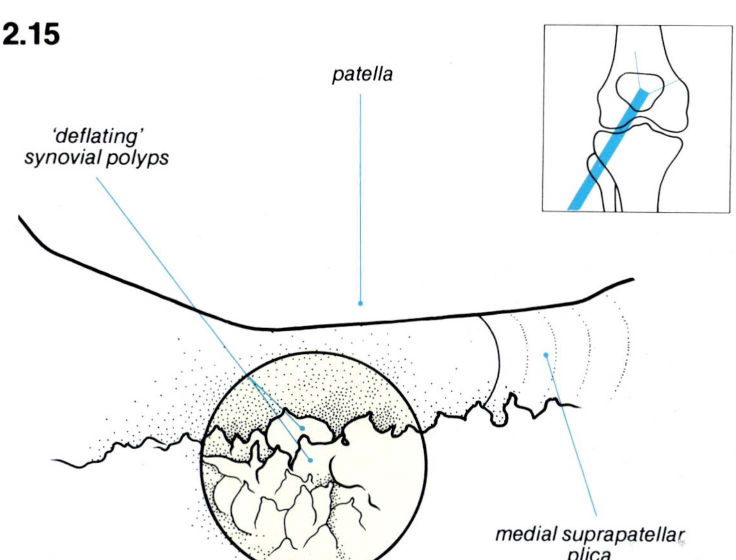

difficult to identify. Figs.2.16 and 2.17 show the typical synovial changes of rheumatoid arthritis. The synovial fronds, or polyps, have a slightly stiff and bloated appearance when compared with those of Fig.2.13 and vascular markings are not seen. Fig.2.17 shows a clump of polyps in the suprapatellar pouch. The polyps did not move as freely in the saline flow as those in Fig.2.16 and, although the synovium in the background is apparently

2.16

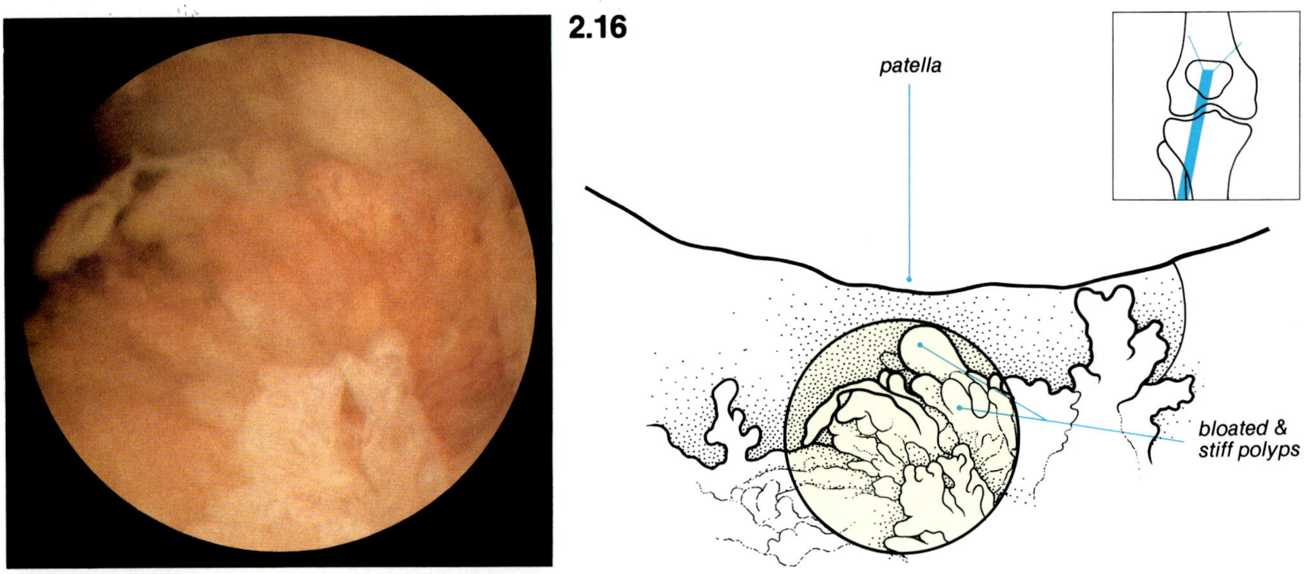

2.17

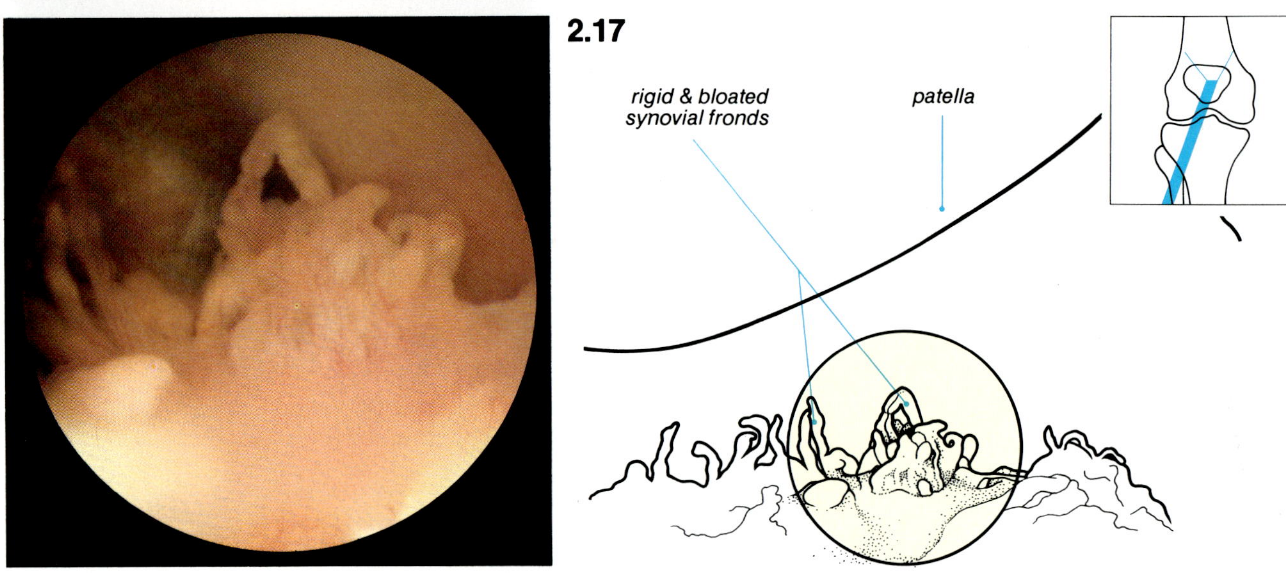

2.18

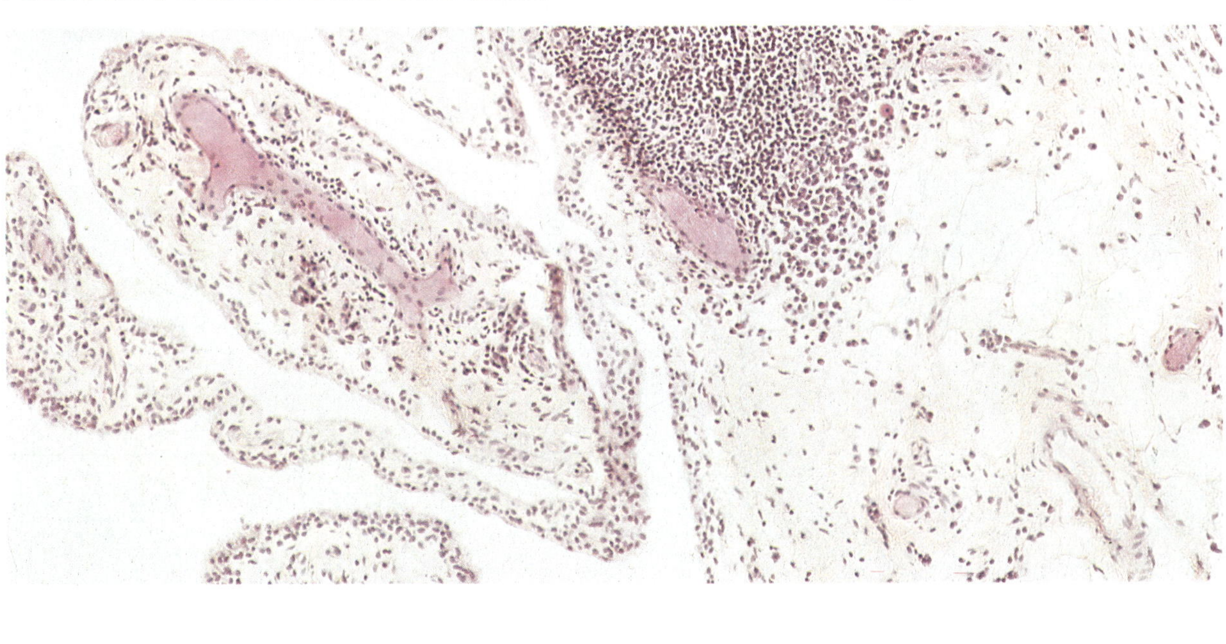

normal, other areas of the medial wall of the joint had the typical rheumatoid appearance. Histological examination of the synovium (Fig.2.18) showed hyperaemia with luxuriant synovial lining cells and oedematous fronds infiltrated by plasma cells and some lymphoid follicles.

Psoriatic arthritis

The appearances of psoriatic arthritis are similar to those of rheumatoid arthritis. It is difficult to distinguish between the two on arthroscopic grounds only, but the vascular markings of the synovium in psoriatic arthritis are generally more exaggerated than in rheumatoid arthritis and the synovial polyps are less rigid. Fig.2.19 is from a young man with swelling of one knee only and a history of a twisting injury that could have caused a meniscal tear. The patient also had mild psoriasis which had given him little trouble for several years. At arthroscopy no meniscal lesion was identified but the synovium was intensely inflamed with increased vascular markings. The histological appearance (Fig.2.20) was of a hypoplastic synovial lining with an infiltration of lymphocytes, neutrophil polymorphs and some plasma cells.

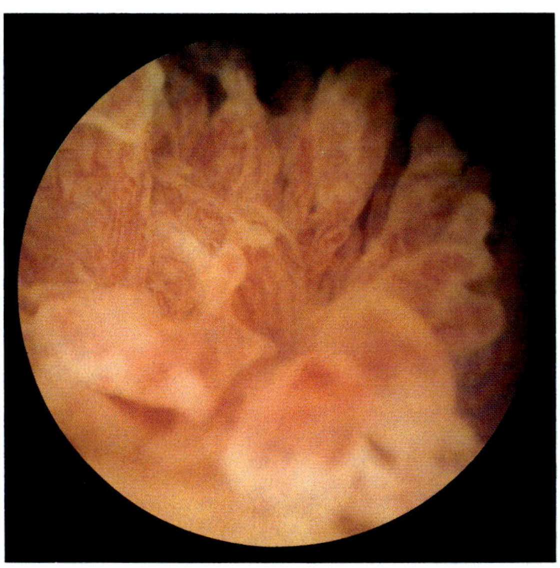

2.19

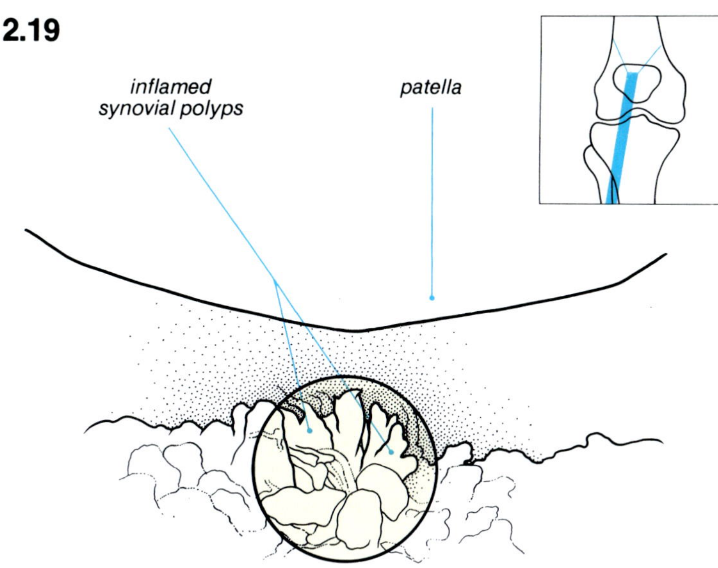

2.20

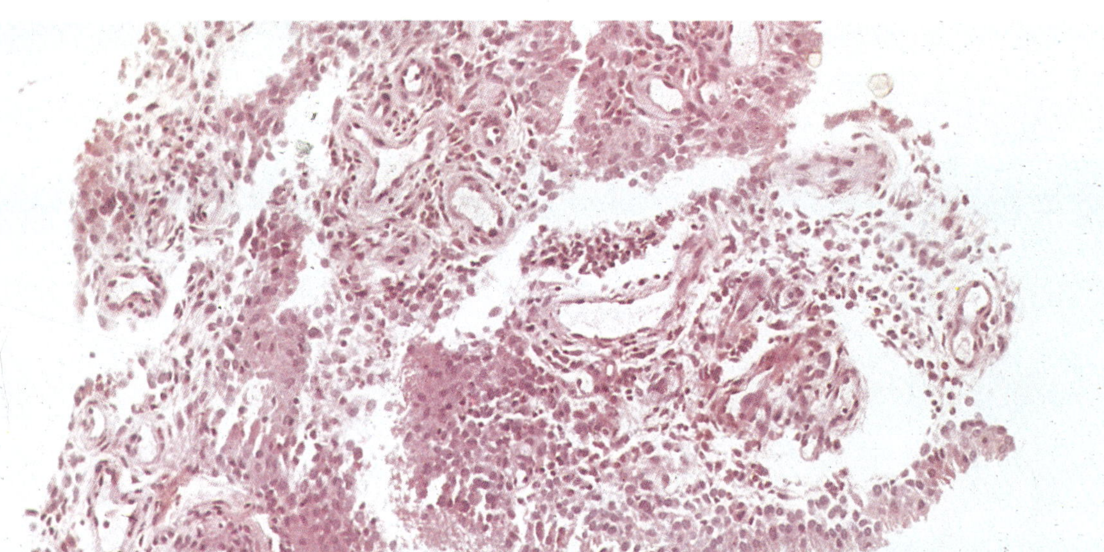

It is probably unwise to attach too much diagnostic importance to the finer points of synovial morphology seen through the arthroscope. Fig.2.21 is of a patient who had psoriatic arthritis but who was also affected by osteoarthritis. Much articular cartilage debris was present in the joint and some fragments had become attached to the synovium. Although it is very likely that much of the synovitis is the result of the patient's psoriasis, at least some must have also been the result of irritation from the debris. The histological appearance (Fig.2.22) was similar to that of Fig.2.20.

Miscellaneous

Fig.2.23 shows the knee of a patient during an acute episode of Behçet's disease. The knee was swollen, tender and warm. At arthroscopy the synovium of the suprapatellar pouch appeared to have been shed, revealing the underlying fibres of the joint capsule denuded of all synovial covering. A few patches of necrotic synovium were found around the joint, but no normal synovium could be seen. The appearance of Fig.2.23 is entirely consistent with the changes in the mouth and other serous membranes.

Fig.2.24 has a slightly similar appearance to that of Fig.2.23, but the clinical picture was much more complicated. The patient had acute systemic lupus erythematosus and was being treated with steroids. The knee was also infected with *Salmonella paratyphi*, making it difficult to distinguish the changes due to the systemic lupus erythematosus from those of the infection. The synovium had been shed from the capsule throughout the knee. Fig.2.24 shows the posterior cruciate ligament from the posteromedial approach with a few flimsy patches of necrotic synovium adherent to it. Some articular cartilage had also been shed (see Fig.3.17).

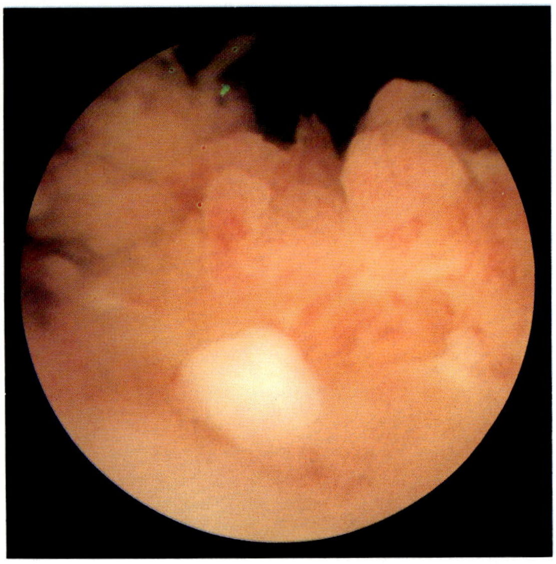

2.21

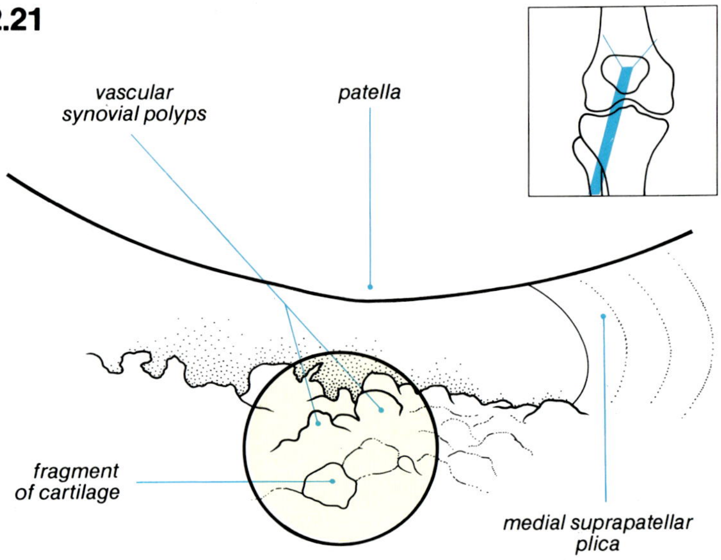

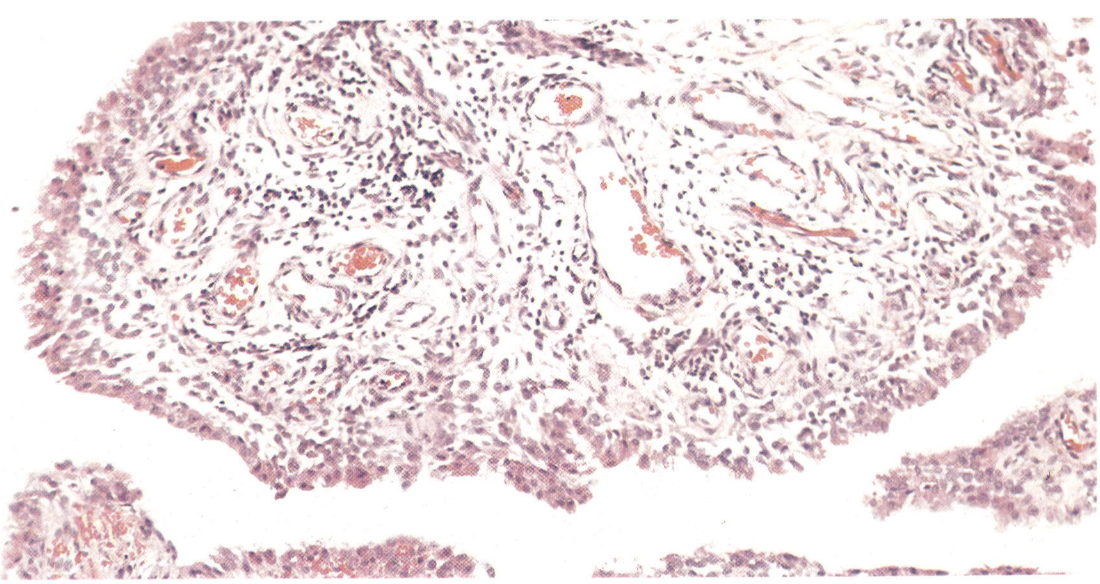

2.22

Crystal synovitis

Crystals are often associated with synovitis, particularly in the older patient with degenerative osteoarthritis. The crystals are sometimes deposited within the synovial tissue but are also seen around the margins of degenerate articular cartilage and on the fringes of damaged menisci.

In Fig.2.25 a chalky mass of calcified material protrudes from beneath the medial meniscus and other calcified deposits are seen on the surface of the meniscus itself.

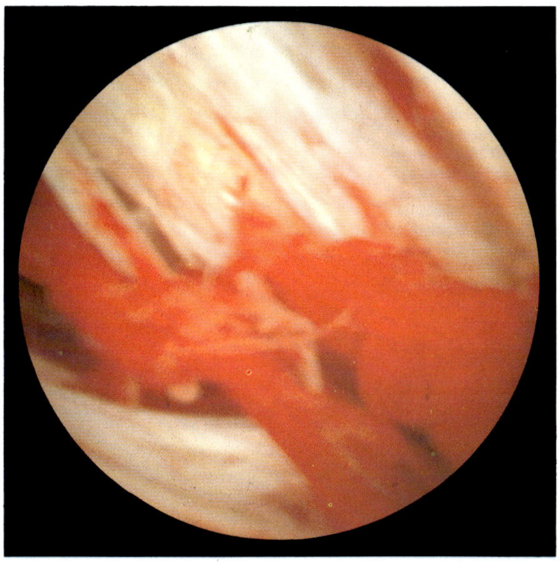

2.23

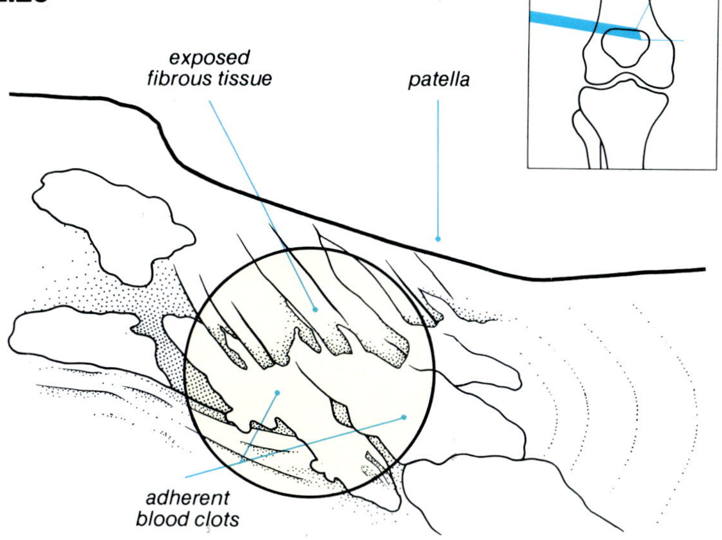

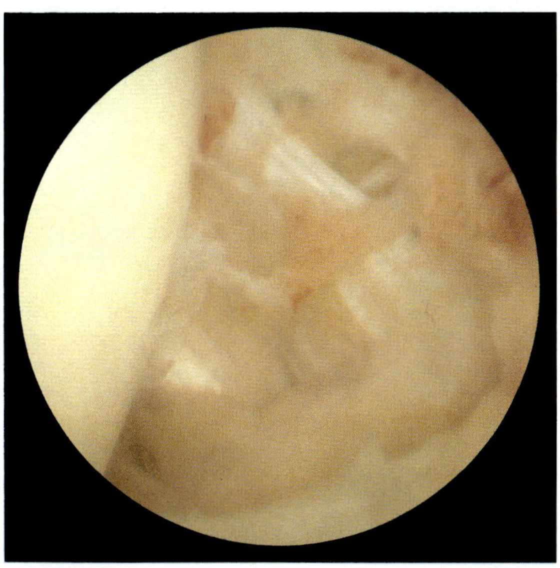

2.24

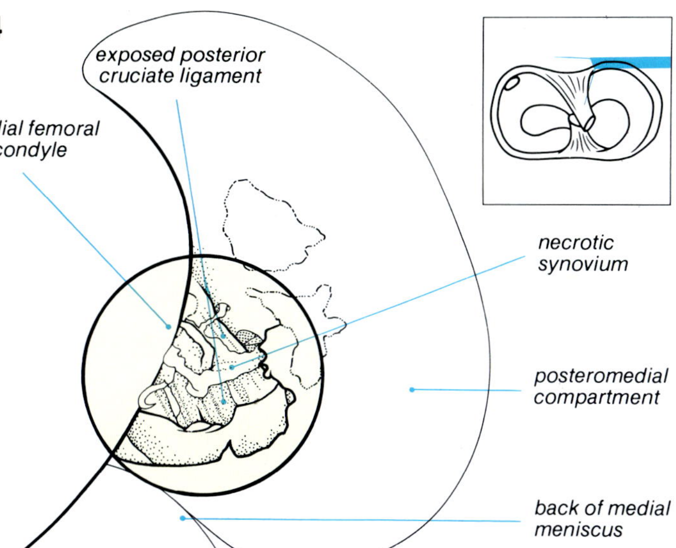

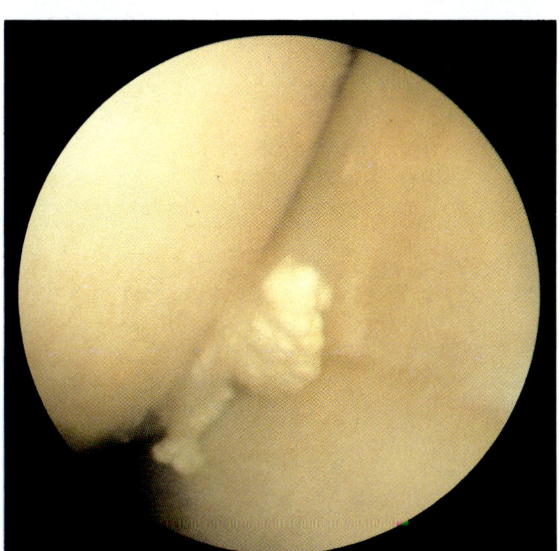

2.25

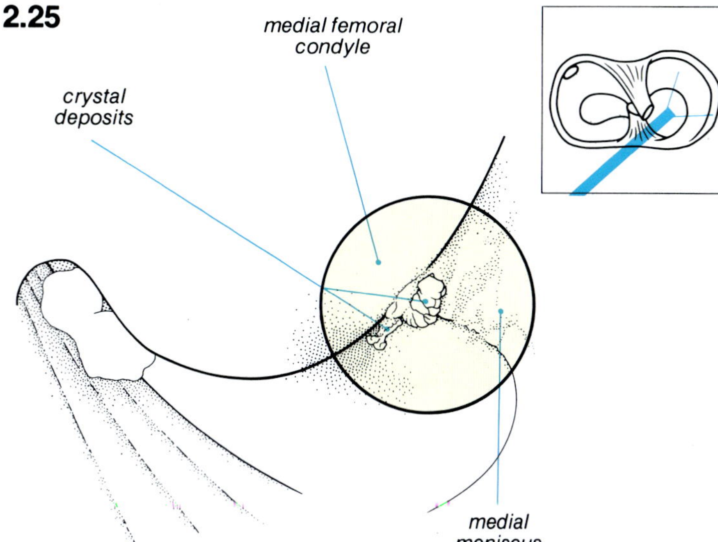

Radiography (Fig.2.26) showed calcification within the meniscal substance of all four menisci as well as a foreign body, a piece of lead shot. There was no major meniscal tear.

Fig.2.27 shows crystal deposition on fronds of degenerative articular cartilage on the back of the patella. A layer of translucent soft tissue surrounds the crystal deposit, suggesting that the crystals are deposited inside the tissue rather than upon it.

There is considerable discussion about the exact nature of the calcium salts and compounds involved in this so-called crystal synovitis. Calcium hydroxyapatite, calcium pyrophosphate and brushite can be found in the deposits but there does not appear to be definite evidence to suggest that different types of crystals or calcified deposit are associated with any specific arthroscopic appearances or clinical presentation.

Although it is possible that some metabolic abnormality may give rise to early deposition of calcium in the younger patient, in the elderly it is perhaps more probable that the calcium is deposited on any irregular or abnormal surface and that the calcification is no more specific than that seen in the pelvic veins, the costal cartilages or the great vessels.

Fig.2.28 shows superficial calcification on soft tissue debris in the intercondylar notch. The crystals have been deposited over the anterior horn of the medial meniscus but the synovial fronds themselves are free of calcium. Fig.2.29 shows a medial meniscus with many strands of degenerate and macerated meniscal tissue. Calcified deposits are seen on several of the strands, yet the articular surfaces are in good order. Both Figs. 2.28 and

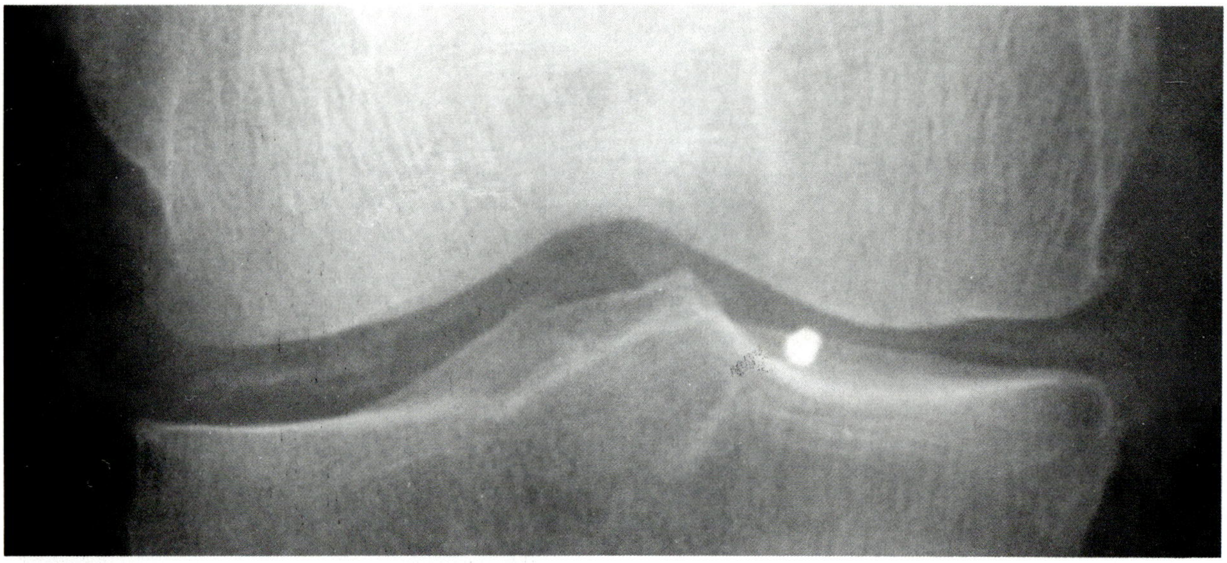

2.26

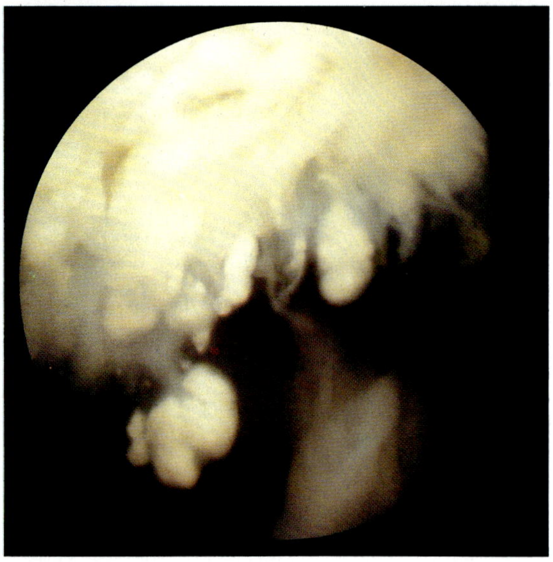

2.27

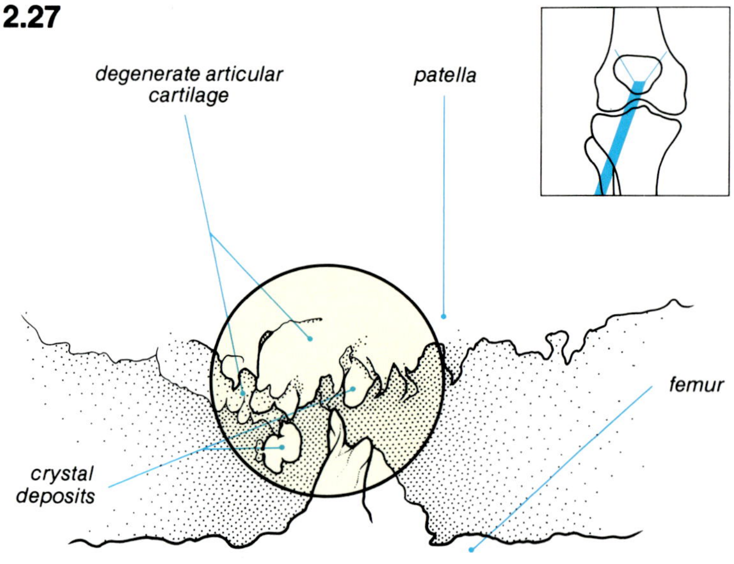

2.29, taken from different patients, show the deposition of calcium on irregular and degenerate surfaces rather than within the tissues as in Fig.2.27.

Fig.2.30 shows a large bucket handle fragment of the lateral meniscus, itself degenerate, lying in front of the lateral compartment of the knee. In the centre of the meniscal fragment there is a calcified area which is well demarcated and surrounded by soft tissue. Fig.2.30 shows the lateral compartment of the same knee as in Fig.2.28. In the latter the calcification is superficial while in Fig.2.30 the calcification is deep within the meniscal fragment.

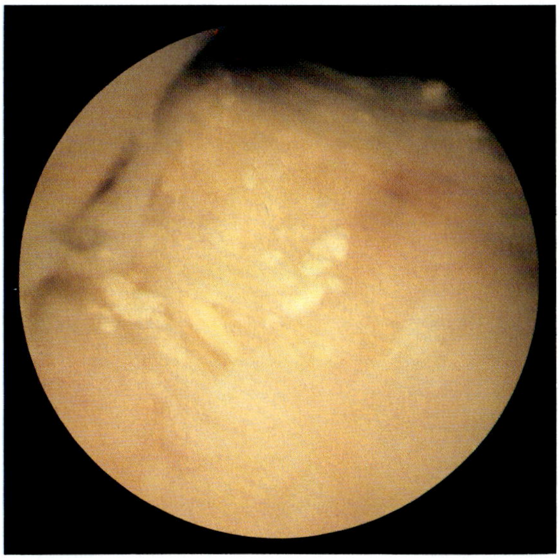

2.28

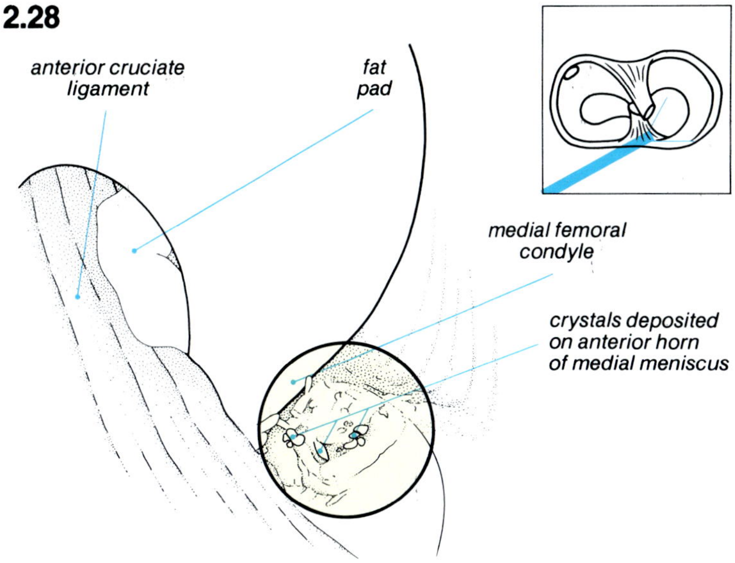

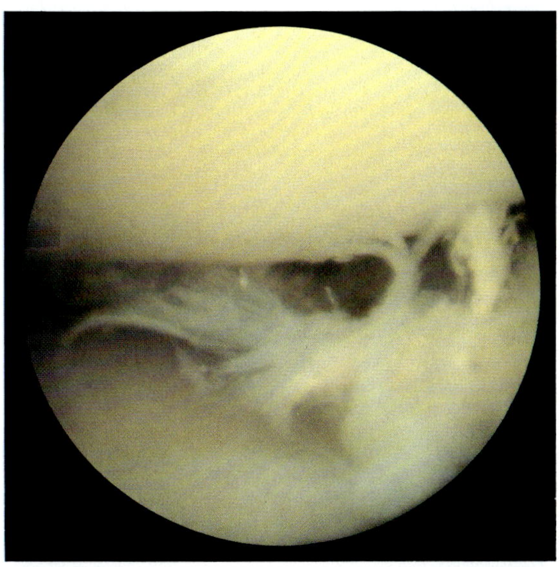

2.29

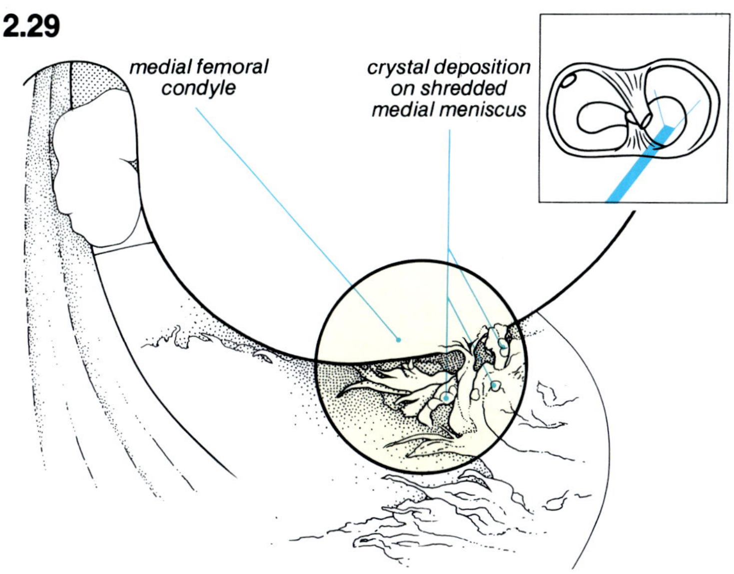

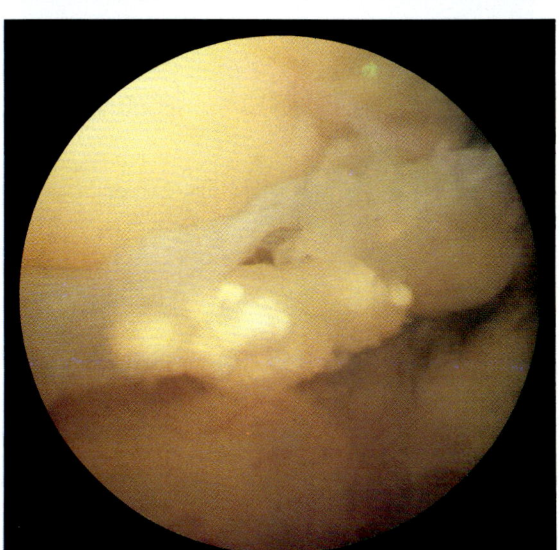

2.30

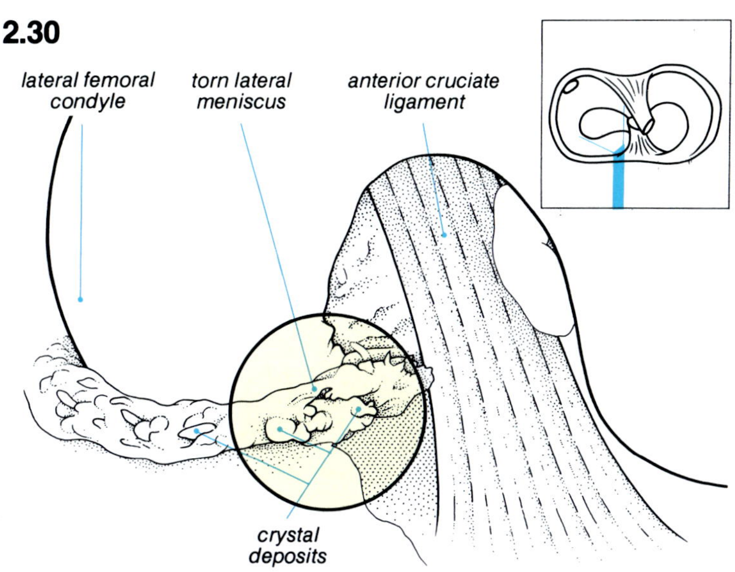

Fig.2.31 is of a younger patient, a 44-year-old woman, who developed acute pain and swelling after a comparatively minor twisting injury sustained while playing tennis. On clinical examination there was an effusion, synovial thickening and tenderness. Radiography showed no abnormality and no calcific deposits. At arthroscopy there was generalized synovitis, and a few crystals were noted. There was also the curious appearance (Fig.2.31) of a fold of synovium at the front of the joint with small wedge-shaped haemorrhages at its periphery. The distribution of these wedges suggests the possibility of embolism but, although the concept of calcified material occupying the capillaries and producing localized necrosis is attractive, it is probably far too naive and simplistic to be correct. The histology (Fig.2.32) showed a hypoplastic synovial lining with no cellular infiltrate. The patient was greatly improved by irrigation of the knee and the administration of non-steroidal anti-inflammatory drugs.

Synovial chondromatosis

This condition can present in many ways and has many arthroscopic appearances. In some patients the knee is filled with a mass of cartilaginous debris while in others, mature cartilage forms within the substance of the synovium. The differences between these appearances are so great that there may well be several disease processes involved.

Fig.2.33 shows a mass of loose granular material in the lateral gutter of the knee which on close inspection proved to be a collection of translucent loose bodies. The radiograph showed no abnormality and the patient

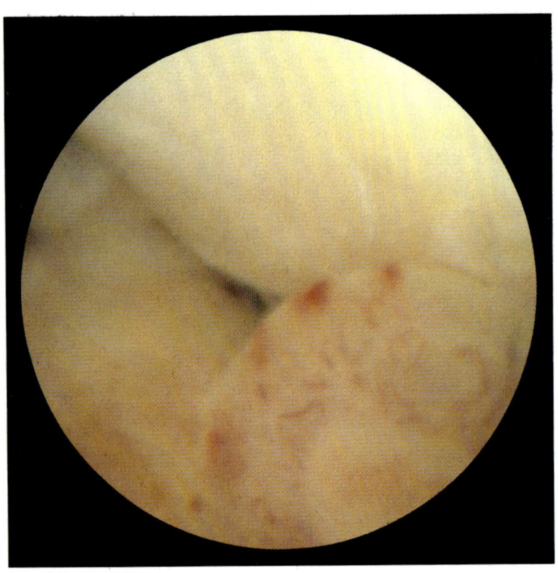

2.31

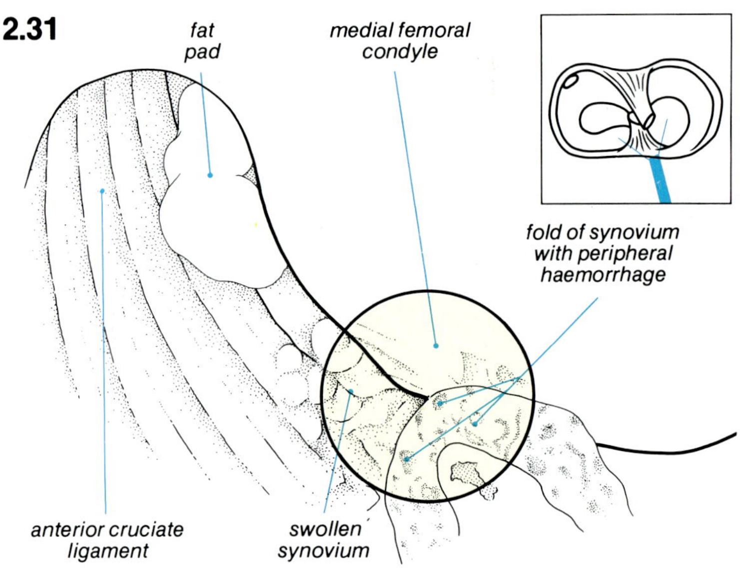

2.32

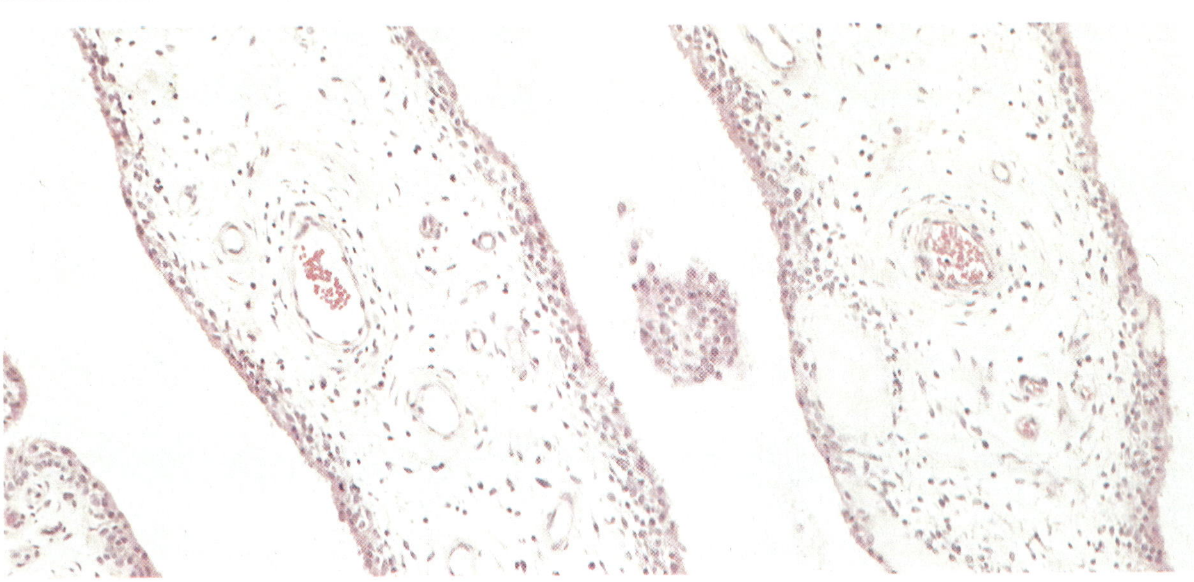

presented with a persistent effusion. At arthroscopy the debris would obstruct vision by floating in front of the lens and blocking the irrigation needle, thus occluding the drainage channel and making it difficult to achieve a clear view. The source of the loose bodies (Fig.2.34) was the synovium of the suprapatellar pouch. There was no normal synovium to be seen, the whole surface being covered with rounded polyps containing cartilaginous deposits.

A very different appearance (Fig.2.35) is presented when loose bodies, each about 1cm in diameter, lie free in the synovial cavity of the suprapatellar pouch. The loose bodies are surrounded by highly vascular and luxuriant synovial fronds which are remarkably free of

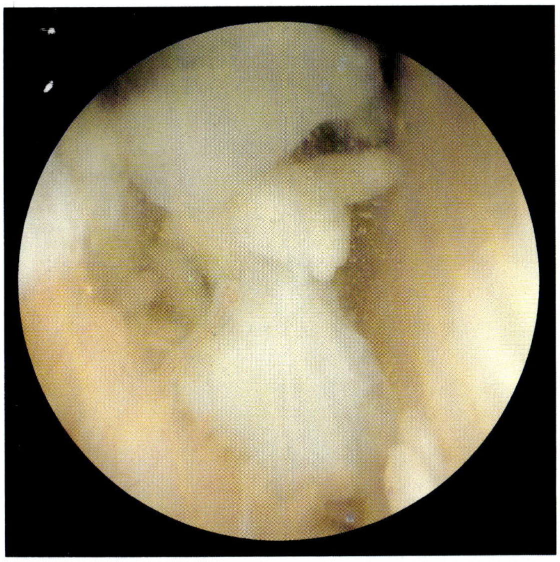

2.33

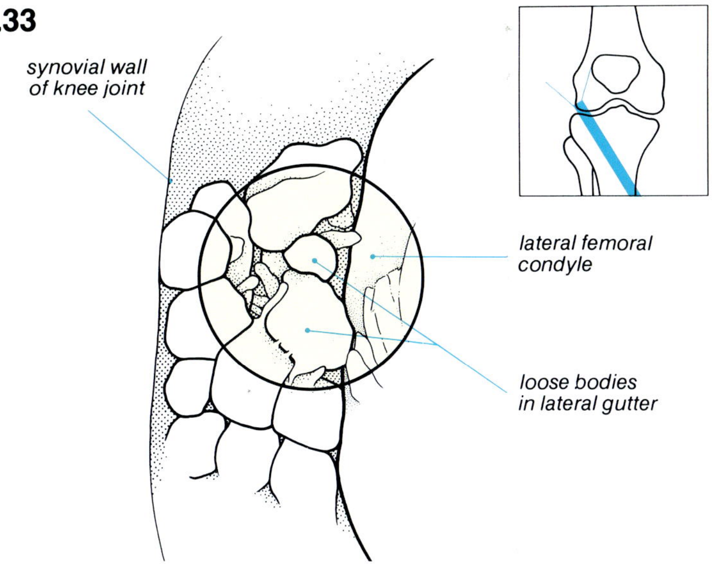

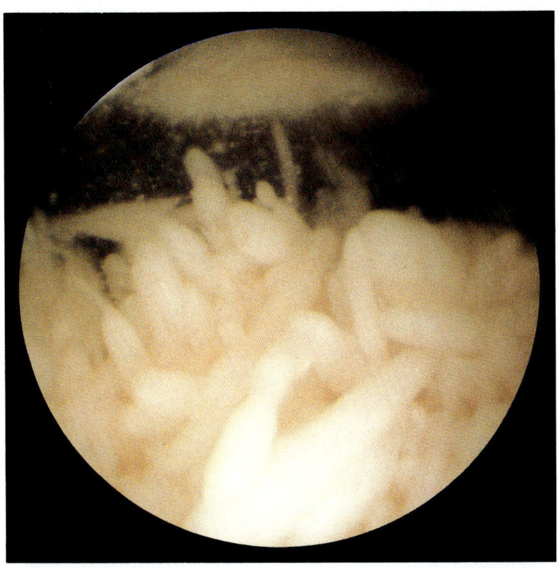

2.34

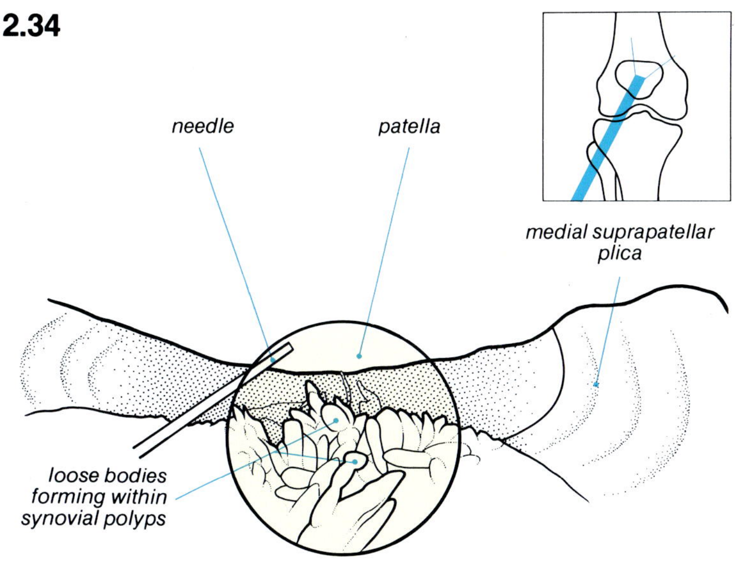

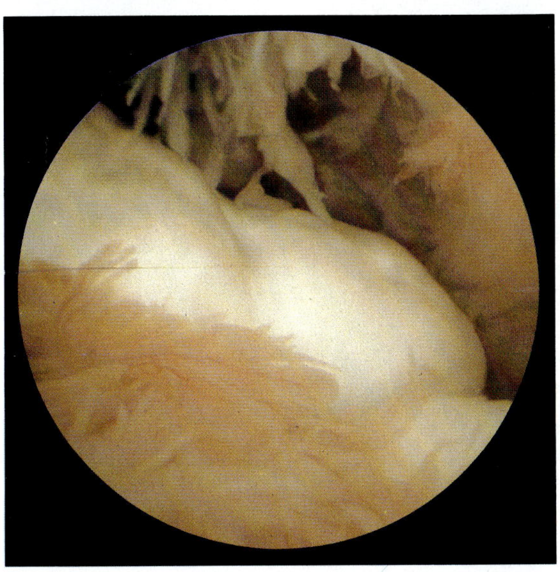

2.35

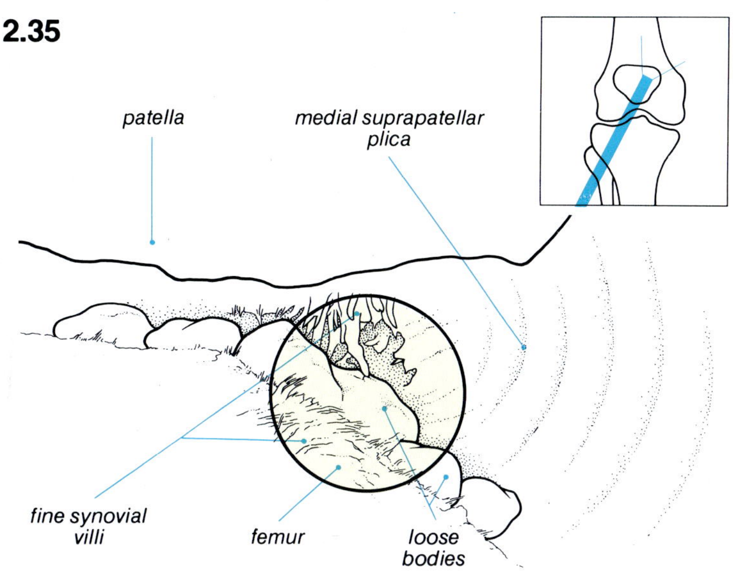

cartilaginous deposition. Two of the loose bodies are seen in Fig.2.36. The uppermost has a pedicle which has become twisted. It is easy to imagine how torsion of this pedicle could lead to its necrosis and liberate the cartilaginous deposit into the synovial cavity. The synovium in between these two loose bodies is strikingly normal apart from the synovitis, suggesting that only some areas of the synovium are involved in the disease process with intervening areas remaining normal.

Further differences were seen in the radiological appearances. The knee in Figs.2.33 and 2.34 showed multiple loose bodies while Fig.2.37, the same knee as in Figs.2.35 and 2.36, shows a mass of well circumscribed loose bodies in all areas of the joint, including the posterior compartments.

The difference between the various types of synovial chondromatosis is important from the therapeutic standpoint. Patients with many large pedunculated lesions and loose bodies can be helped by removal of the loose bodies under arthroscopic control, but those whose deposits are more deeply seated and not lying in the synovial cavity itself require a total open synovectomy.

Figs.2.38 to 2.40 are of synovial chondromatosis with neither loose bodies nor a synovial effusion. The deposits lie beneath a thin layer of synovium. In Fig.2.38 the deposits are flat, giving a cobble-stone appearance. The synovium is free of both fronds and polyps. Fig.2.39 shows an elongated cartilaginous deposit which is distorting the meniscosynovial junction by lying partly

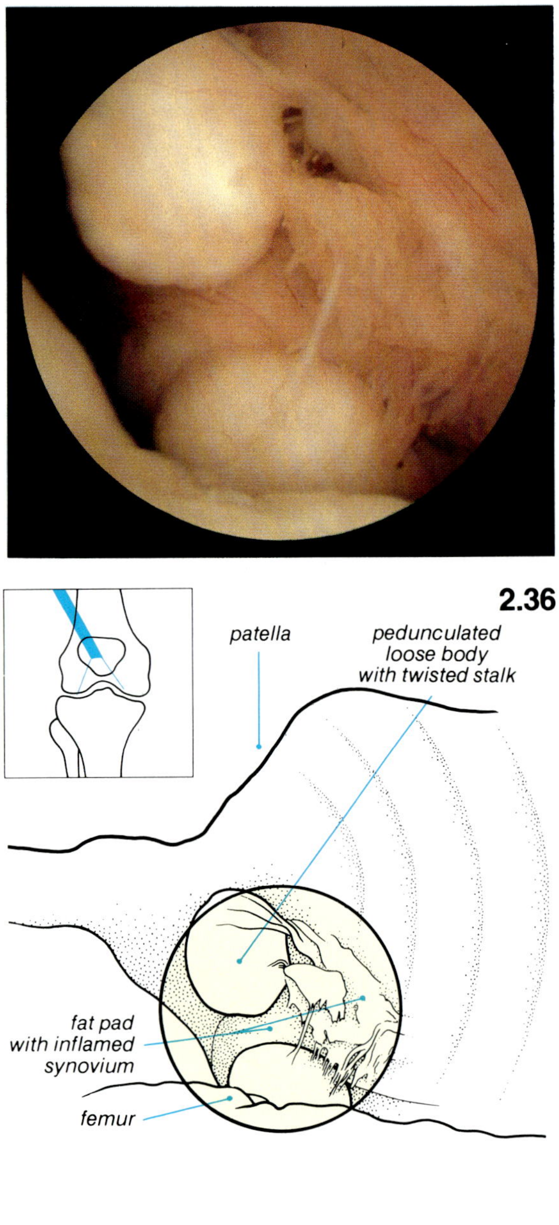

2.36

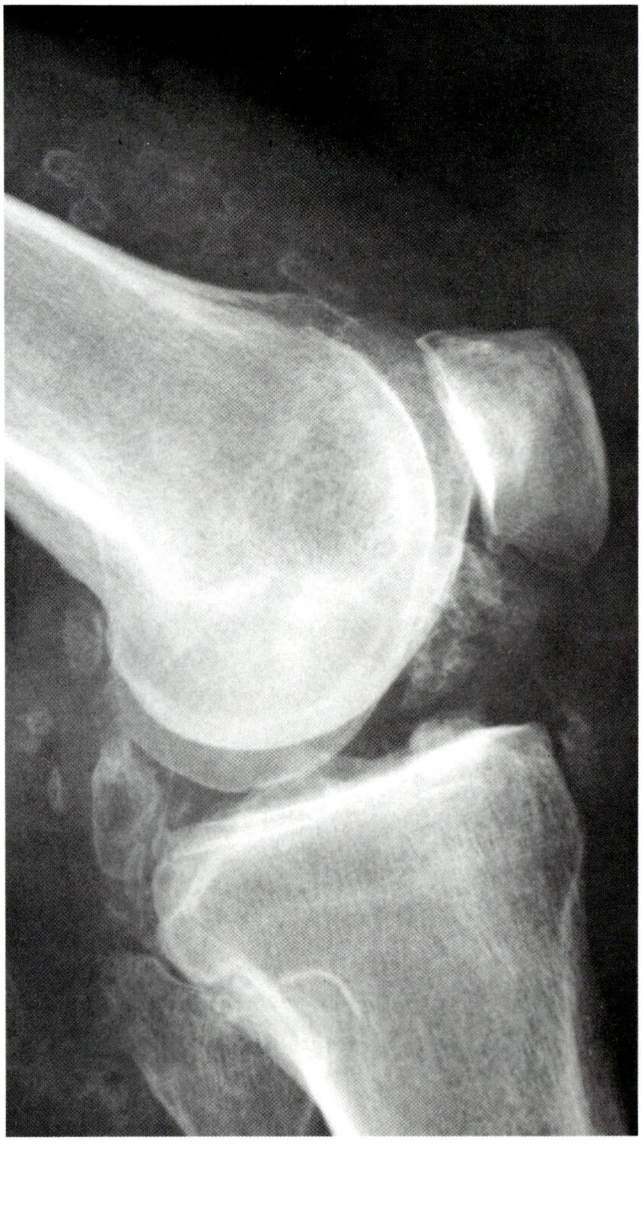

2.37

beneath the meniscus and partly beneath the synovium. Even when quite large, there is no tendency for these deposits to form pedicles or be shed into the knee as loose bodies. Fig.2.40 shows a subsynovial deposit more than 1cm in length lying in the medial gutter with no sign of pedicle formation. The vessels in the synovium

2.38

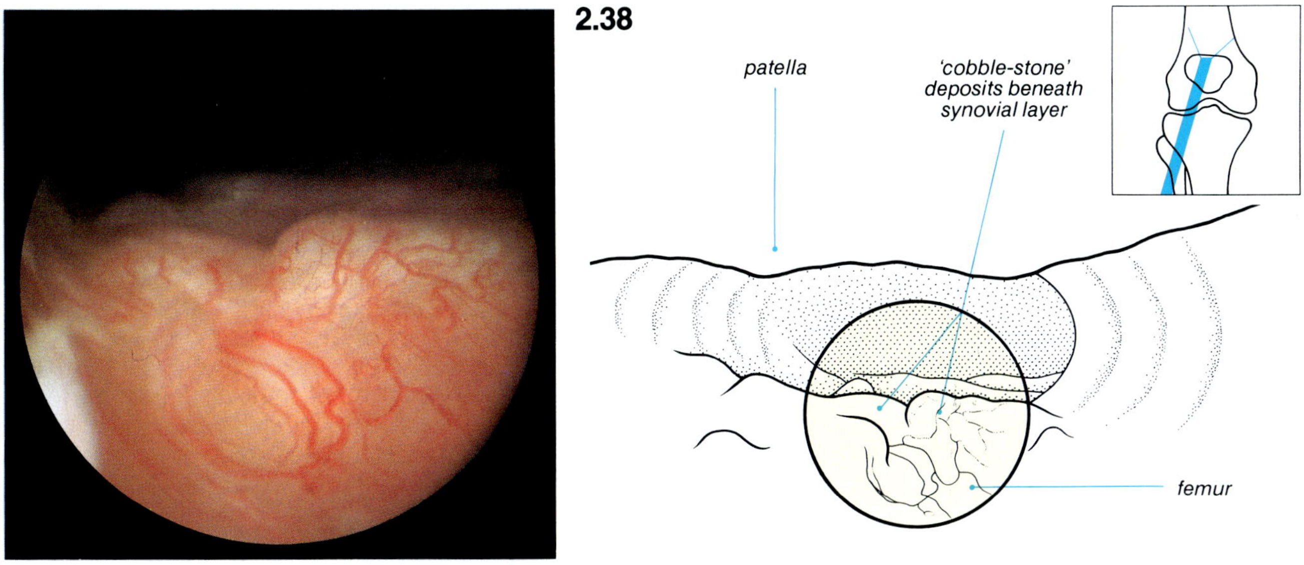

2.39

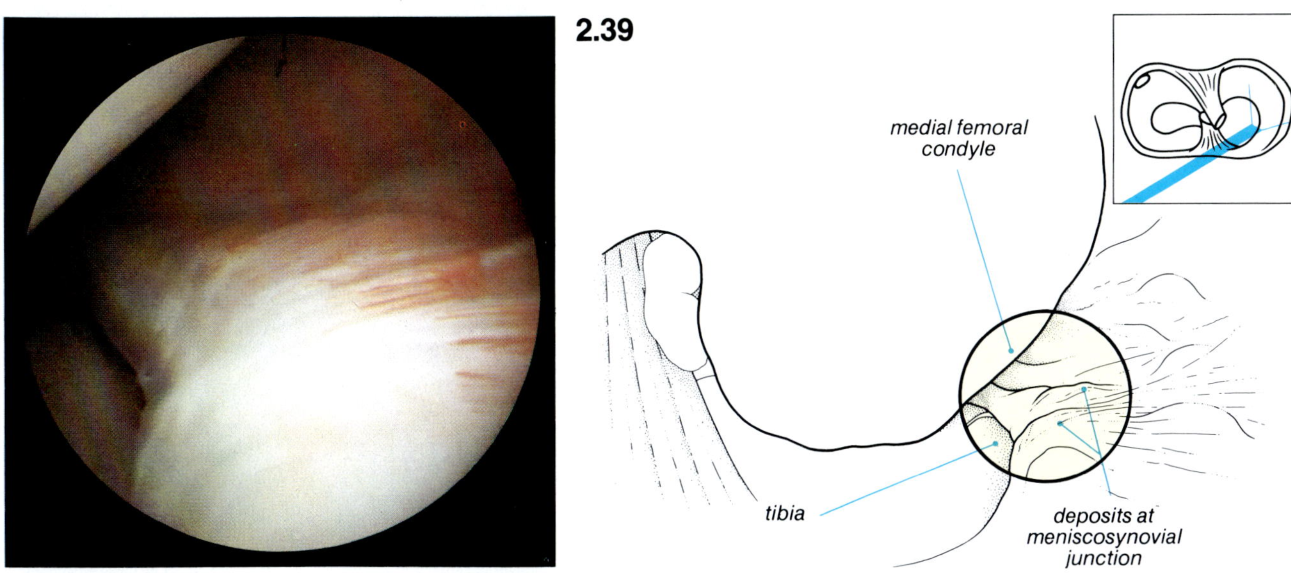

2.40

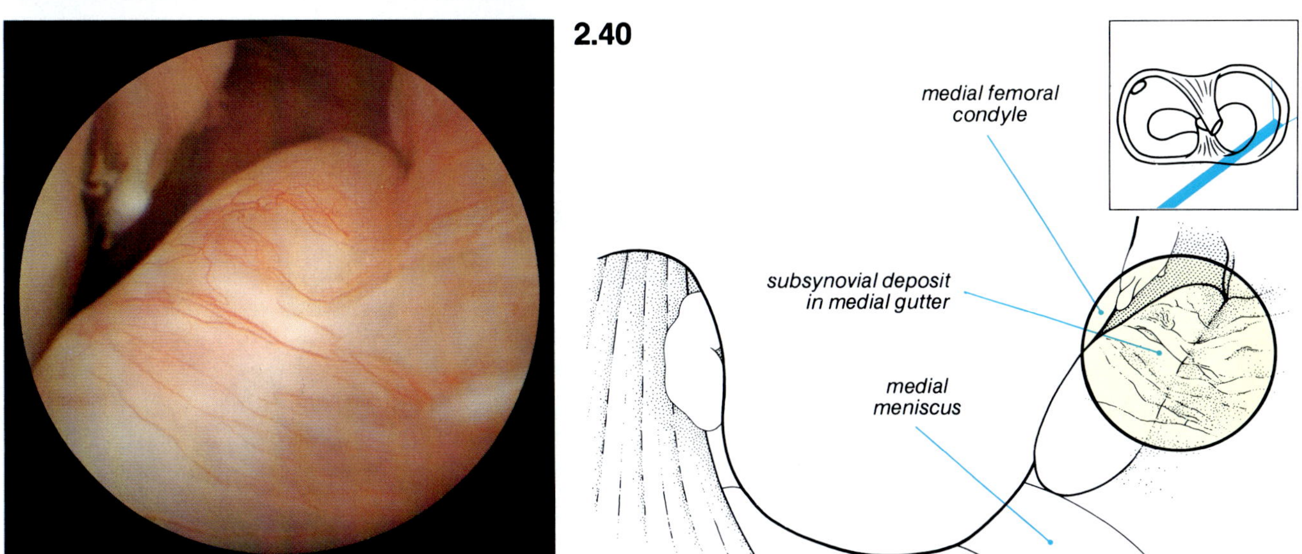

overlying the lesion are easily seen but there are no synovial fronds. Radiography (Fig.2.41), however, demonstrated calcified lesions around the knee that were very similar to those in Fig.2.37 but were perhaps less well circumscribed.

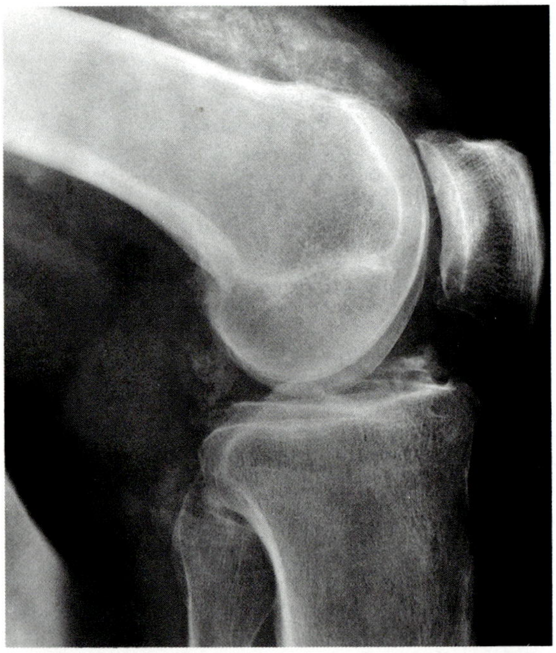

2.41

A fourth variety of synovial chondromatosis is seen in the knee of a 12-year-old girl (Fig.2.42). No radiographic abnormality was detectable at the time of presentation, but specks of calcification later became visible on a plain radiograph (Fig.2.43). At arthroscopy the appearance was of pearl-like beads of cartilage strung on a loose lacework of delicate synovial fronds. Fig.2.6 also showed the suprapatellar pouch with a loose body in the foreground and small beads of cartilage attached to the synovium in the background. Unfortunately, still photographs do not convey fully the rather beautiful appearance of this condition. Histological examination (Fig.2.44) showed fragments of cartilage and little abnormality apart from hyperaemia.

Benign tumours

Soft tissue lesions of the synovium can present as pedunculated tumours and are often found as incidental findings. Fig.2.45 shows a small pigmented pedunculated polyp lying just lateral to and above the medial synovial shelf. The lesion was approximately 4mm in diameter and did not appear to be giving rise to symptoms. The patient had previously undergone an arthrotomy and it is possible that the lesion represented the contracted stub of a ruptured adhesion, a speculation for which there is no evidence whatsoever apart from the appearance of the lesion.

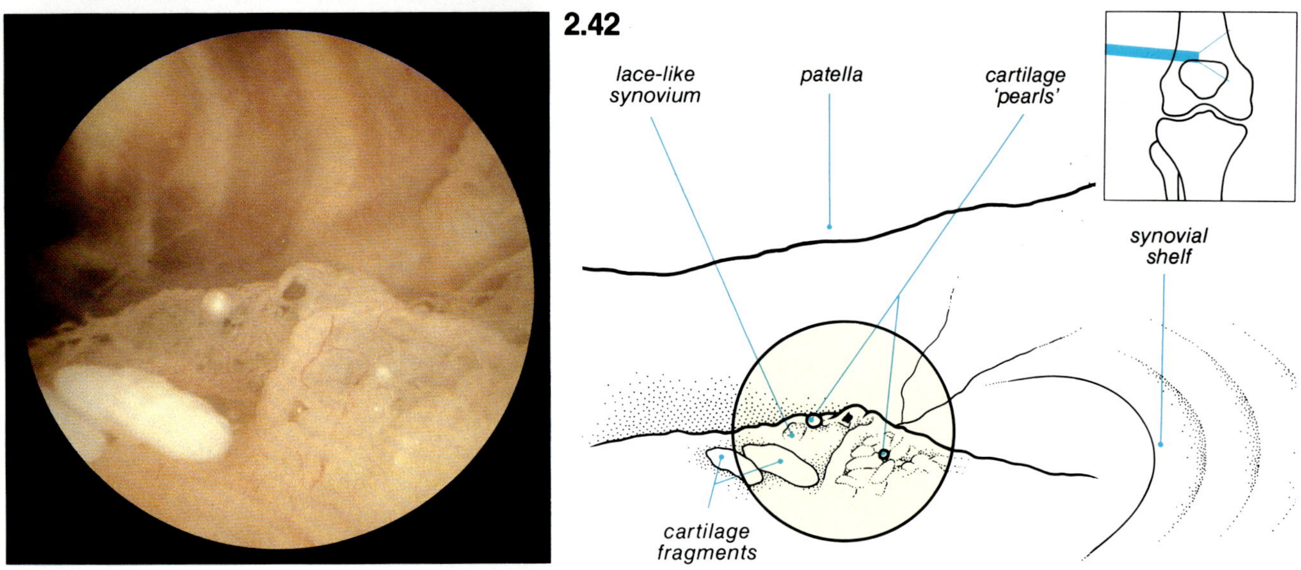

2.42

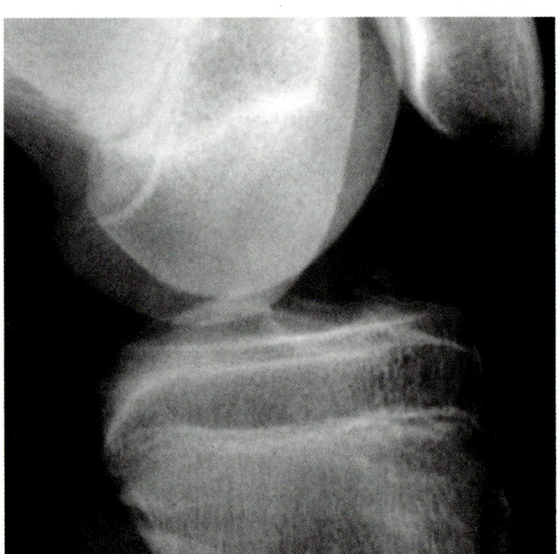

2.43

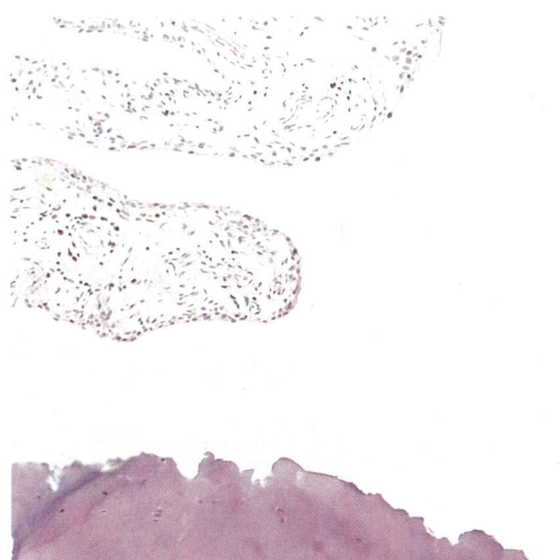

2.44

Pedunculated tumours (Fig.2.46) are also found in the knee. This example measured approximately 2cm in diameter and was lying in the medial gutter attached to the synovium by a narrow pedicle. Histological examination of the lesion (Fig.2.47) showed many vacuolated cells, probably lipid-filled, with haemosiderin present in one area. Before operation, the lesion could be felt in the medial gutter and was thought to be a detached bucket handle fragment of the medial meniscus lying mobile in the medial gutter, tethered at its anterior limit. The patient's symptoms, which consisted of pain and tenderness over the lesion as well as a sensation of something moving within the joint on the medial side, were relieved by arthroscopic excision of the tumour.

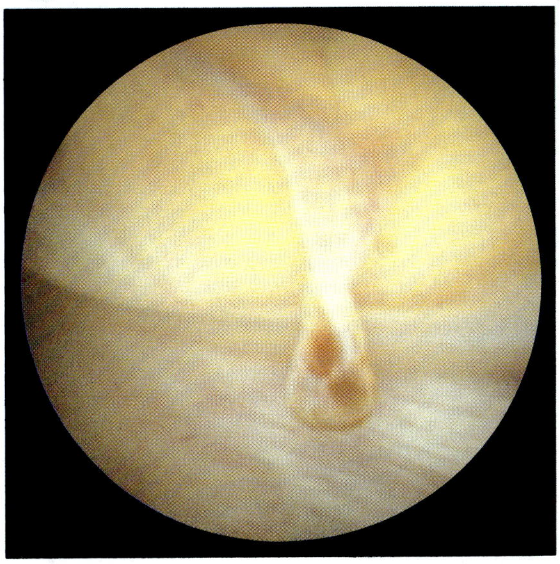

2.45

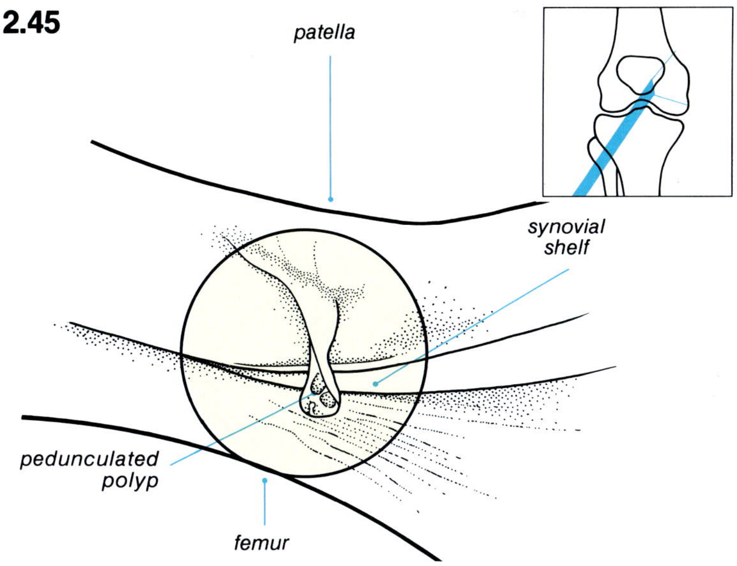

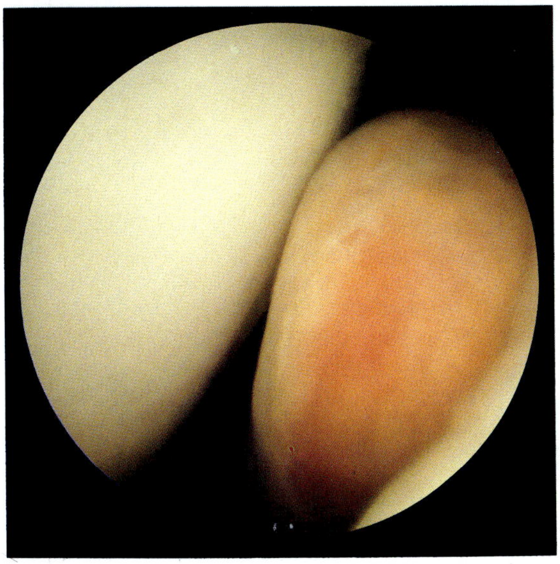

2.46

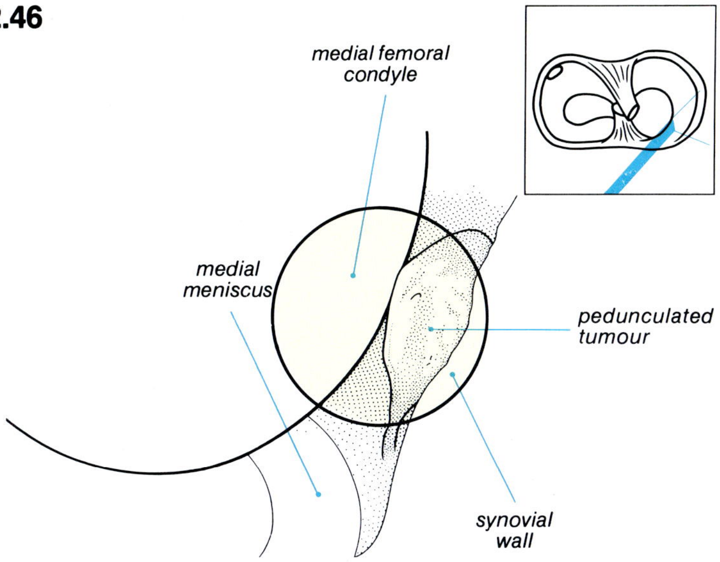

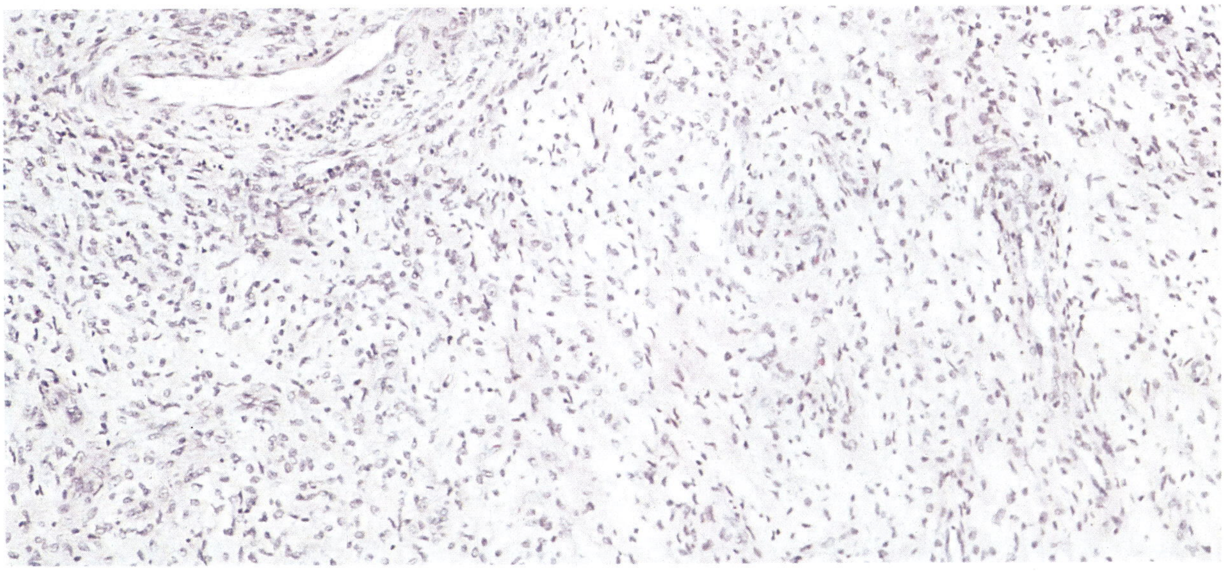

2.47

Fig.2.48 shows the posterior part of the intercondylar notch of a patient who presented with diffuse thickening of the synovium and a small effusion. There was no history of injury and no episode of mechanical locking. Serological examinations were normal and there were no symptoms or signs of joint disease elsewhere. At arthroscopy masses of soft friable tissue were found with small random petechial haemorrhages in all areas of the knee. The structure shown in Fig.2.48 was found emerging from the synovial tunnel that surrounds the posterior cruciate ligament, the rim of which it is distending. The histological appearances (Fig.2.49) were

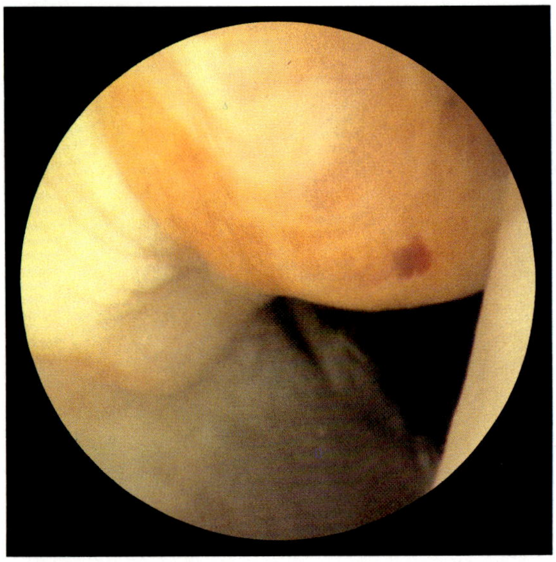

2.48

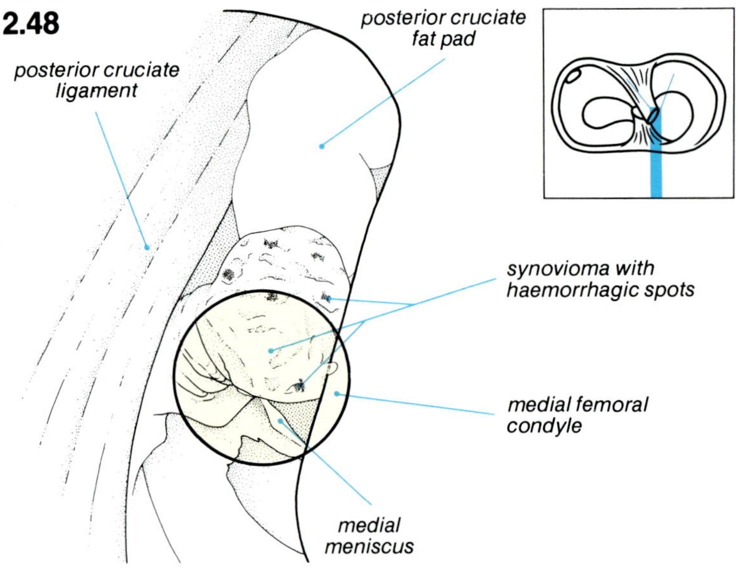

2.49

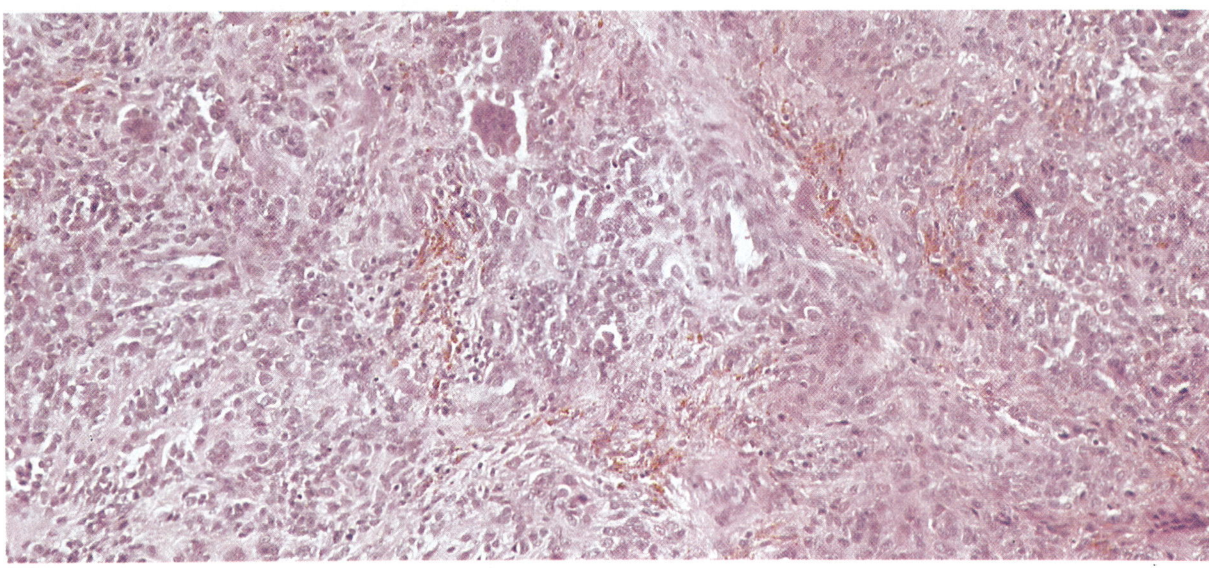

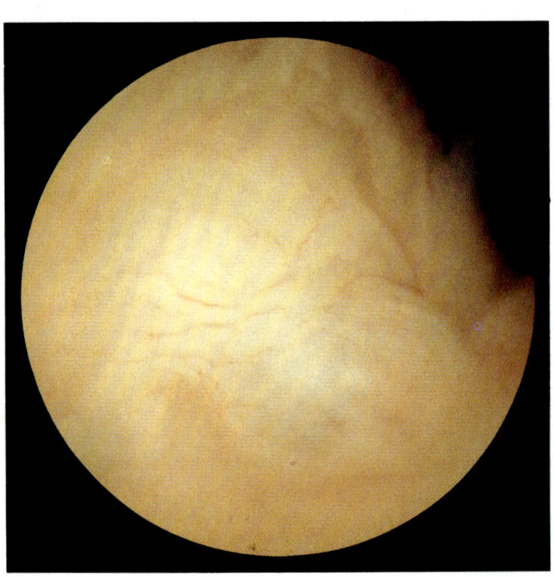

2.50

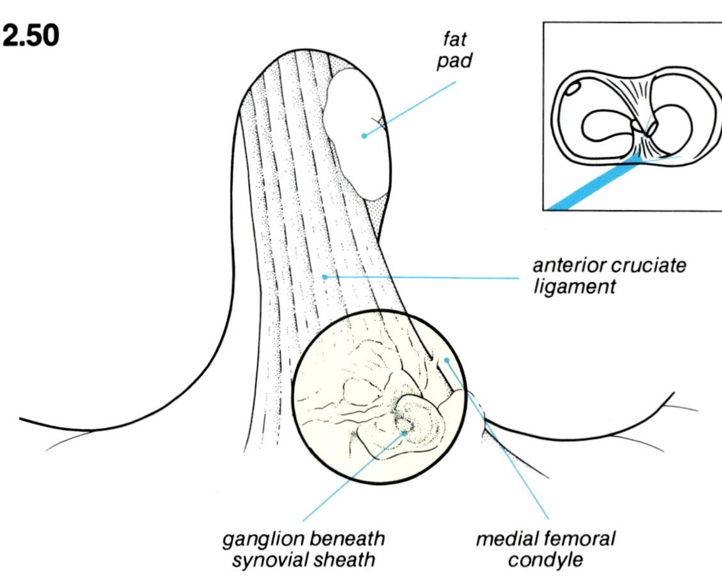

those of a benign synovioma with pigmentation. As much as possible of this tissue was removed and the patient's symptoms were improved though not abolished.

Ganglia can occur inside the knee joint and give rise to symptoms. Ganglia lying beneath the synovium overlying the anterior cruciate ligament (Fig.2.50) may be compressed as the knee is extended and cause pain on full extension. The patient in this case complained of pain on full extension of the knee and was thought on clinical grounds to have a torn medial meniscus. Arthroscopy revealed the ganglion lying between the synovium and the anterior cruciate ligament. The ganglion was easily excised under arthroscopic control and the symptoms were relieved. Histological study confirmed that the lesion was a synovial cyst or ganglion.

Pedunculated ganglia can also occur over the base of the anterior cruciate ligament and in other parts of the knee. Fig.2.51 shows a small cluster of ganglia immediately above the posterior horn of the lateral meniscus. The patient's symptoms were pain at the front of the knee on full extension, following a direct blow to the front of the knee and forced flexion of the joint. A mass of inflamed synovium was found at the front of the intercondylar notch (Fig.2.51) but the cluster of ganglia in the background was also noted. The inflamed synovium and the cluster of ganglia were removed and the patient's symptoms slowly improved.

Ganglia may also form in the degenerate stubs of ruptured anterior cruciate ligaments. An unusual site for a ganglion is seen in Fig.2.52 which shows a spherical cyst protruding through the posterior wall of the posteromedial compartment. Whether this lesion represents an early popliteal cyst or is simply an extra-articular ganglion is not known, but the latter seems more likely because popliteal cysts are relatively common and are seldom visible arthroscopically. Attempts to identify the openings of tunnels leading into popliteal cysts from the knee have been unsuccessful.

The cyst in Fig.2.52 was opened under arthroscopic control from the posteromedial approach and its interior examined. The appearances were those of a synovial cyst or ganglion. Before operation the patient had complained of pain on full flexion of the knee, and the discovery of a lesion that might be compressed on full flexion was therefore enthusiastically welcomed at the time of operation. Excision of the cyst, however, did not relieve the patient's symptoms and no other explanation for them has been found.

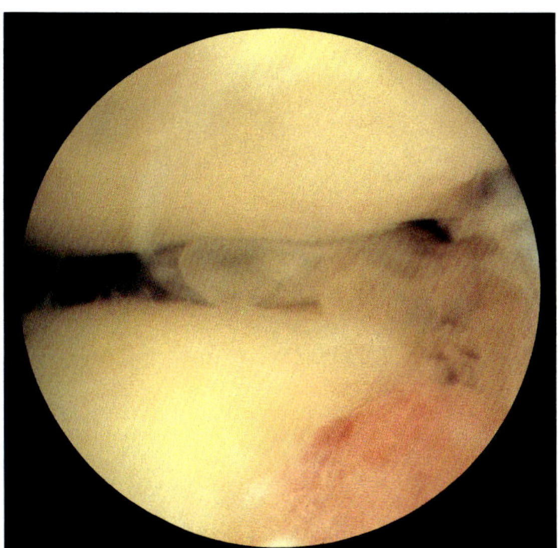

2.51

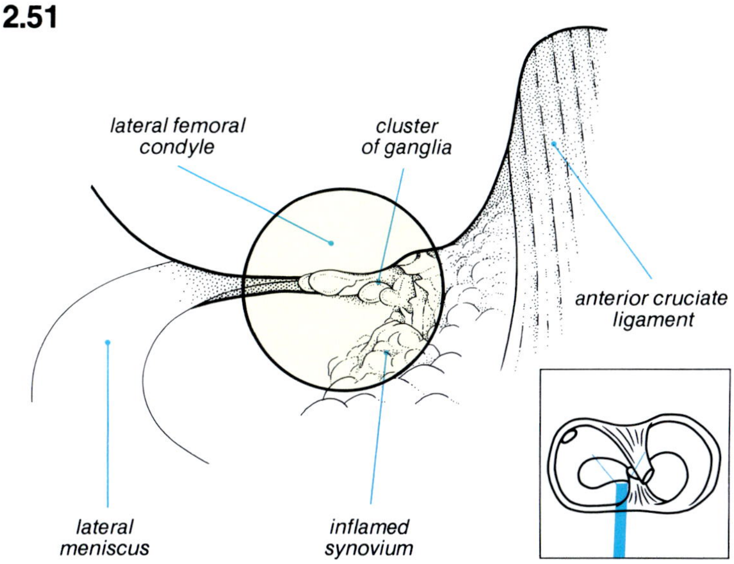

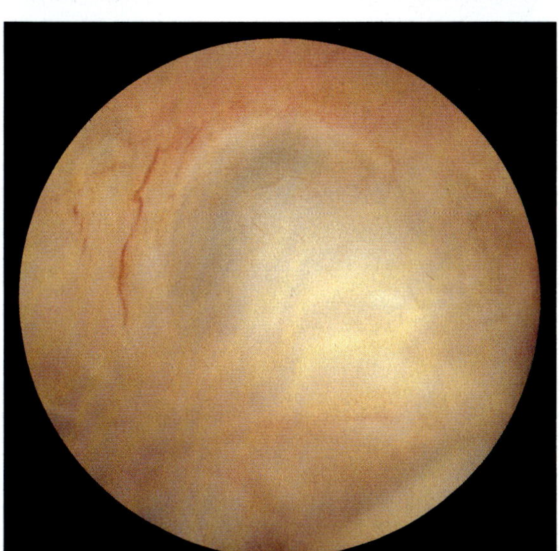

2.52

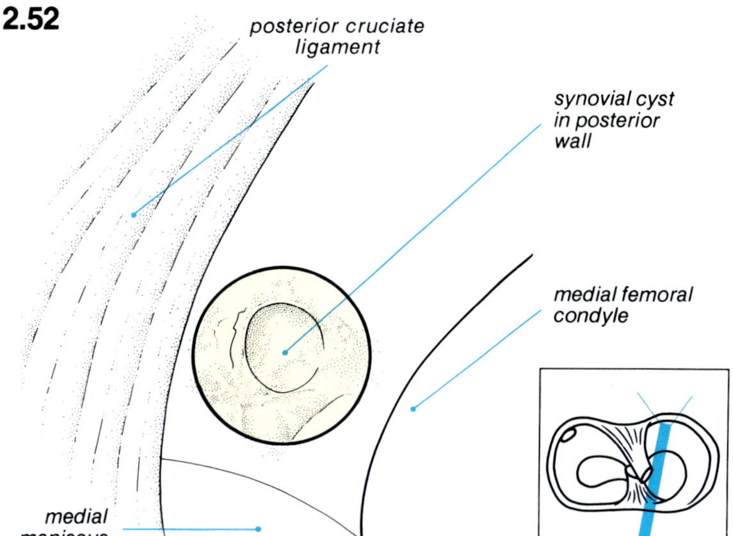

Haemangioma of the synovium is a rare condition, particularly in children. The synovium of a 13-year-old boy who had suffered recurrent bleeding into the knee since the age of 6 and had previously undergone an open partial synovectomy is seen in Fig.2.53. There was no abnormality in the clotting mechanism. Between episodes of bleeding the knee was never entirely normal but was warm, with an effusion and synovial thickening. A knot of distended vessels is seen in the centre of the picture, apparently lying unprotected in the synovial cavity. Many such vascular lesions were present and the remaining synovium was pigmented, with prolific synovial fronds. The appearances of the synovium are suggestive of pigmented villonodular synovitis superimposed on the haemangioma.

Pigmented synovitis

Fig.2.54 shows the synovium of the same knee as in Fig.2.53. The changes are more typical of chronic pigmented villonodular synovitis, but a knot of vessels is also visible. In addition to the pigmentation, the villi and the haemangioma, the patellar surface is irregular which must offer a poor prognosis for a boy only 13 years old. The colour of the synovium is a dusky brown, best appreciated by comparison with the red of the vascular lesion. The vessels of the haemangioma inevitably collapsed after excision while the more solid synovium did not. As a result, synovitis and massive iron deposition were the dominant features on histological examination (Fig.2.55) and special search had to be made for the vascular wall of the lesion. The pigmented villonodular

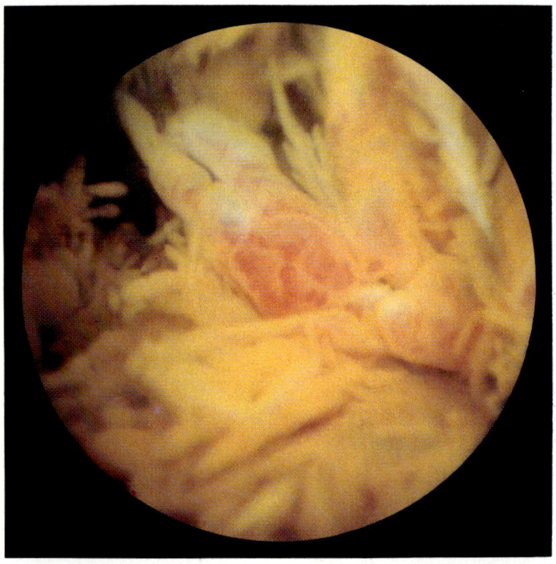

2.53

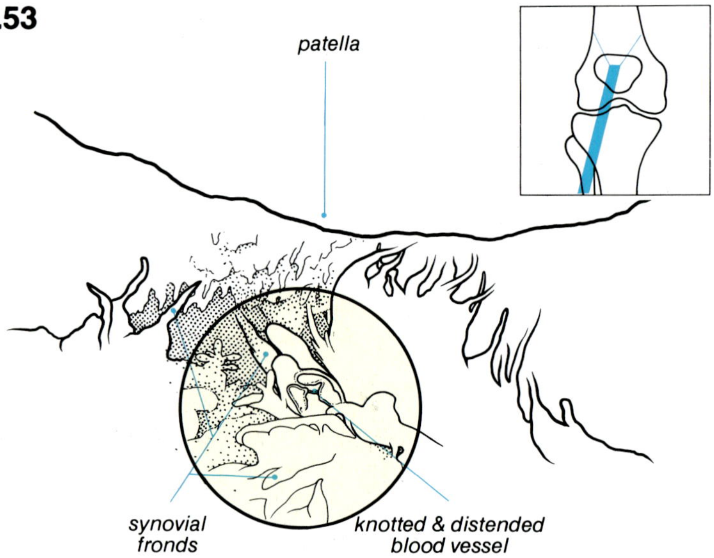

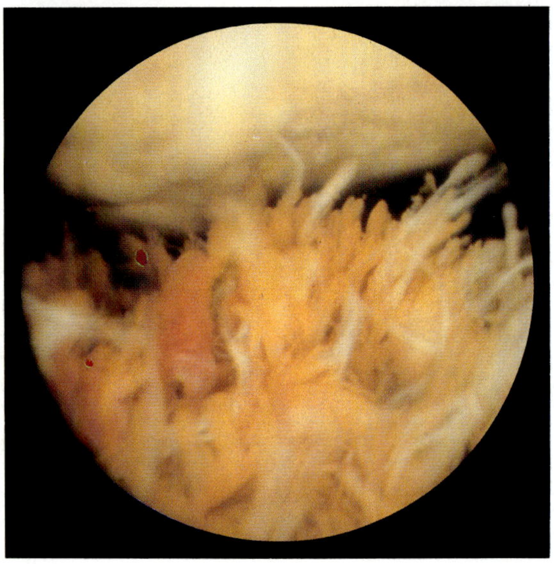

2.54

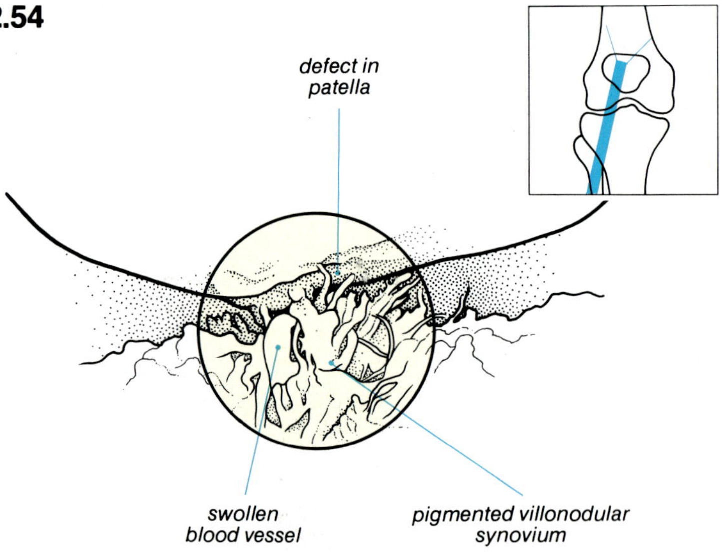

synovitis was almost certainly the result of repeated intra-articular haemorrhage. Pigmented synovitis is almost invariably secondary to some other condition and is probably not a disease in its own right.

The histological appearances of the synovium in Fig.2.56 were of pigmented villonodular synovitis (Fig.2.57) but with less superficial iron deposition (see Fig.2.55). At arthroscopy the lesions were best seen in the lateral gutter. The synovium bore nodules, villi and was pigmented but these observations do not explain why the condition occurred. The patient had an unstable anterior cruciate ligament with repeated episodes of collapsing followed by repeated haemarthrosis which may well have contributed to the pigmentation and perpetuation of the synovitis.

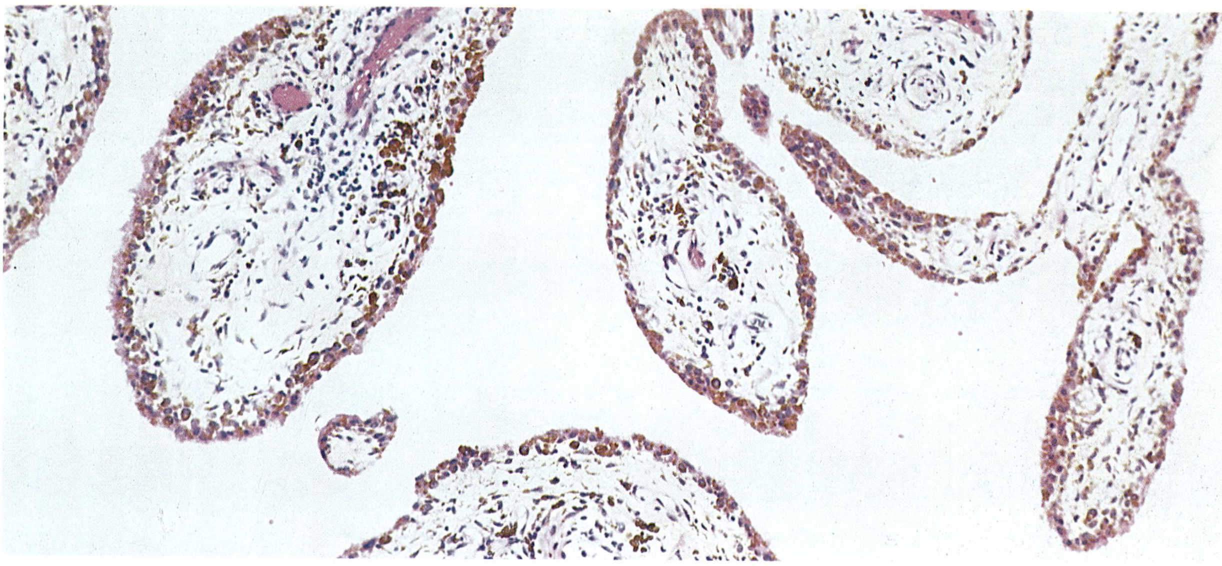

2.55

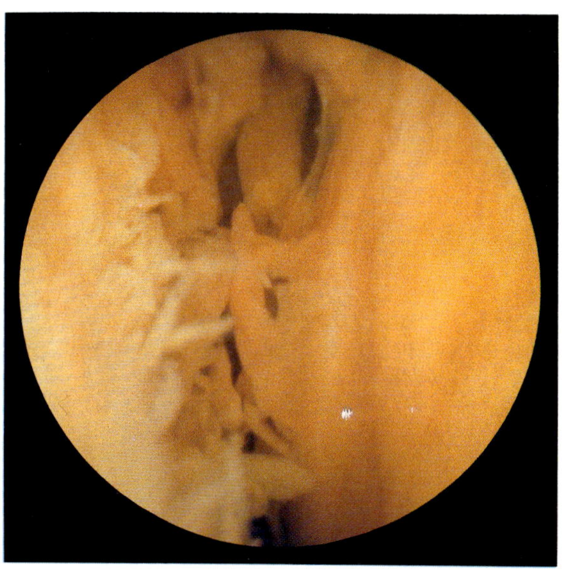

2.56

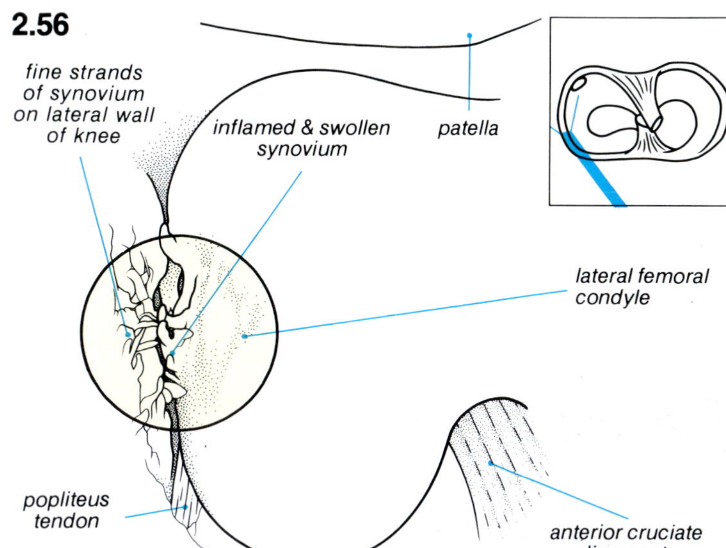

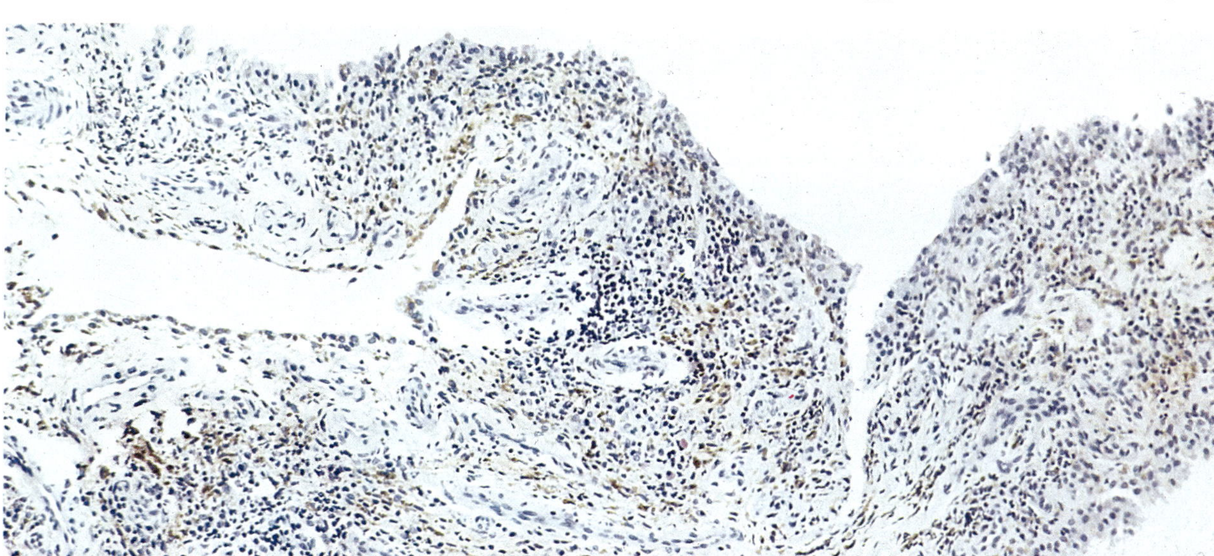

2.57

Haemophilia

Haemophilia produces a great range of appearances in the knee but the predominant changes are chocolate-brown pigmentation, synovial thickening, and a profusion of polyps and filiform fronds. The articular surface becomes pitted, perhaps due to the action of intra-articular enzymes. Fig.2.58, from a 14-year-old boy, shows thickened polyps of synovium and, in the foreground, a large rounded osteophyte. This knee (see also Fig.3.30) was grossly abnormal. Plain radiography (Fig.2.59) shows irregularity of the articular surfaces with narrowing of the joint space.

Removal of the prolific synovium with an arthroscopic shaver exposed the underlying tissue (Fig.2.60) and the trabeculated appearance of the joint lining, suggesting the presence of intracapsular fibrosis. This appearance,

2.58

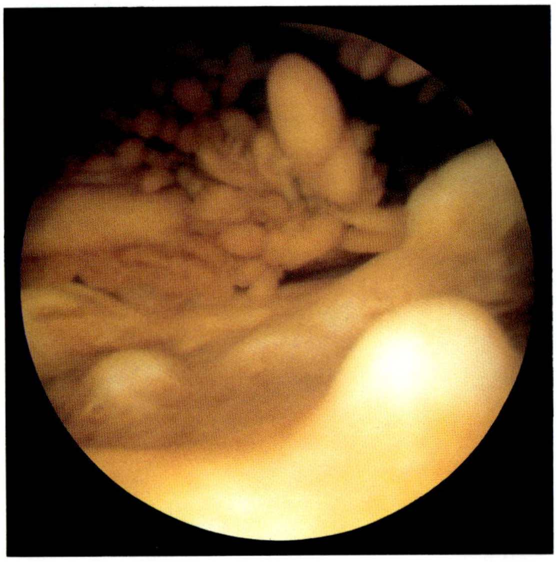

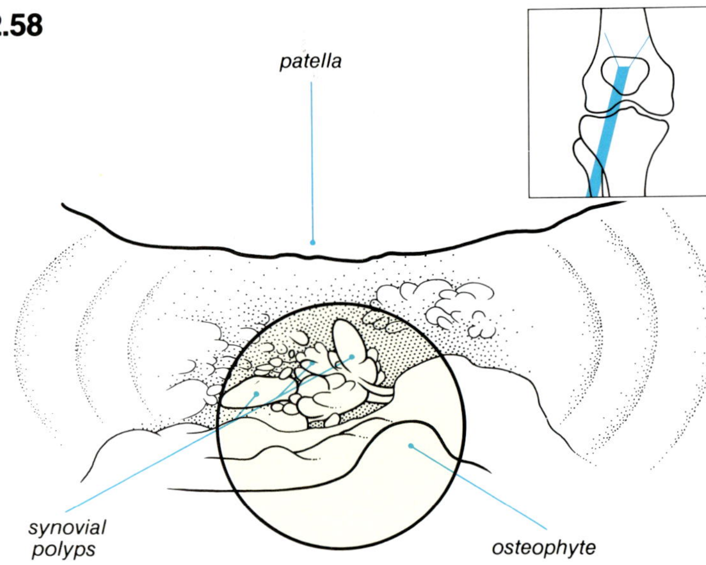

2.59

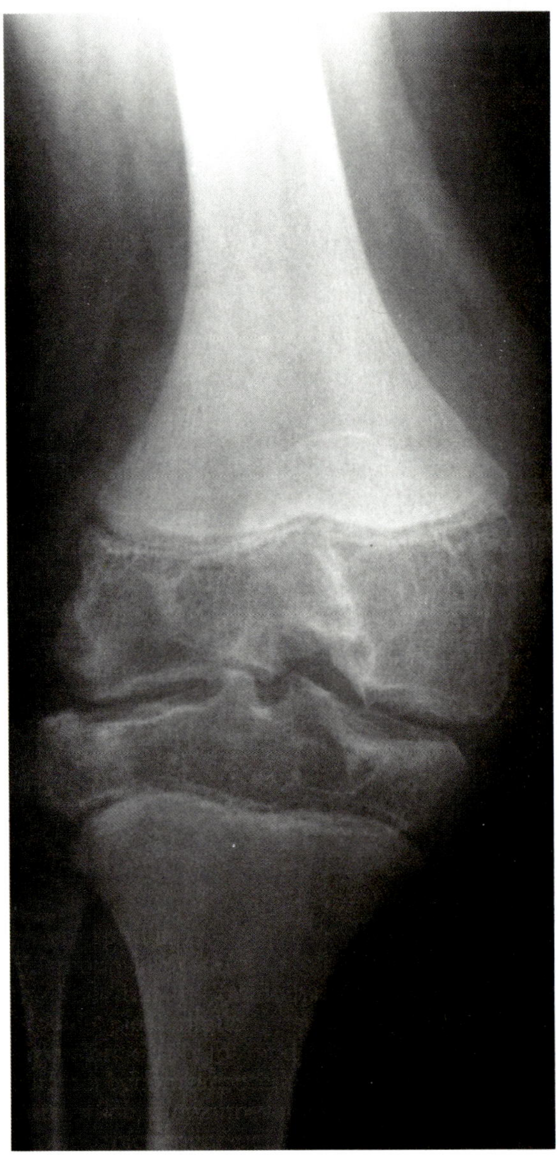

2.60

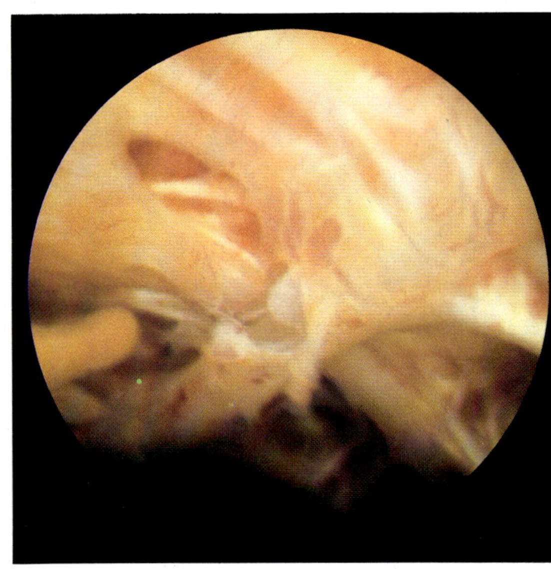

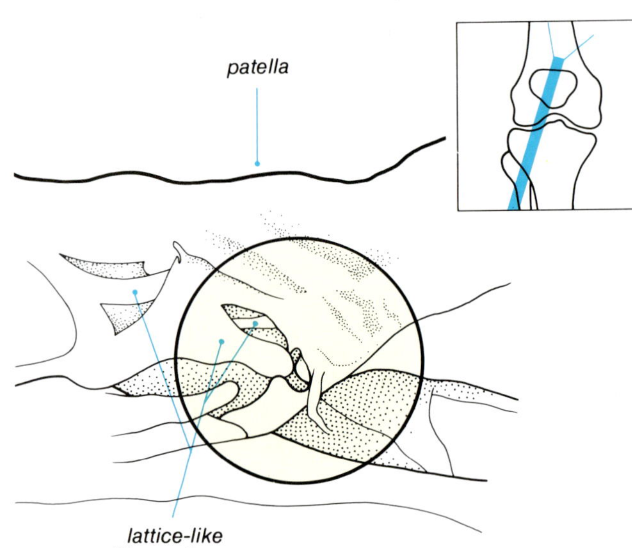

together with the presence of bony irregularity, suggests that the pathology of haemophilia may differ not only in degree but also in nature from that of pigmented villonodular synovitis and other conditions in which there is repeated haemorrhage into the joint. The histological appearances of the synovium (Figs.2.61 & 2.62) are of widespread iron deposition and thickening of the stroma.

From a practical standpoint, it should be noted that the deep chocolate-brown pigmentation of the synovium in haemophilia makes photography in the joint, particularly in the suprapatellar pouch, exceedingly difficult.

The appearances of synovitis do not always fall easily into a category or type. In Fig.2.63, for example, a fringe of intensely inflamed synovium is seen along the medial border of the patella, but the rest of the synovium is

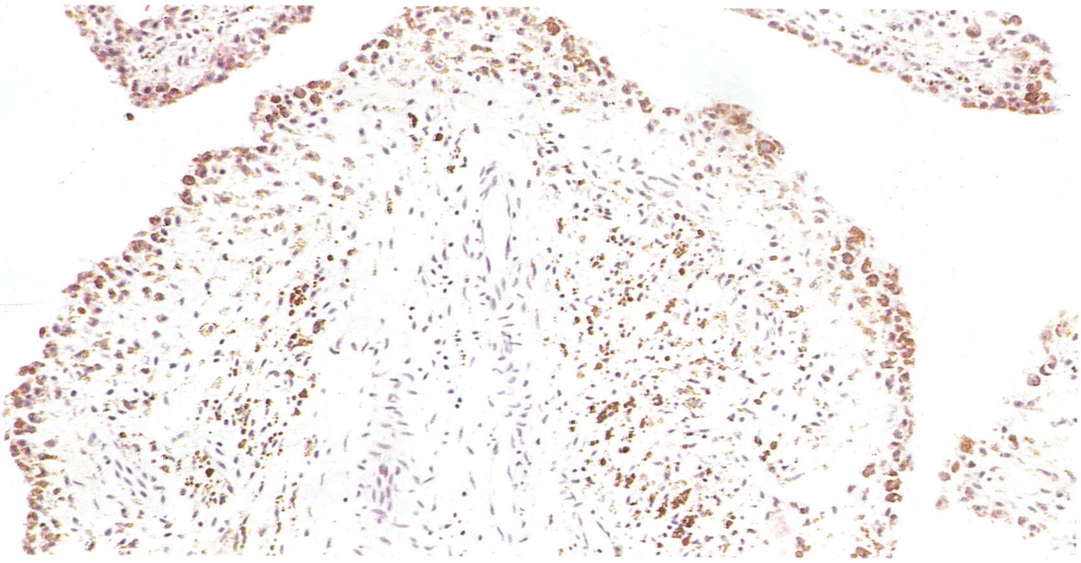

2.61

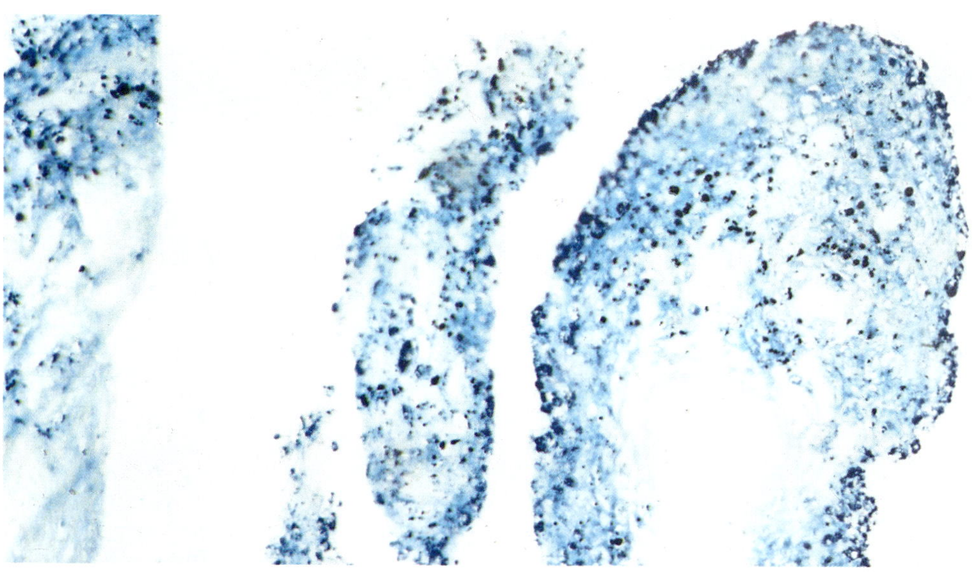

2.62

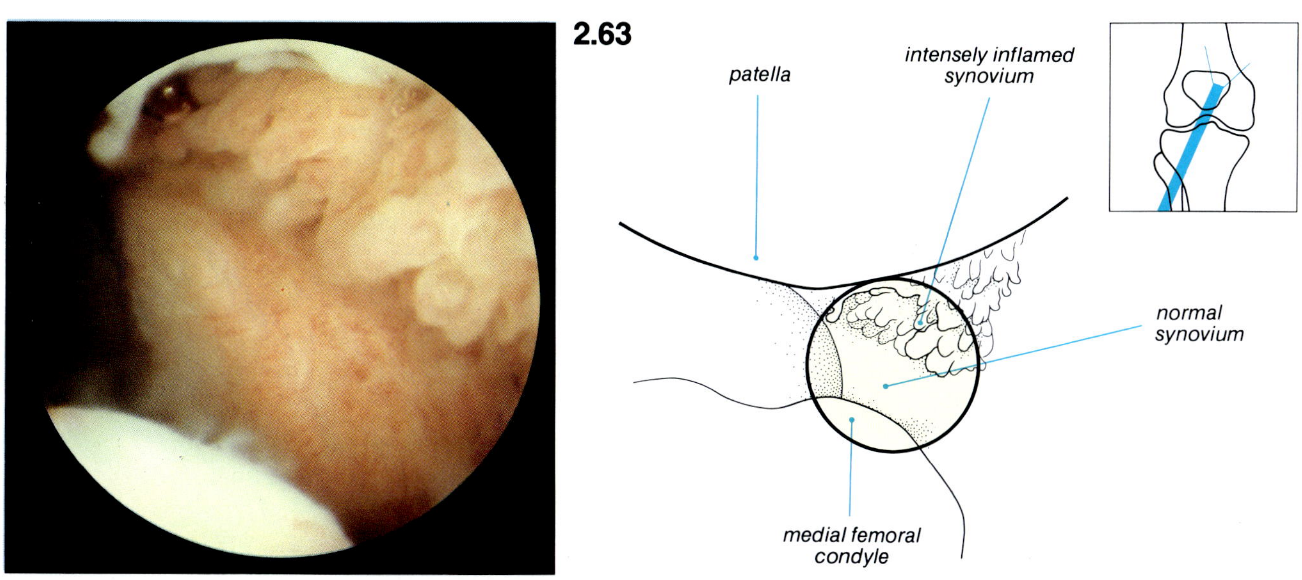

2.63

entirely normal. The patient had a ruptured anterior cruciate ligament with repeated collapsing episodes but no pigmentation or villi were found, and the appearances were quite different from those of Fig.2.56. No serological abnormality was found on investigation and no explanation could be found for the curious appearance of the synovium.

Alkaptonuria

Fig.2.64 shows a knee of a patient with alkaptonuria. The synovium throughout the suprapatellar pouch bears many black needle-shaped crystals of homogentisic acid mostly lying on the surface. Histological examination (Fig.2.65) showed ochronosis of the cartilage. Alkaptonuria has a destructive effect on other tissues as well, for example, in the lateral femoral condyle and lateral meniscus (Figs. 3.54 & 3.55). As with haemophilia, the pigmentation of the knee is so dense that photography is difficult and requires more light than usual.

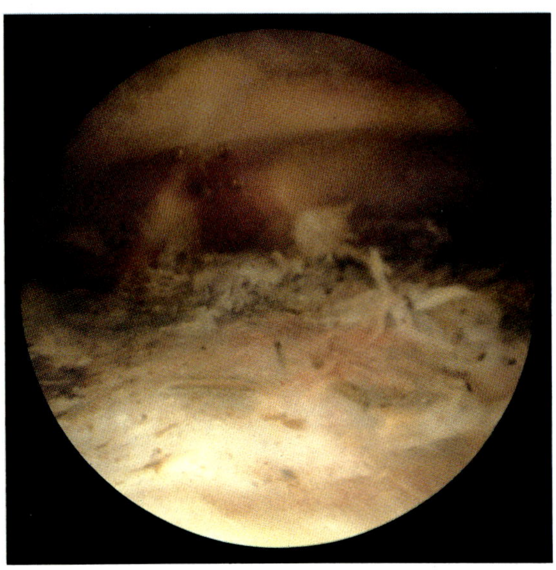

2.64

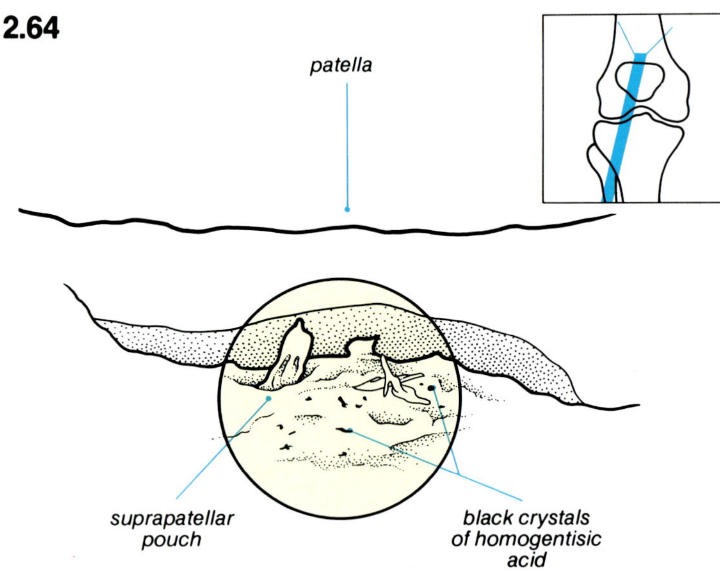

2.65

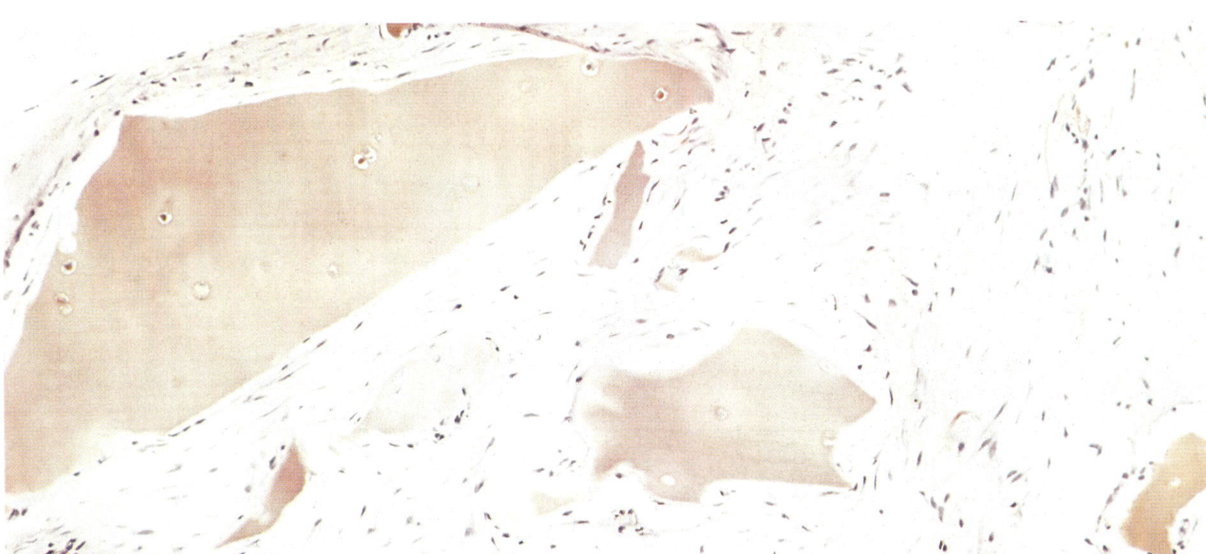

3

Lesions of Bone and Articular Cartilage

Trauma

Acute osteochondral fractures of the patella and lateral femoral condyle can occur with surprisingly little trauma, particularly in the adolescent. Any adolescent presenting with a haemarthrosis and intact ligaments after a twisting injury of the knee should be suspected of having sustained an osteochondral fracture of the lateral femoral condyle. Figs. 3.1 and 3.2 are of an acute osteochondral fracture of the lateral femoral condyle of a sixteen-year-old boy who twisted sharply on the extended knee while throwing a cricket ball. The boy felt a sudden crack in the knee and arrived at the emergency department with an acute haemarthrosis. Radiographs showed an osteochondral fracture of the lateral femoral condyle. The lesion was identified at arthroscopy after thorough irrigation of the joint to remove blood. Fig.3.1 shows the osteochondral fragment lying free in the joint. The cancellous surface of the fragment is facing downwards and the smooth articular cartilage is above. Fig.3.2 shows the bed of the lesion from which the fragment arose. The defect has a clear 'punched-out' margin and is filled with blood clots. The surrounding articular surface is normal.

Osteochondritis dissecans

A different type of lesion is seen in Fig.3.3. The patient attended hospital with pain and catching in the knee and had no memory of past injury or, indeed, any sudden pain or swelling in the knee. The radiological appearances (Figs.3.4 & 3.5) were similar to those of classical osteochondritis dissecans except that the defect involved the weight-bearing surface of the femoral

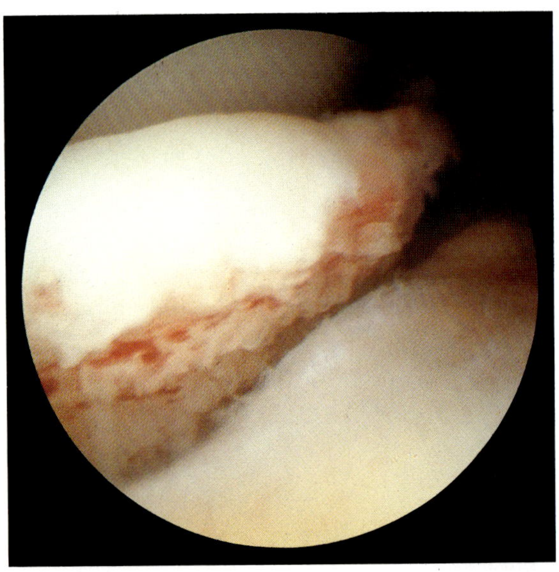

3.1

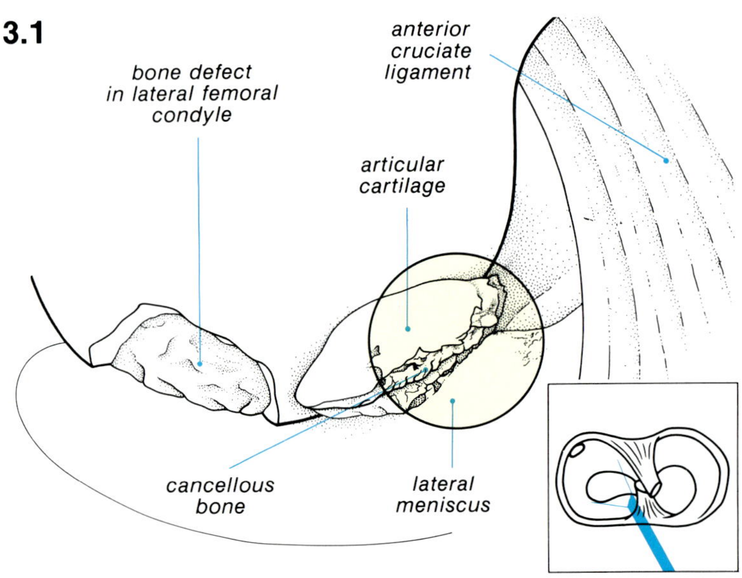

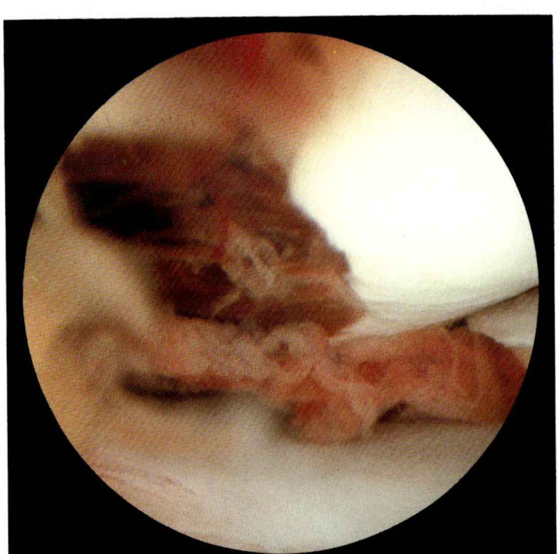

3.2

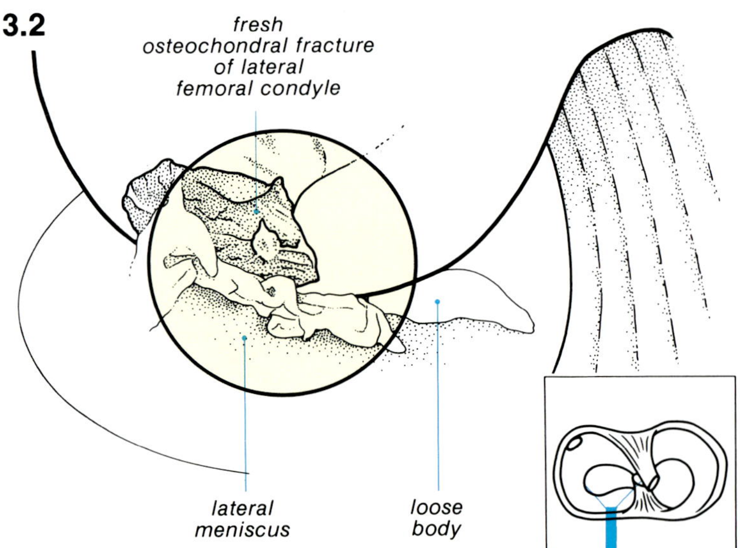

condyle. Arrangements were made for removal of the fragment of bone but it had already separated by the time the patient was admitted.

At arthroscopy the femoral condyle showed a shallow bony defect with a rounded margin of articular cartilage. The floor of the defect was uneven but did not have the appearance of recently exposed cancellous bone. The lesion had not healed and it was concluded that the fragment had separated gradually from its bed over a long period of time, having been held only at the margin of the articular cartilage which eventually fractured, releasing the loose body.

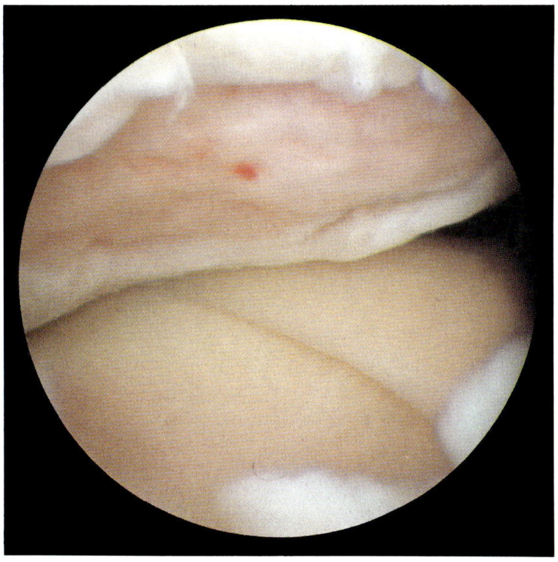

3.3

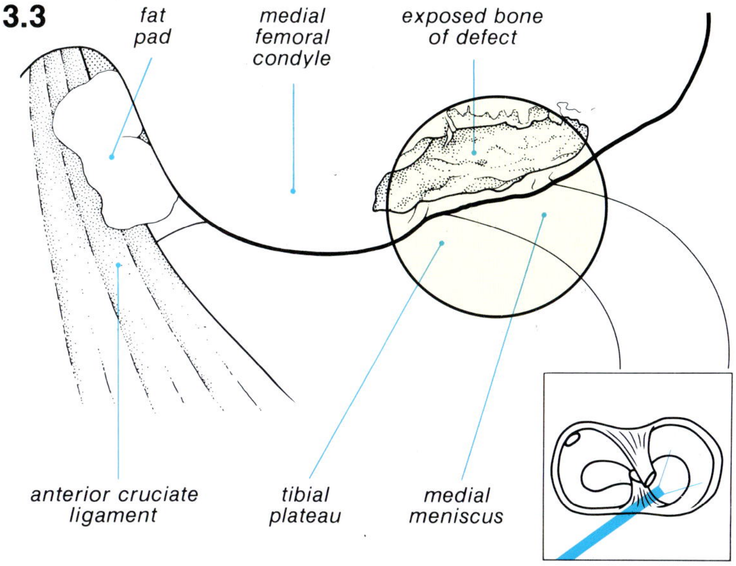

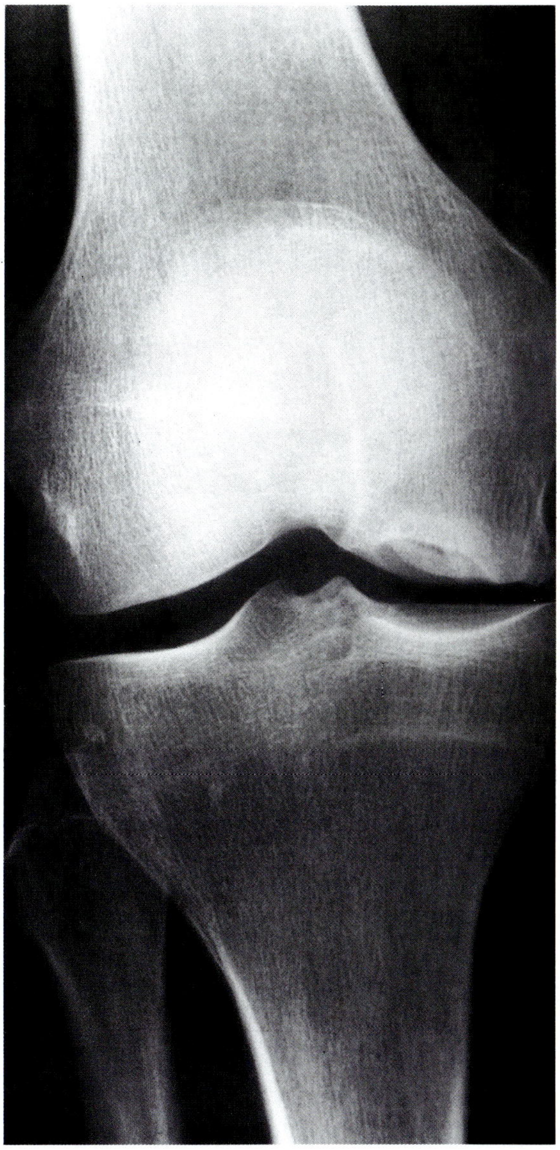

3.4

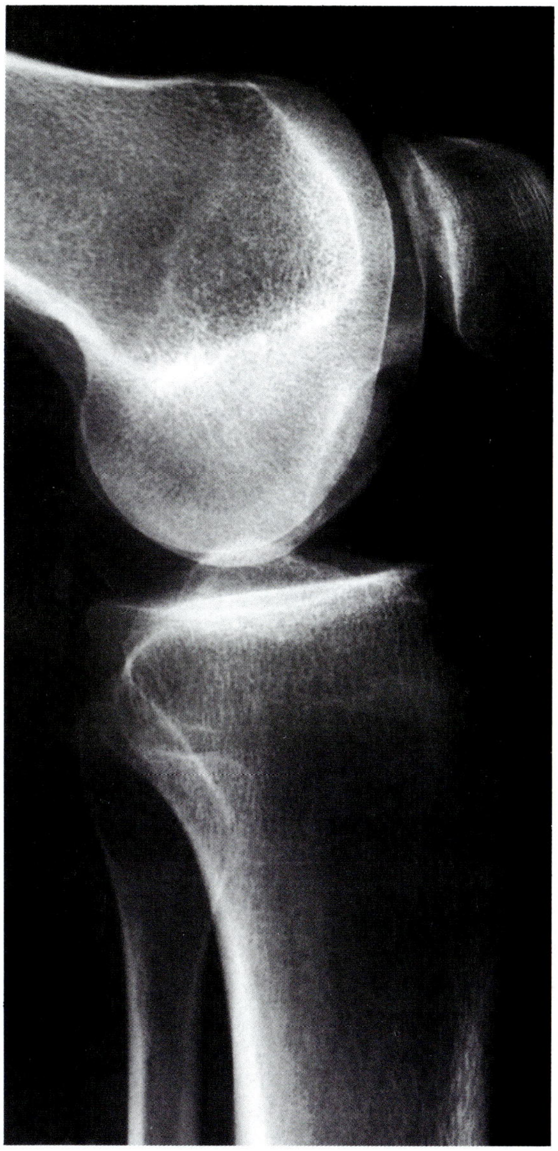

3.5

Fig.3.6 shows an osteochondritic lesion in which a fragment has just been shed into the knee as a loose body (Figs.3.7 & 3.8). The appearances in Fig.3.6 are more typical of the condition than that in Fig.3.3. The bed of the lesion is sclerotic and has vertical sides, as if the loose body had been truly dissected out of the bone. As in Fig.3.3, the appearance of cancellous bone is not fresh and there is no sign of healing with fibrocartilage.

Once the osteochondritic fragment has been shed, the defect will usually fill with bone and fibrocartilage, leaving a smooth surface. Fig.3.9 is of a 49-year-old patient who had suffered from a loose body in the knee for many years. The lesion, which was on the medial femoral condyle at the classical site of osteochondritis dissecans, is smooth but lacks the brilliance or shine of a normal femoral condyle; the wearing properties of such a

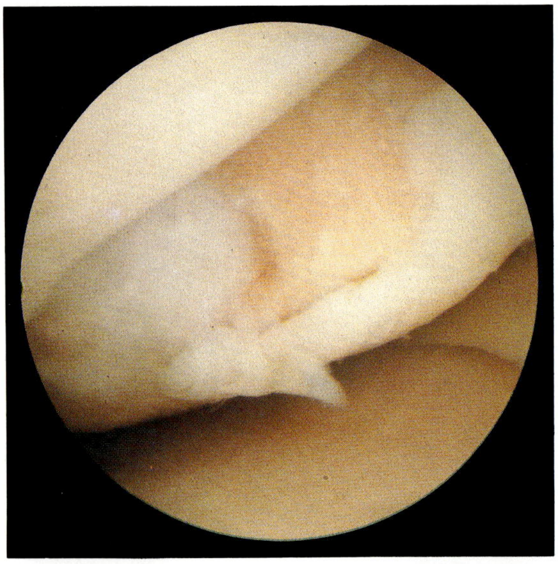

3.6

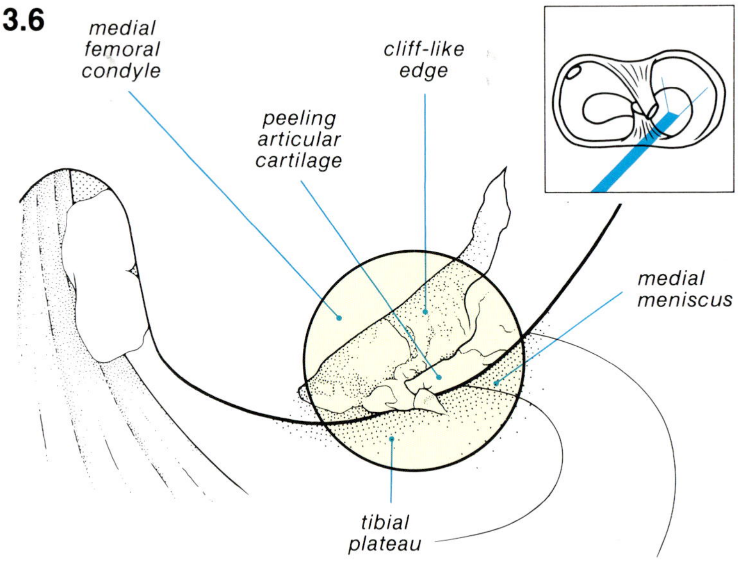

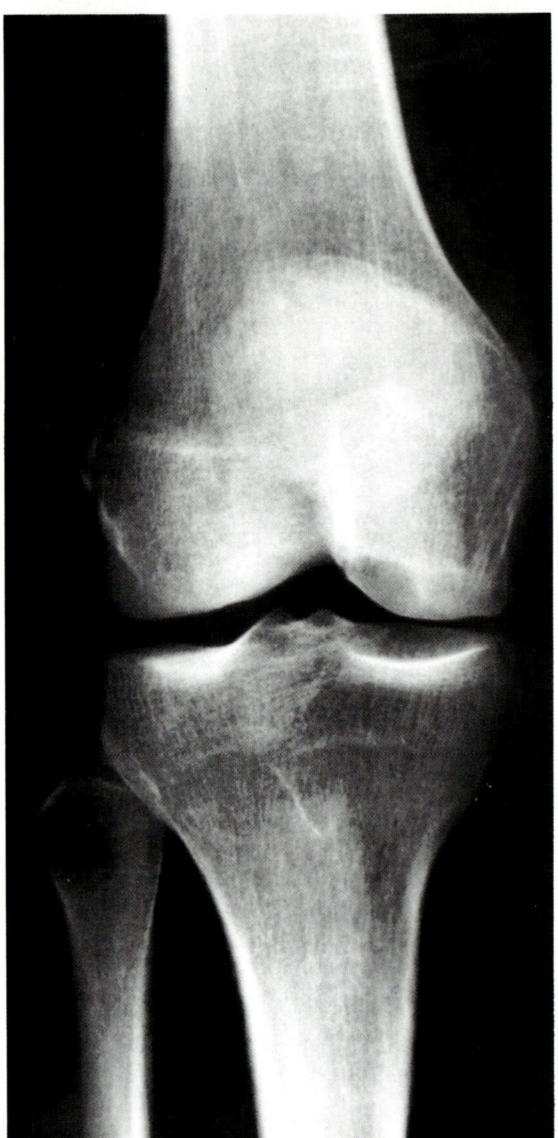

3.7

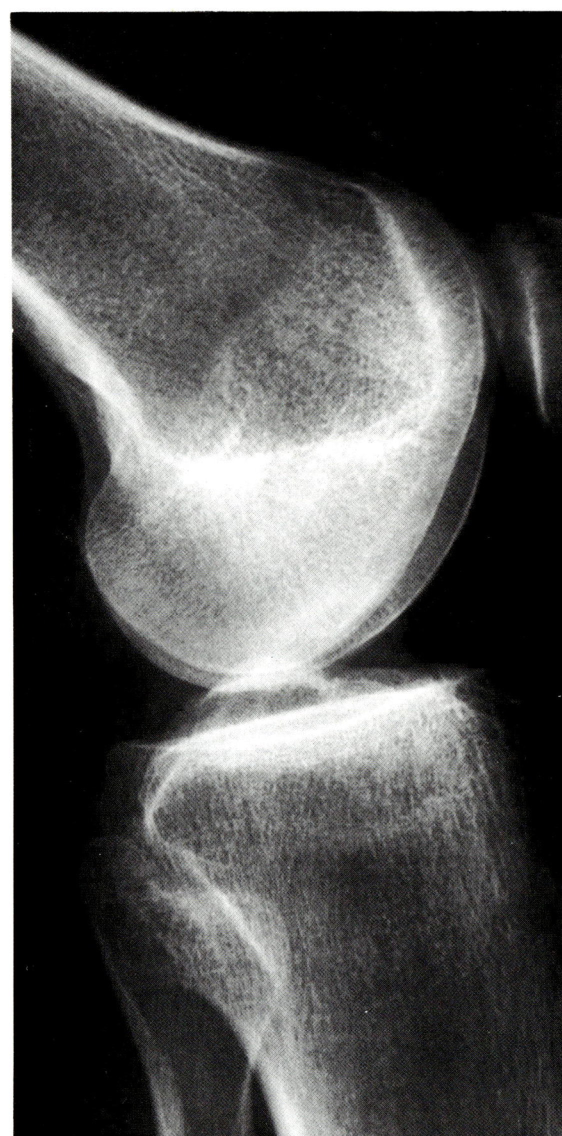

3.8

condyle are almost certainly imperfect. There is a small irregularity of the medial meniscus, but it was considered that the meniscus was still able to protect the articular surface and was therefore left untouched.

Lesions of the femoral condyle do not always heal as well as that in Fig.3.9, particularly if the lesion is on the central part of the weight-bearing arc. Fig.3.10 shows a medial femoral condyle from which a loose body had arisen, but the defect has not healed with firm fibrocartilage. The lesion is irregular; the joint surface is shaggy as if in the process of breaking down and there is a small patch of exposed subchondral bone in the centre of the defect. Degenerative osteoarthritis would seem to be an inevitable consequence of such a lesion on the weight-bearing arc of the femoral condyle.

Fig.3.11 shows the intercondylar groove of a knee from

3.9

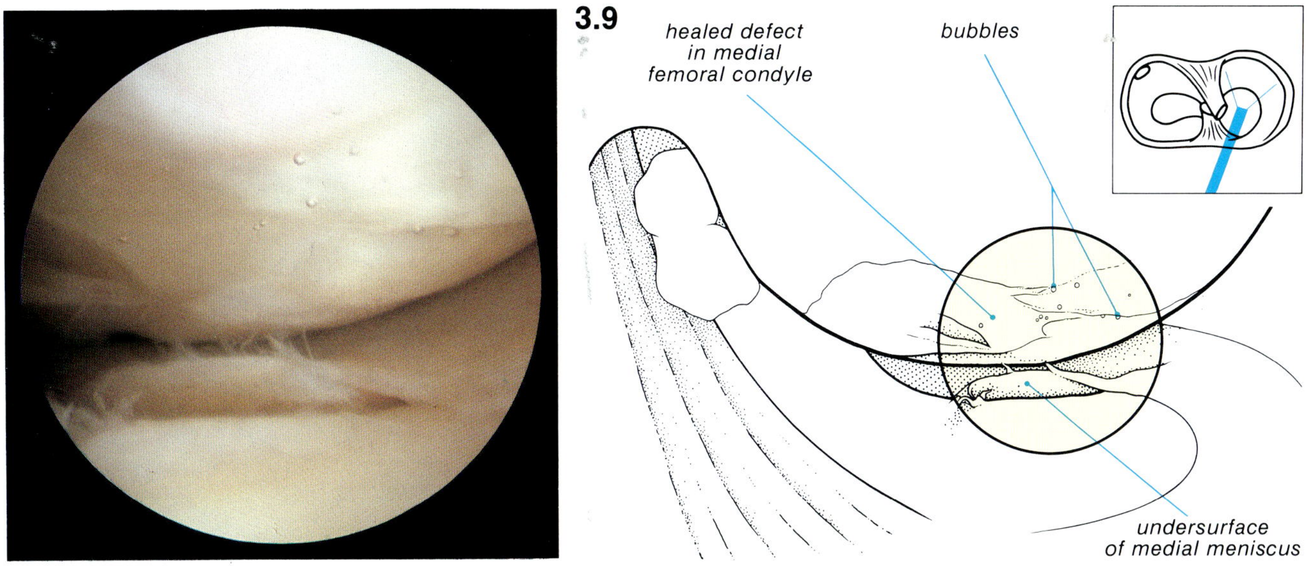

3.10

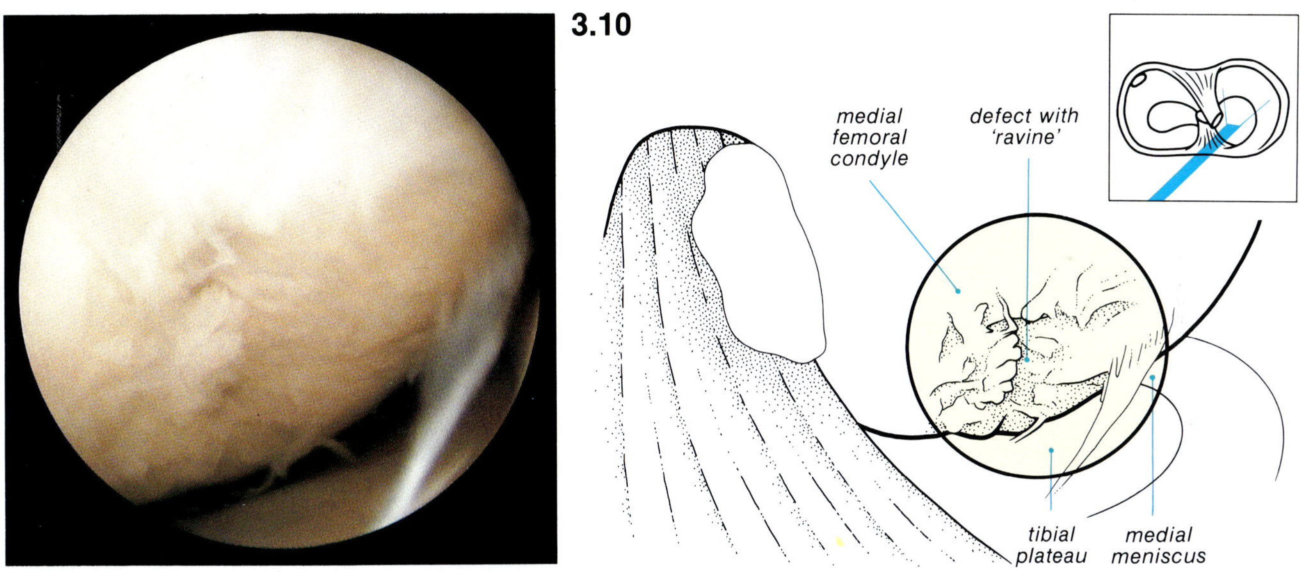

3.11

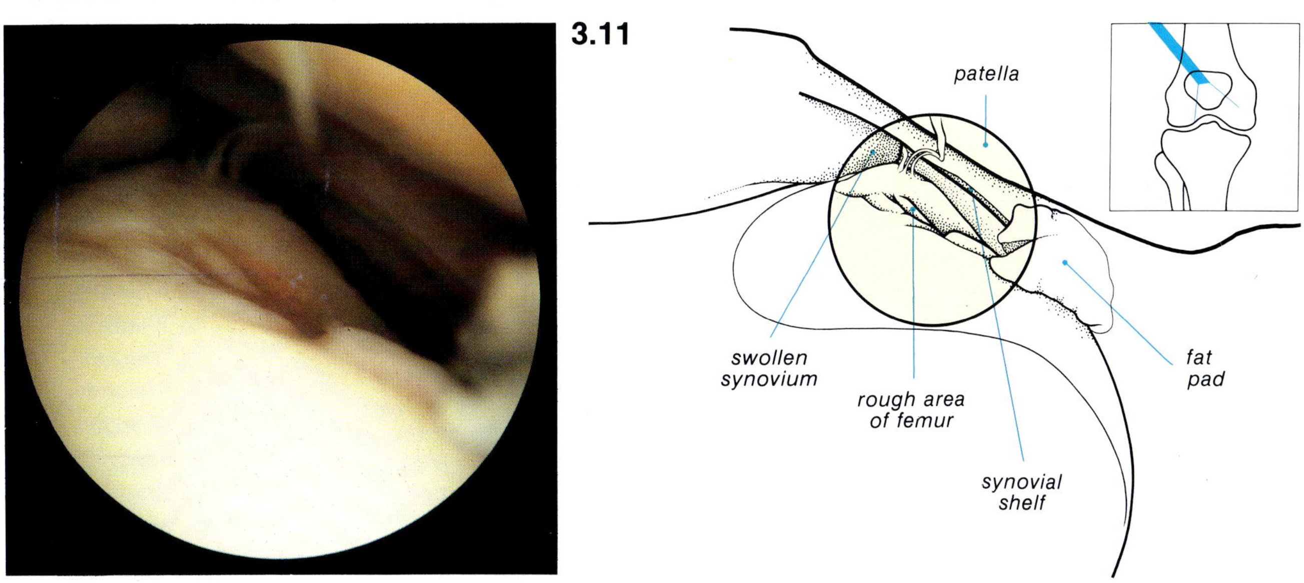

which a loose body measuring 2 x 3cm had been removed. The loose body consisted of cancellous bone on one surface and articular cartilage on the other. The only articular cartilage defect found is seen from the lateral suprapatellar approach. There was no history of direct injury to the knee although the lesion lay directly beneath the patella at ninety degrees of flexion. Lesions at this site are most unusual.

Chondral separation

In the adolescent knee, twisting upon the knee under load can produce osteochondral fractures (see Figs.3.1 & 3.2). In the adult, a more likely consequence is separation of a fragment of articular cartilage without damage to the underlying bone. Fig.3.12 shows a lesion of the medial femoral condyle caused by a sharp twisting injury with the knee under load. The patient felt

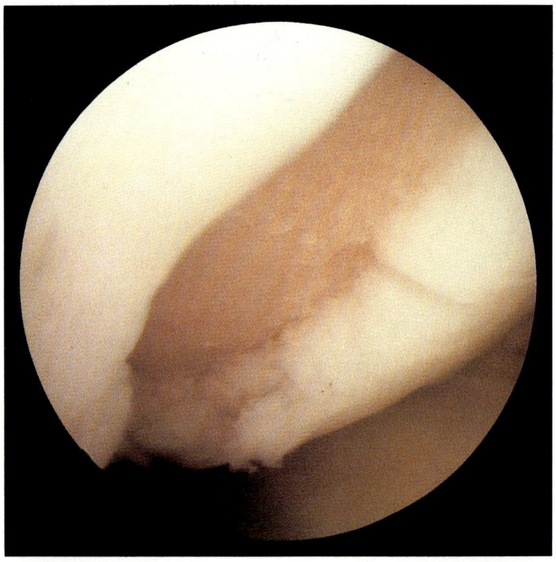

3.12

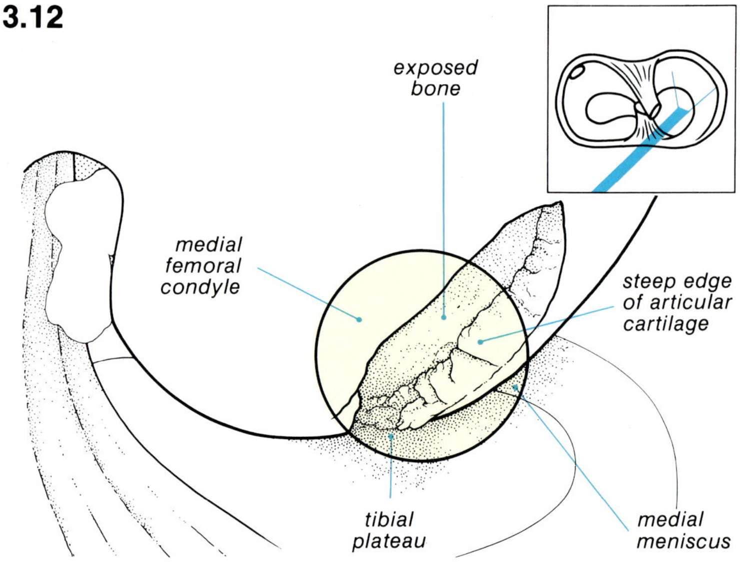

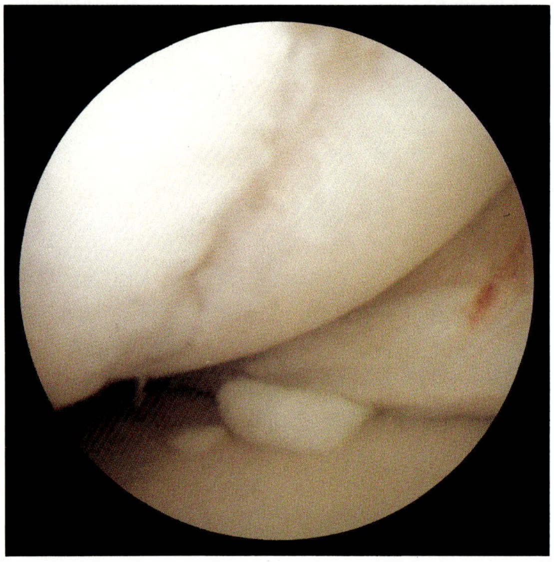

3.13

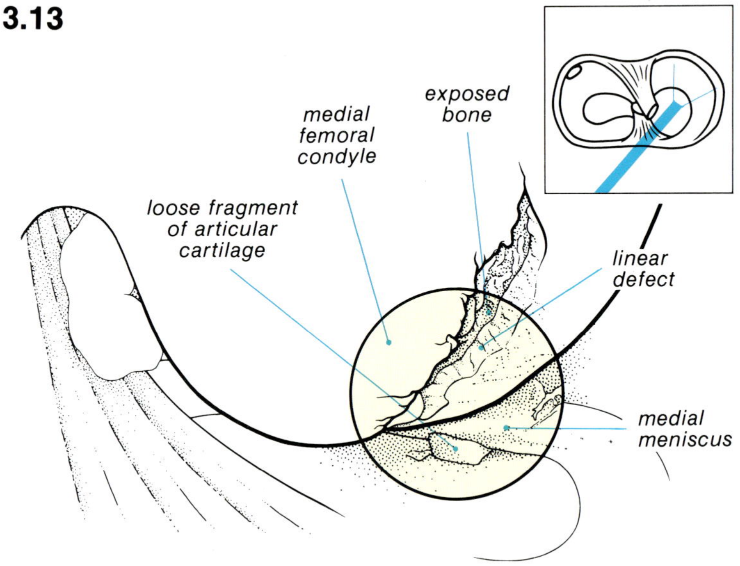

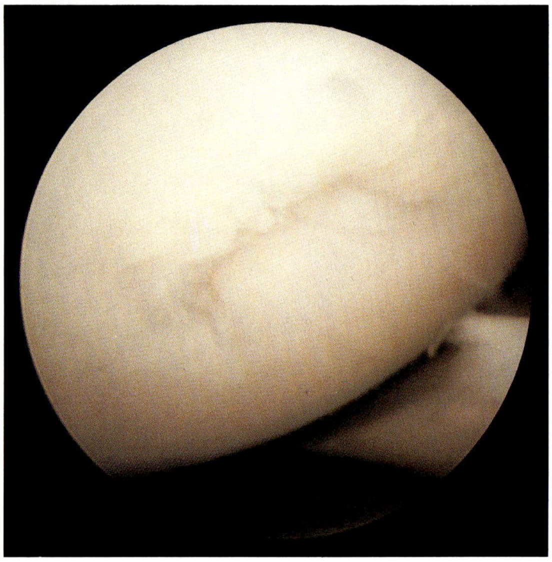

3.14

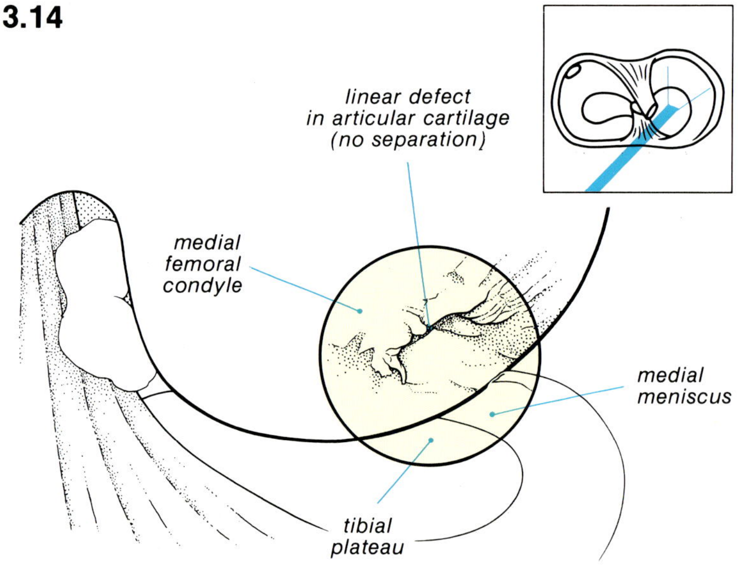

something crack inside the joint and later noticed swelling due to an effusion of fluid. A loose body was identified in the medial gutter and a lesion of the medial meniscus was diagnosed.

At arthroscopy one week later, the fragment could not be found but there was much articular cartilage debris free in the joint. The appearance (Fig.3.12) was that of a chondral separation which has resulted in the shedding of a plaque of articular cartilage from the subchondral bone. The characteristic features of these lesions include the steep cliff-like margins of articular cartilage surrounding the defect and the smooth floor of fresh subchondral bone.

In some patients chondral separation has a curious linear appearance in which a strip of subchondral bone is exposed. In Fig.3.13 a small fragment of articular cartilage can be seen lying adjacent to the medial meniscus. These linear lesions always appear to run in an anteroposterior direction in the centre of the weight-bearing arc of the condyle. Why this specific pattern of lesion should occur is not clear; perhaps the articular cartilage at one end of the lesion becomes separated and then acts as a rasp to scrape at the strip of cartilage behind it each time the knee is flexed.

Fig.3.14 shows a more unusual type of lesion; there is neither exposed bone nor cliff-like edges around the lesion. There is, instead, a depression in the articular surface, as if it has been struck sharply with a blunt square-ended object. There was no history of trauma to account for this lesion.

A much larger chondral separation is seen in Fig.3.15 in which the cleavage between the bone and articular cartilage is obvious. The lesion was at least six months old and the smooth surfaces of subchondral bone do not look as fresh as in Figs.3.12 and 3.13. Also, the margins of the defect are not clean and sharp but rounded. The line of cleavage between articular cartilage and femur suggests that the basic pathology lies perhaps in a failure of adhesion between the articular surface and the underlying bone rather than in trauma alone. These lesions are difficult to manage by any technique, but removal of loose articular cartilage in an attempt to confine the lesion and prevent enlargement may prove helpful.

Fig.3.16 shows an incidental finding in an older patient. A loose flap of articular cartilage is seen on the medial femoral condyle, based medially and lying adjacent to the anterior cruciate ligament. No symptoms could be attributed to this lesion but the appearances are very suggestive of a healed chondral separation with a flap of loose articular cartilage at its posterior limit. Such lesions are not uncommon, but it is not known if they are simply

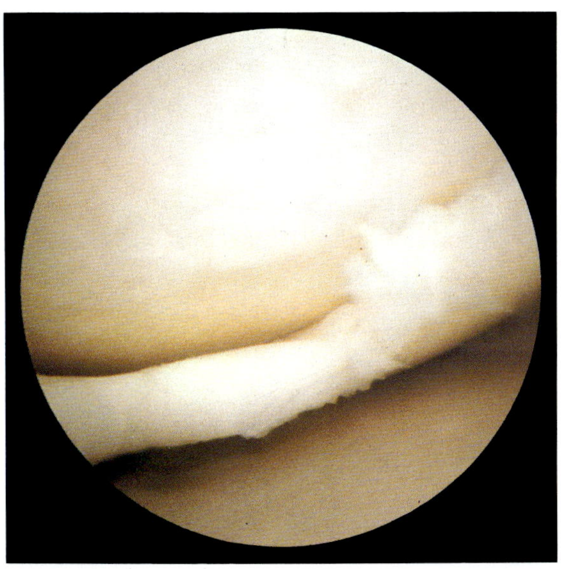

3.15

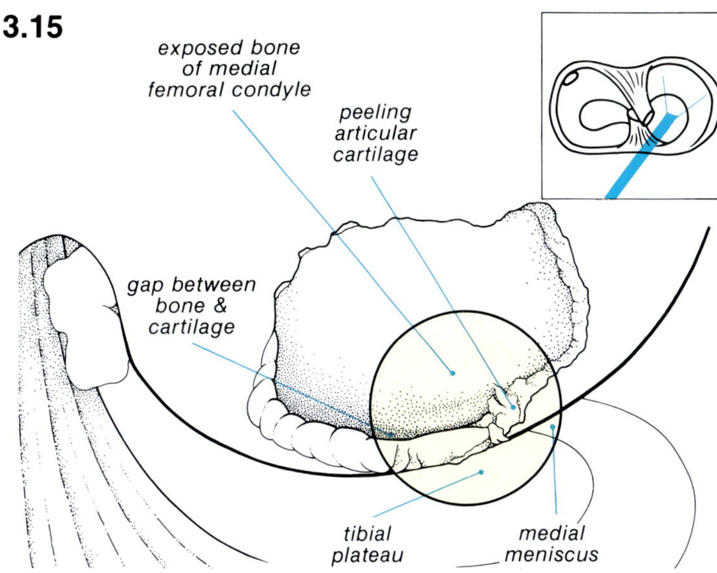

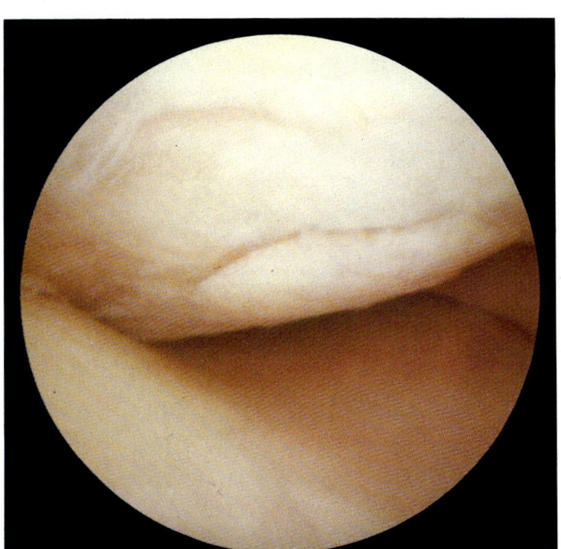

3.16

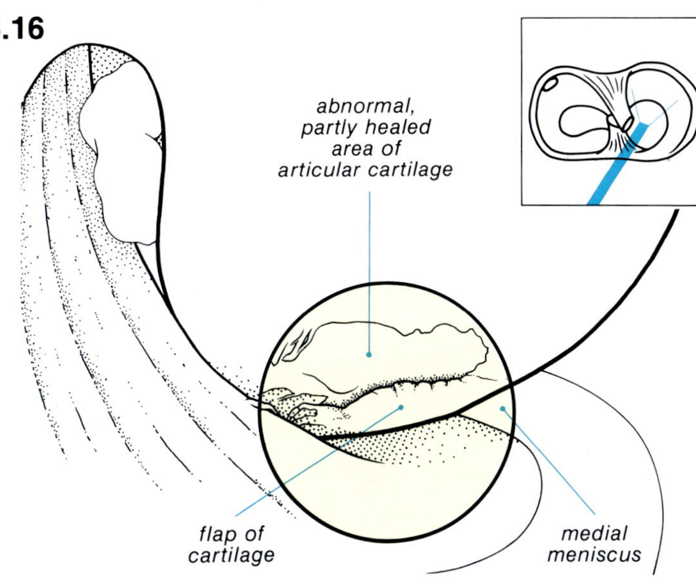

due to contact between the anterior cruciate ligament and the femoral condyle in full extension or if they represent a healed chondral separation.

Fig.3.17 shows the knee of a patient who had systemic lupus erythematosus with superimposed *Salmonella paratyphi* infection. (The posteromedial compartment of this knee is shown in Fig.2.24). There is a large area of denuded subchondral bone with flakes of thin articular cartilage at the margin of the lesion. The articular fragments removed from this knee were soft, friable and almost fibrous in nature. The flimsiness of the normally firm articular cartilage may have been due to the systemic lupus erythematosus, the *Salmonella* infection or simply to the steroid medication that the patient was receiving. Although the patient's symptoms improved remarkably following the irrigation of debris from the joint and control of the infection, the long-term prognosis for such articular surface damage and so much exposed subchondral bone must be poor.

The tibial plateau is less often affected by chondral separations than the femoral condyles. Fig.3.18 shows the knee of a 30-year-old footballer who had a lesion of the medial meniscus which consisted of a detached 'bucket handle' meniscal fragment lying in the medial gutter. The articular surface of the tibia had separated to expose subchondral bone. The margins of the defect were loose. There was an irregularity on the medial femoral condyle at the point of contact with the tibial defect but the articular surface had not separated from the femur. Despite a clear explanation of this poor prognosis, the patient continues to play football. The opportunity for a further arthroscopic examination has not occurred.

Fig.3.19 shows chondral separation caused by a sudden twisting movement under stress similar to the lesion of the medial femoral condyle seen in Fig.3.12, except that here the lesion lies on the lateral margin of the femoral condyle. The patient had an effusion, was tender on the joint line and the clinical diagnosis was a tear of the lateral meniscus. Arthroscopy showed that the lesion lay just above the anterior horn of the lateral meniscus. The bed of the lesion, which was two weeks old, was already covered with loose fibrinous material and the articular margins had begun to round off.

Chondral separations can also occur in older patients. Fig.3.20 shows a normal meniscus with degenerative changes on the tibia. The femoral condyle lacked an articular surface and was similar to that in Fig.3.19. The symptoms began, accompanied by sudden pain and effusion, following a twisting movement of the knee under load during a game of golf. The fragment from this defect was identified and removed as a loose body.

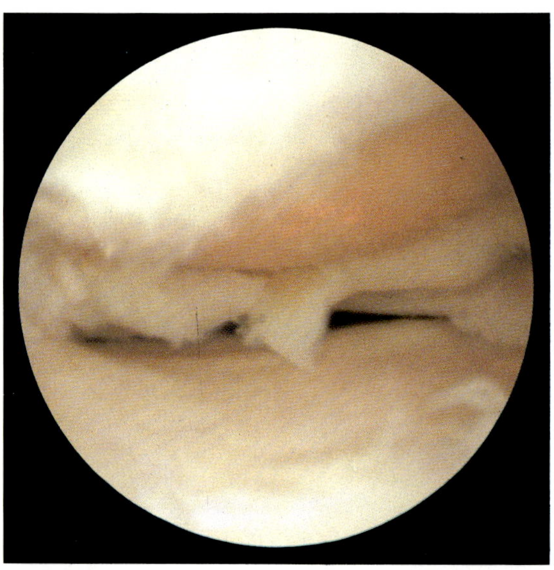

3.17

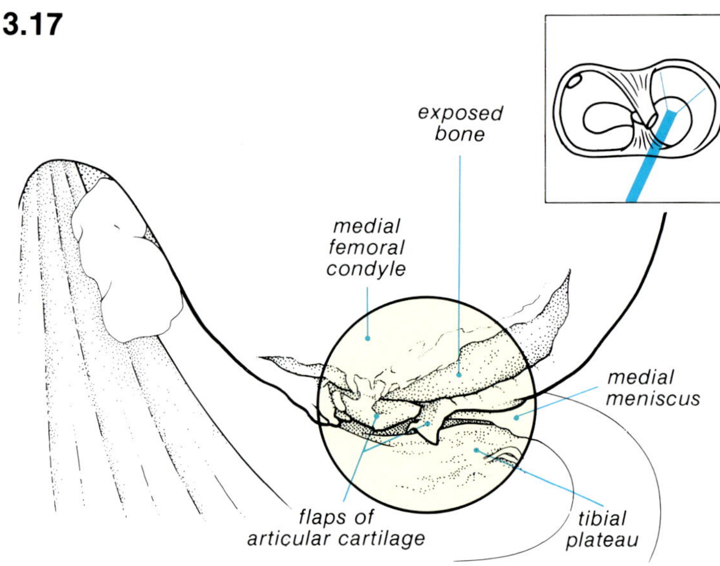

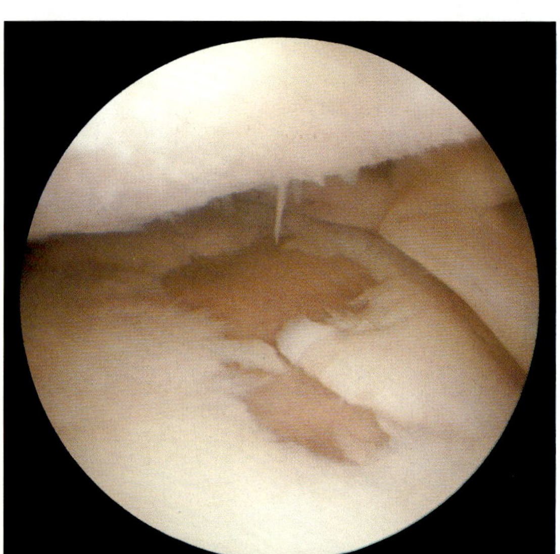

3.18

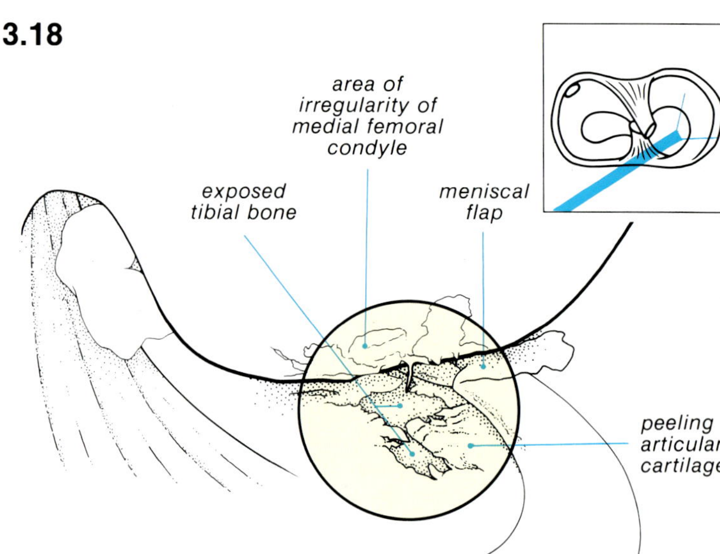

Although the patient continues to play golf, the prognosis for such a knee with damage to both articular surfaces must be poor. The patient was thought, on clinical grounds, to have a tear of the medial meniscus but arthroscopy demonstrated that the meniscus was in fact the only healthy structure in the medial compartment.

Not all chondral separations have clearly defined margins. Fig.3.21 shows a medial femoral condyle in which the defect in the articular cartilage has cracks radiating from its centre. The pattern of these cracks might suggest that the surface of the joint has sustained a direct blow, but no history of such an injury could be obtained from the patient. The triangular articular

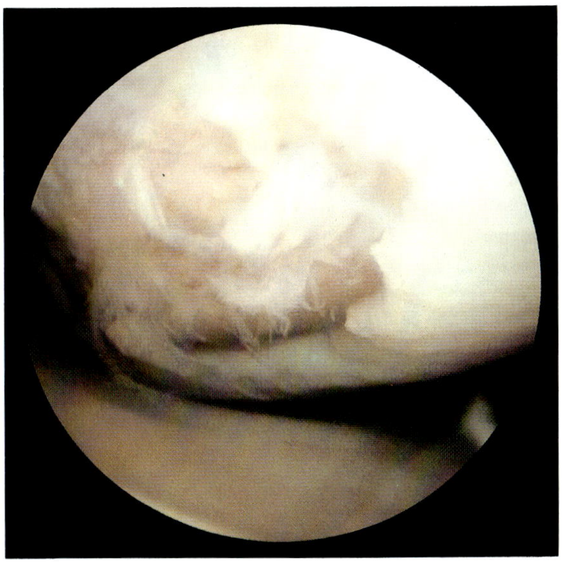

3.19

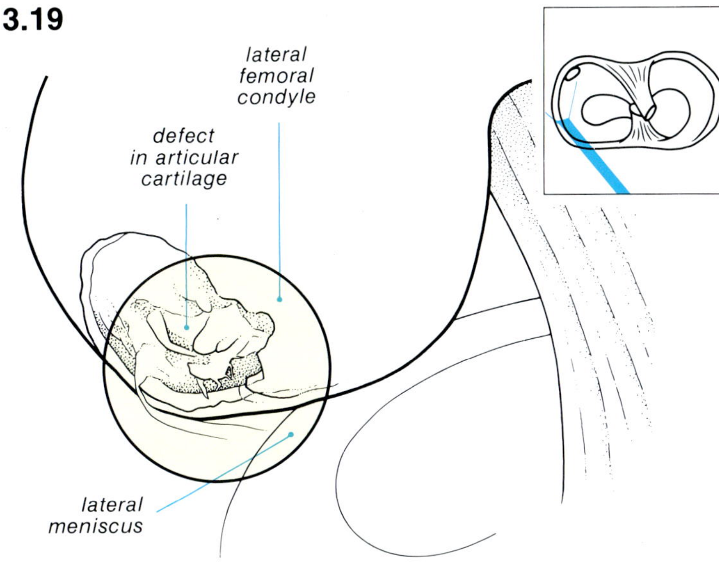

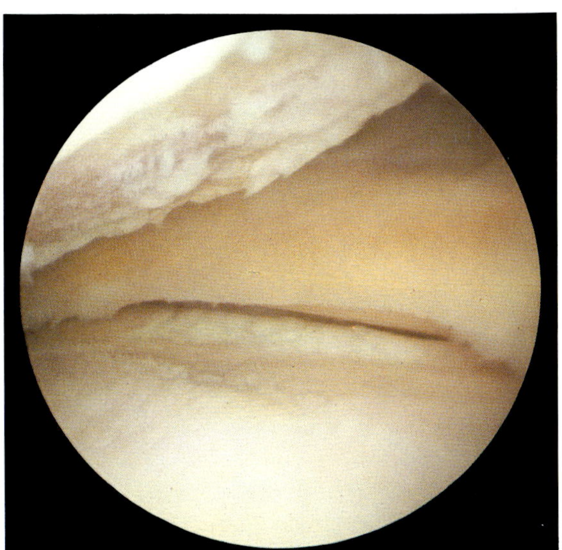

3.20

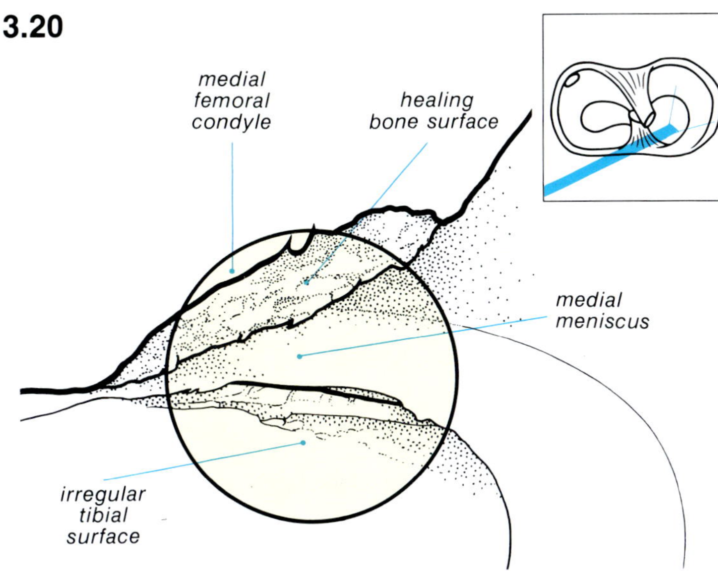

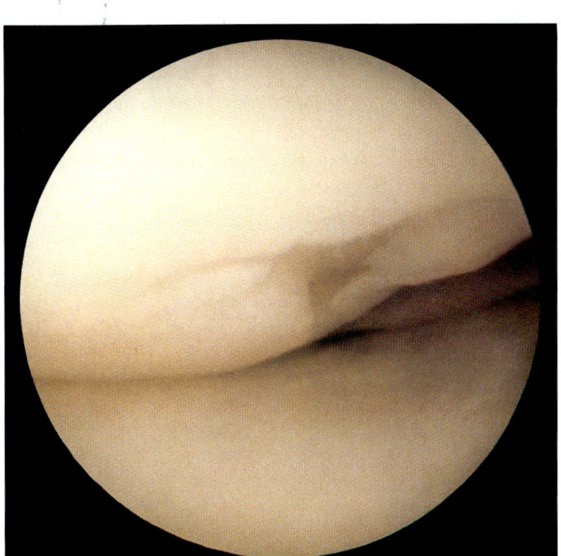

3.21

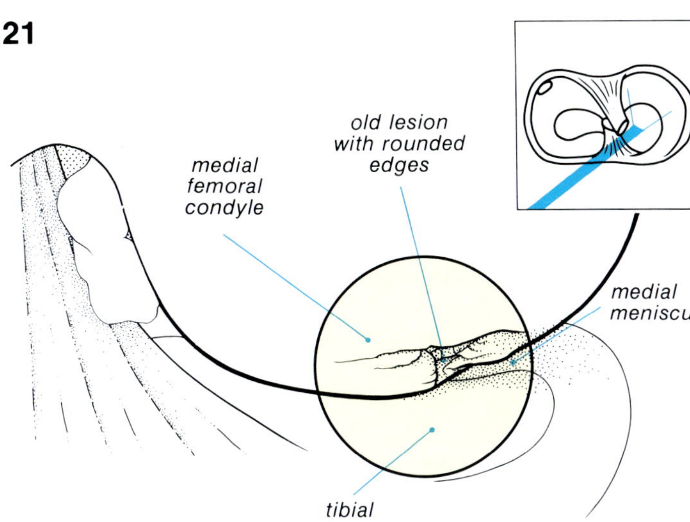

cartilage flaps at the margin of the lesion were loose and, if these flaps had separated, the appearances would have been those of the more typical chondral separations (see Fig.3.13). As it is, Fig.3.21 is similar to Fig.3.14 (see page 3.6). There was no history of injury to account for the appearance. The significance of these lesions is not known, but they may perhaps indicate the start of the process of separation of the articular cartilage from underlying bone that leads to a larger chondral separation.

Not all articular cartilage separations involve the full thickness of the joint surface. Articular cartilage flaps are also found and present a different appearance from full thickness chondral separation. The lesion in Fig.3.22 is a flap of articular cartilage based medially and involving the superficial articular surface only. The symptoms included clicking and catching on rotation of the knee and were very similar to those of a torn medial meniscus except that there were no true locking episodes. The symptoms were relieved by excision of the flap and the patient was able to return to active sport.

Subchondral bone necrosis, in which the bone beneath the articular cartilage is resorbed without damage to the articular cartilage itself, can produce the curious appearance of an unsupported flap of articular cartilage (Fig.3.23). A split in the articular surface opens into the space beneath it. Because there is no cortical bone supporting the articular surface, a mobile segment of cartilage is created that can overlap the normal articular cartilage which is fixed to the underlying bone at the

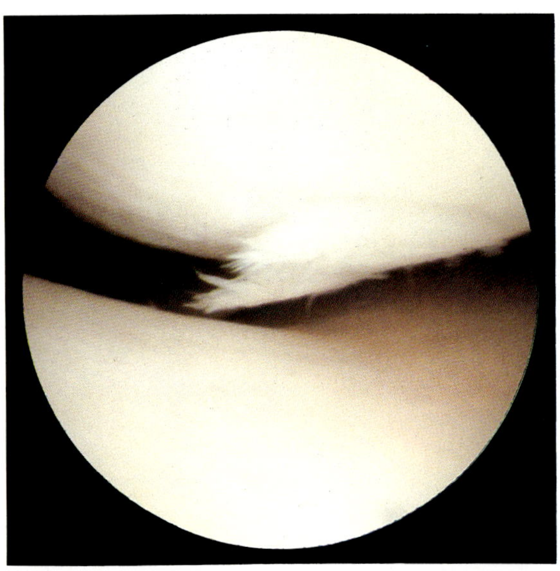

3.22

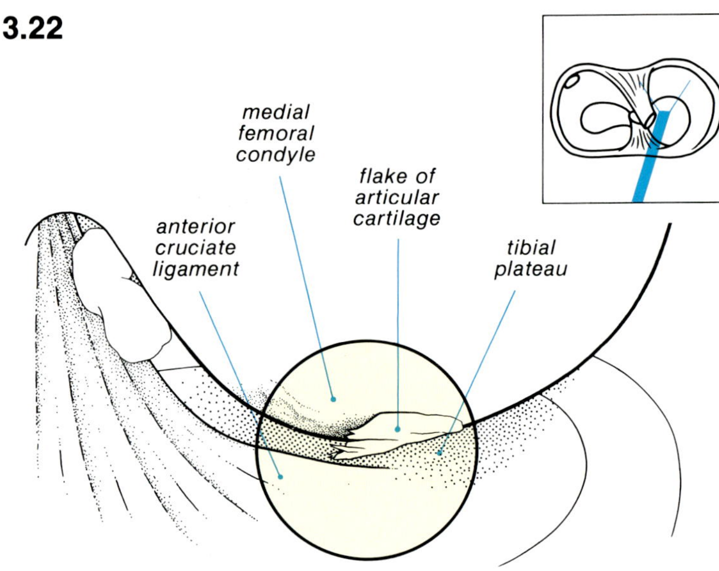

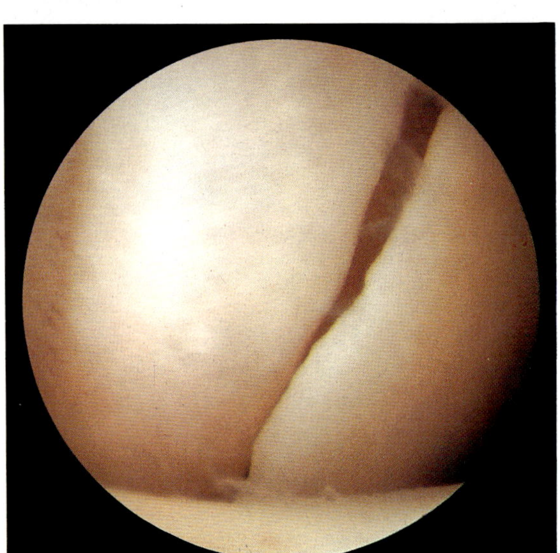

3.23

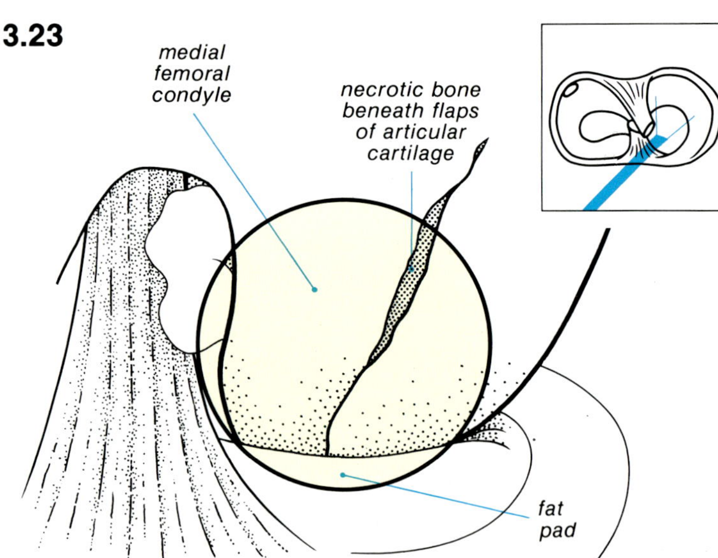

margin of the defect. The radiographic appearance of the lesion is shown in Fig.3.24.

Large defects in bone may be visible on plain radiography with no abnormality being found at arthroscopy. Fig.3.25 shows the radiological features of osteochondritis dissecans yet arthroscopy showed an intact articular surface. The only abnormality found arthroscopically was that, on probing with a blunt hook, the articular surface was softer than usual (Fig.3.26).

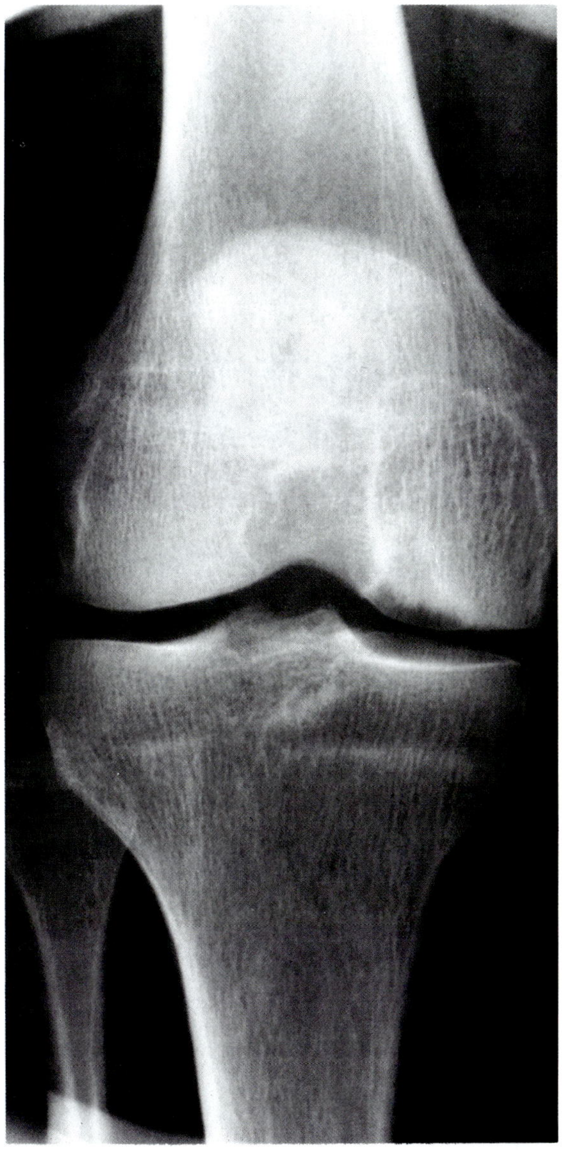

3.24

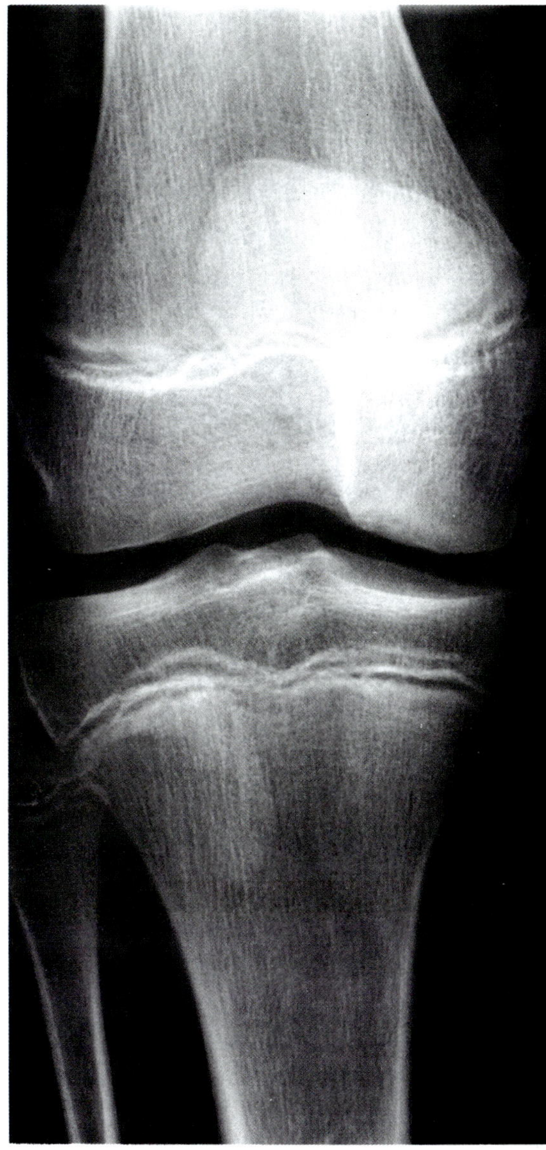

3.25

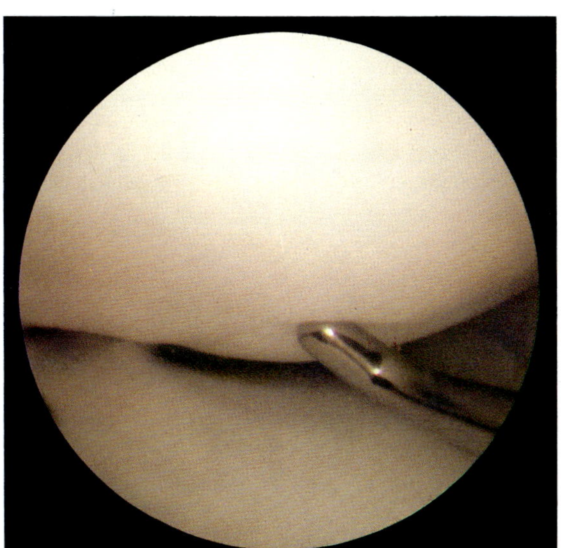

3.26

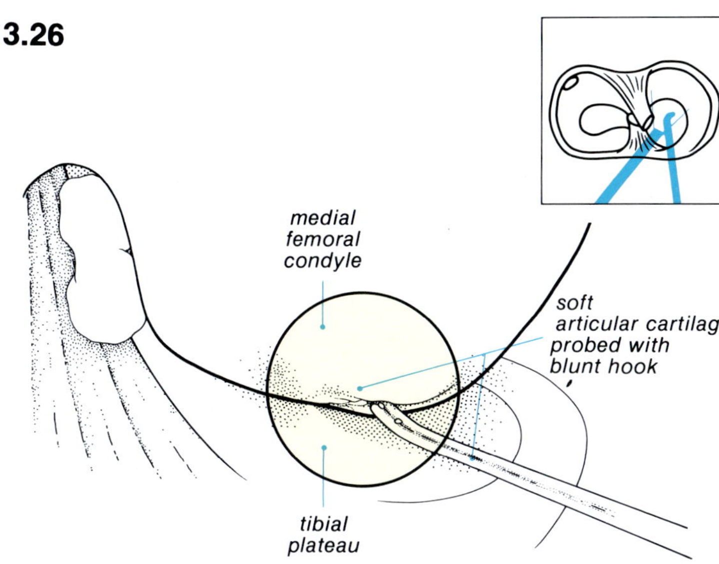

Fractures of the tibial plateau can also lead to dramatic radiological changes, but the arthroscopic changes are often much less obvious. While radiographs showed a depressed fracture of the lateral tibial plateau (Figs.3.27 & 3.28), arthroscopy (Fig.3.29) showed that the defect was filled with firm cartilage that bore a strong resemblance to normal hyaline cartilage. Little irregularity could be seen, apart from a slight change in colour along the fracture line. The medial meniscus sat unusually high above the tibial plateau but was intact. The explanation for its unusual position may be that the distance between its periphery and two tibial attachments had been increased by the fracture.

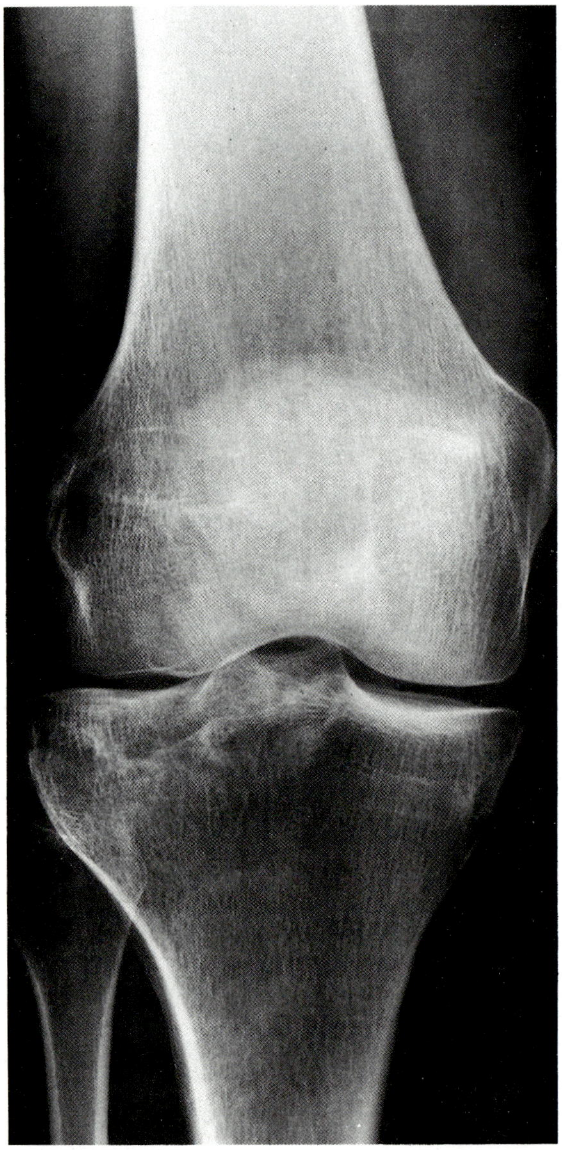

3.27

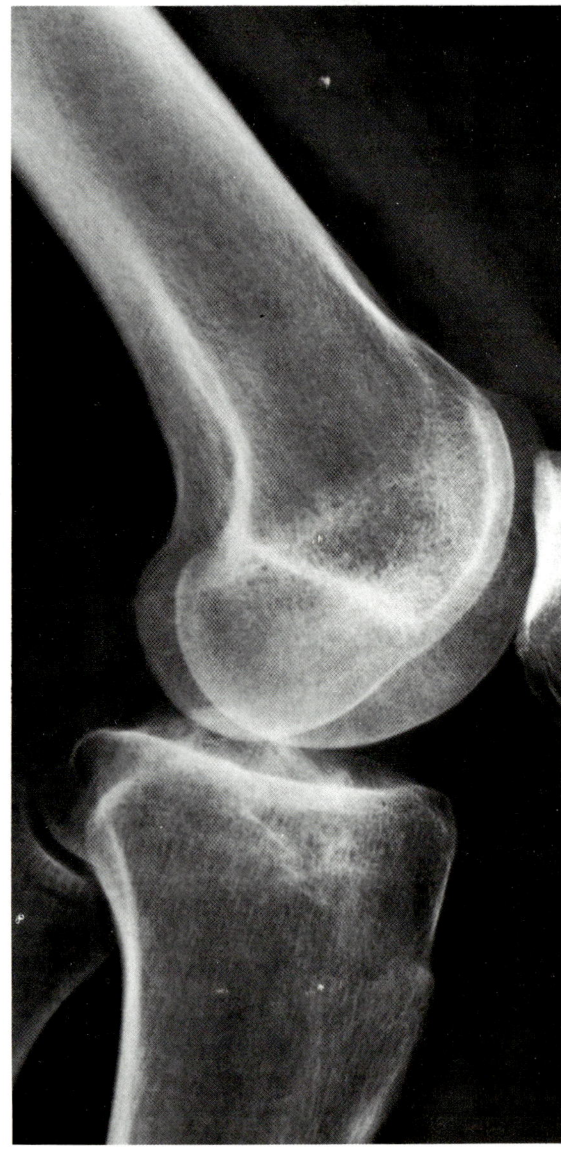

3.28

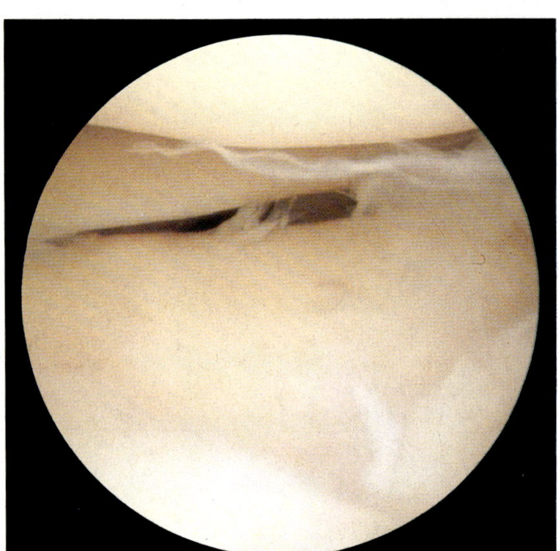

3.29

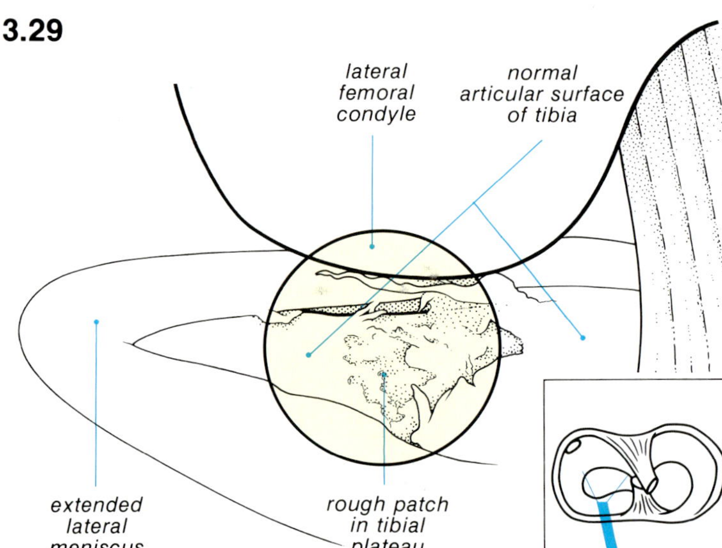

Miscellaneous

Fig.3.30 shows the femoral condyle of a boy with haemophilia (see Figs.2.58 & 2.59 for views of his suprapatellar pouch). The condyle is marked by deep pits which are filled with pigmented synovium, like rock pools filled with reddish-brown seaweed. The articular surface has extensive pannus which is probably responsible for the destruction of the articular cartilage. The pits in the articular surface are quite different from those seen in degenerative osteoarthritis or rheumatoid arthritis.

Bone tumours in the knee joint are rare. Figs.3.31 and 3.32 show a large lesion that proved to be an island of cortical bone. The symptoms were pain and tenderness when the knee was flexed. At arthroscopy the cartilage overlying the lesion was found to be softened and friable

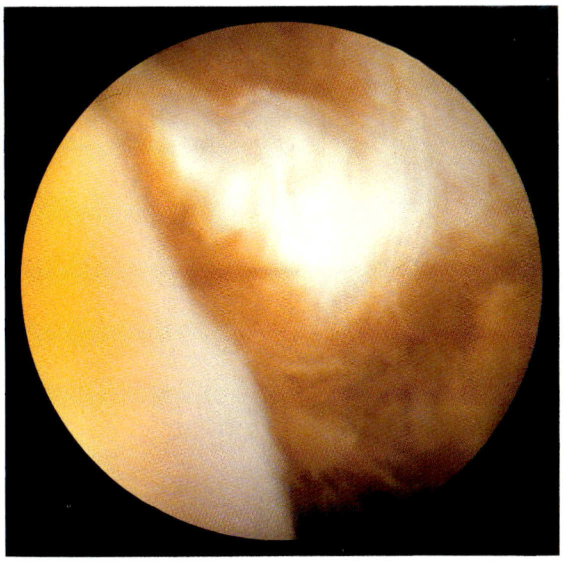

3.30

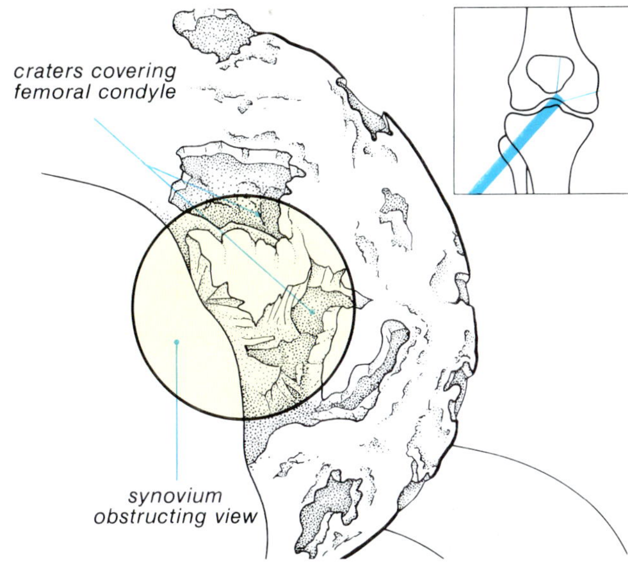

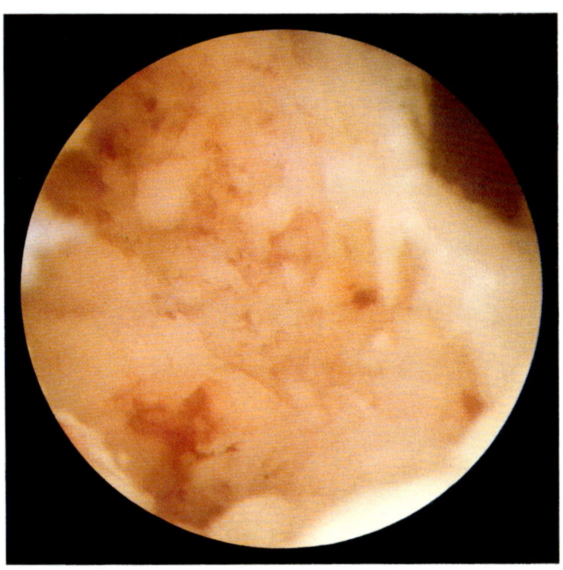

3.31

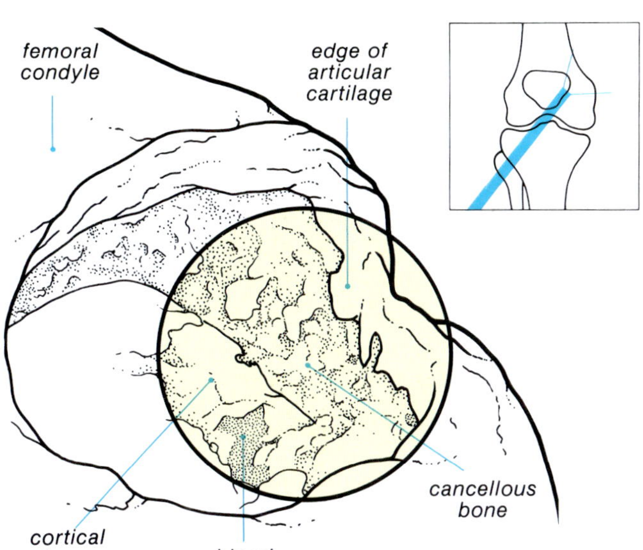

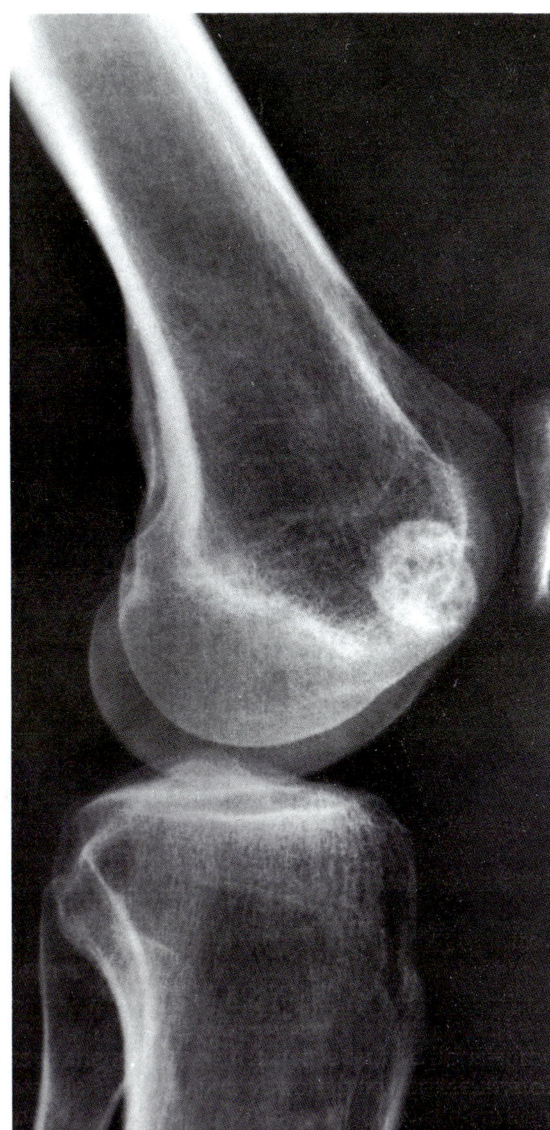

3.32

and came into contact with the medial synovial shelf during flexion. The abnormal cartilage was incised to reveal subchondral bone and a window cut in the bone revealed a mass of hard cortical bone lying within the femoral condyle. The bone island was too hard to be removed arthroscopically, but levelling the raised articular cartilage overlying it was followed by a slow but steady improvement in the symptoms.

Artefacts

Arthroscopy should be an atraumatic procedure but it can result in damage to the articular cartilage. Fig.3.33 shows the damage caused by the tip of an early design of arthroscope, the sheath of which had an unnecessarily sharp edge. Fine shavings of articular cartilage resulted which, although only a few cells in thickness and likely to heal well, are best avoided. Modern designs of

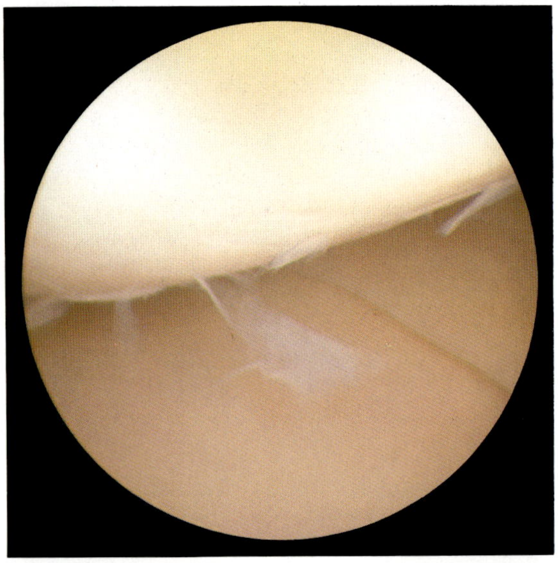

3.33

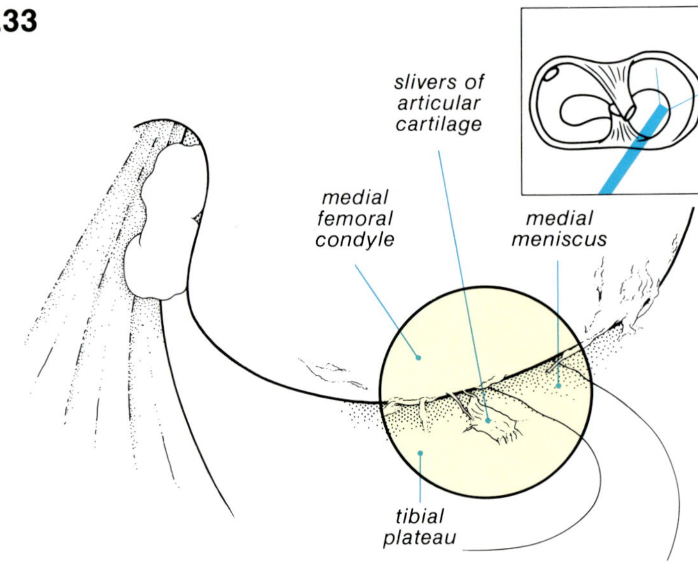

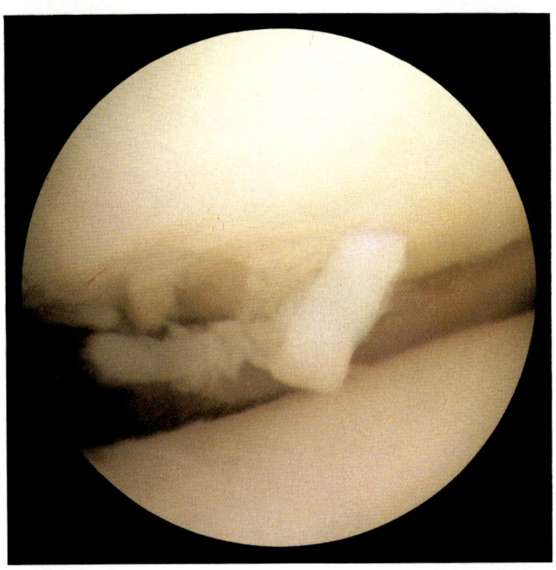

3.34

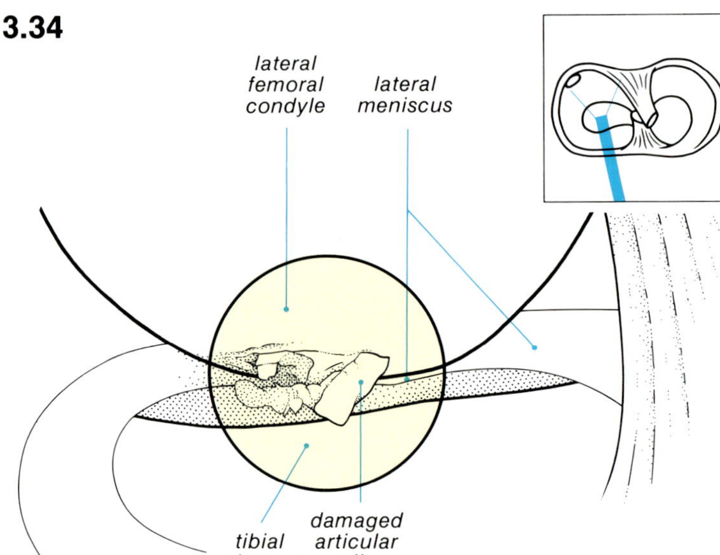

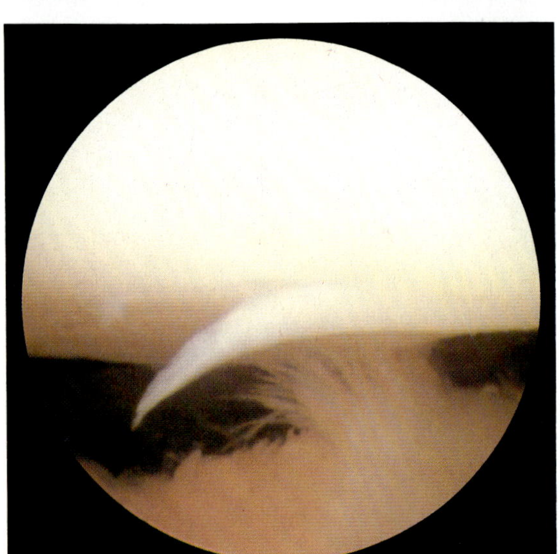

3.35

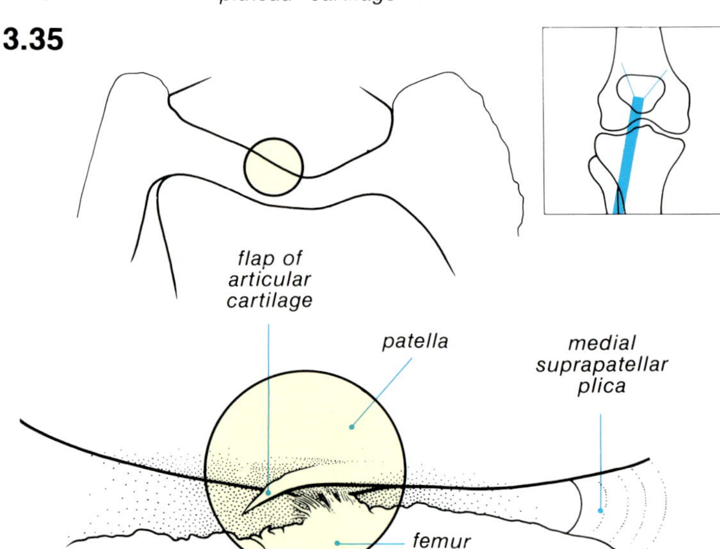

arthroscopes have rounded edges which, together with careful handling of the instrument, should eliminate scuffing of the articular surface during diagnostic arthroscopy.

Damage to the articular cartilage can also occur during arthroscopic surgery through incorrect handling of the instruments. It may be kept to a minimum with careful handling but probably not avoided completely. Fig.3.34 shows damage to the lateral femoral condyle caused by a sharp trocar and cannula inserted as a portal for operating instruments. A divot of articular cartilage left a defect at least 2mm deep. The characteristic appearance of such a lesion, which is fortunately rare, is of a very clean and sharp edge, often with a flake of articular cartilage beside it.

In defence of arthroscopy and arthroscopic surgery it must be stressed that similar damage to the articular surface occurred before the introduction of arthroscopy when operations were done through an open arthrotomy, but then it was much more difficult to see the lesions and they were generally regarded as an accepted, if unusual, hazard of operations upon the knee.

The needle used as an exit for the irrigation system is another potential danger. In Fig.3.35 a flap of articular surface was raised from the patella by the tip of the irrigation needle as it was inserted from the lateral side. The lesion was approximately 1mm in width and the flap 2mm from tip to base but, when seen through the arthroscope, it looks disturbingly large.

Osteoarthritis

In the medial compartment of the knee, degenerative changes are usually first seen at the medial edge of the tibial plateau, in an elongated area adjacent to the medial meniscus similar to the site of the chondral separation of the tibial plateau shown in Fig.3.18. Fig.3.36 shows an oval area of exposed subchondral bone on the tibia with slight involvement of the femur. The degenerative area extends to the margin of the medial meniscus. The meniscus appears to protect the articular surface and is particularly apparent in the early stages of osteoarthritis of the knee. In Fig.3.37 the meniscus of the same knee as in Fig.3.36 is lifted with a needle, showing healthy articular cartilage beneath it. The degenerative changes are confined to the area lacking the protection of the meniscus. These illustrations offer an argument for preservation of the meniscus whenever possible. Medial meniscectomy in the knee shown here can only increase the load upon the vulnerable area of tibial plateau and hasten the development of osteoarthritis.

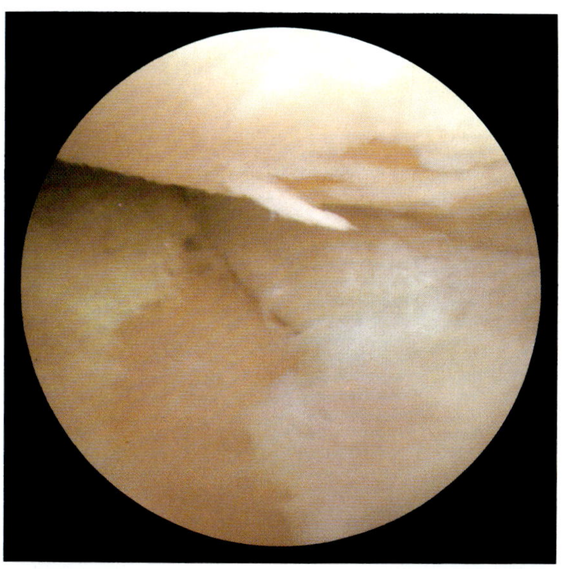

3.36

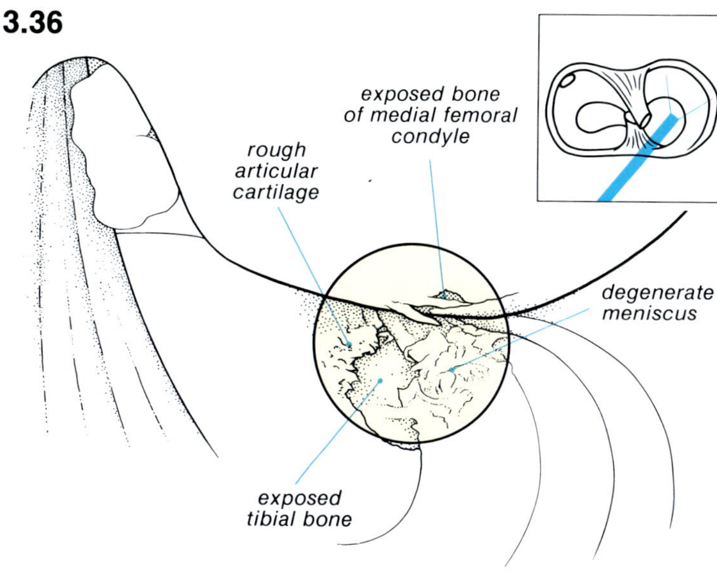

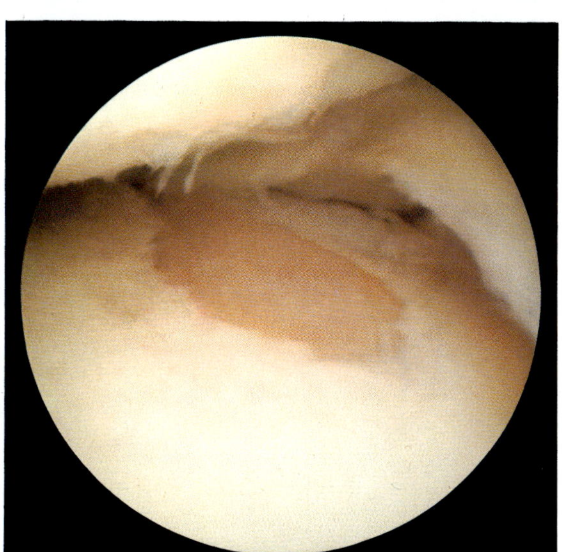

3.37

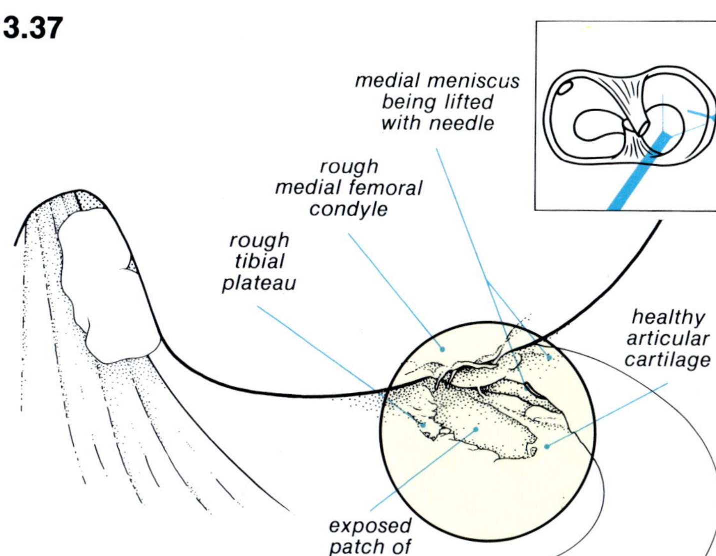

As the degenerative process continues, the area of exposed bone enlarges and the meniscus is gradually removed by attrition. Fig.3.38 shows a larger area of exposed bone on the tibia with involvement of the femoral condyle as well. The meniscus has been abraded but, nevertheless, has a rounded and stable rim. A flap of loose meniscal tissue, which may have contributed to the symptoms of meniscal instability, is lying in the gutter and is no longer offering protection to the tibial plateau. The flap was removed arthroscopically, leaving as much as possible of the intact and stable meniscal rim.

Osteoarthritis of the femoral condyle in its early stages will usually show an irregular and slightly furry appearance (Fig.3.39). Although such changes can be seen on the tibia, they are more common on the femur, perhaps because of the larger articular surface of the femoral condyle. The femoral condyle in Fig.3.39 may to some degree repair itself, but with time and use this repair process will gradually fail, leaving patches of exposed bone with islands of tatty and insubstantial articular surface. A later stage of degenerative osteoarthritis is seen in Fig.3.40 which shows a few strands of articular surface clinging to the subchondral bone. At this stage the knee has probably gone beyond natural repair processes and the prognosis must be poor. As the disease progresses still further, all loose articular surface will be removed by attrition, leaving exposed bone (Fig.3.41) with matching grooves and ridges on the articular surfaces. Only a small rim of insubstantial articular surface remains at the margin of the exposed bone.

In Fig.3.42 the tibial plateau was more severely affected by osteoarthritis than the femoral condyle. As the exposed bone of the femur and tibia became more worn, the ridges of hard eburnated bone of the tibia acted as a rasp, cutting grooves in the otherwise healthy articular

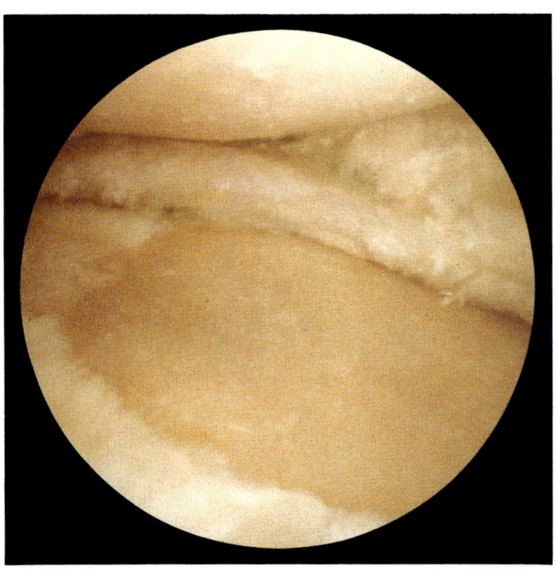

3.38

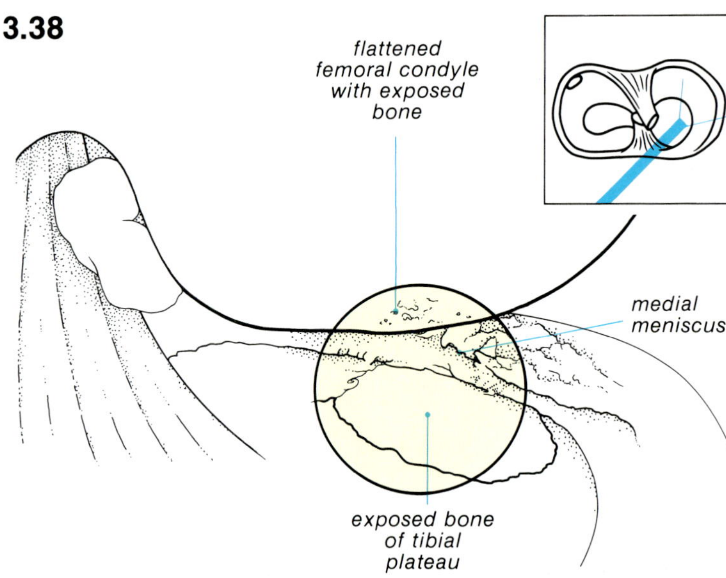

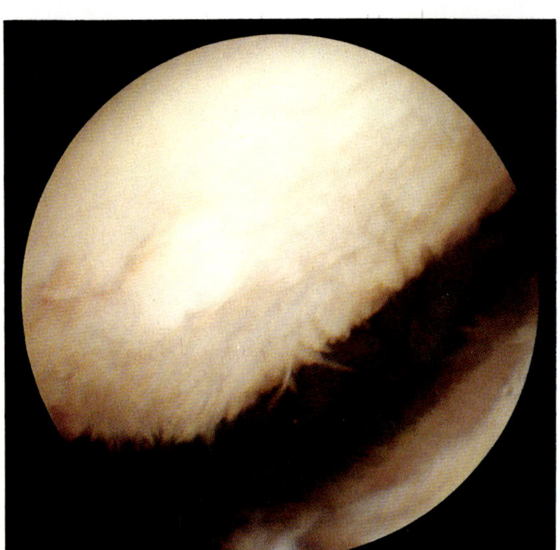

3.39

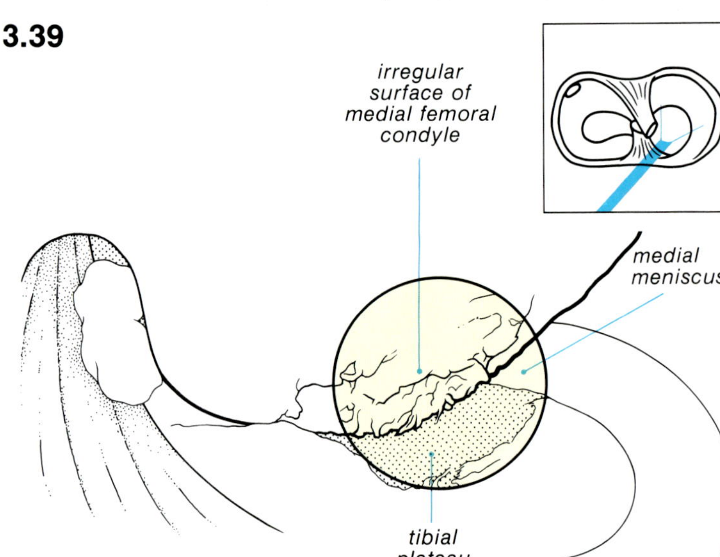

cartilage of the condyle. In this knee there was no intervening band of degenerate articular cartilage between the areas of exposed bone and the healthy joint surface, suggesting an unusually rapid and localized advance of the degenerative process. An explanation for such a rapid advance may be that the subtotal meniscectomy, recently performed as treatment for early osteoarthritis of the knee, had accelerated the degenerative process.

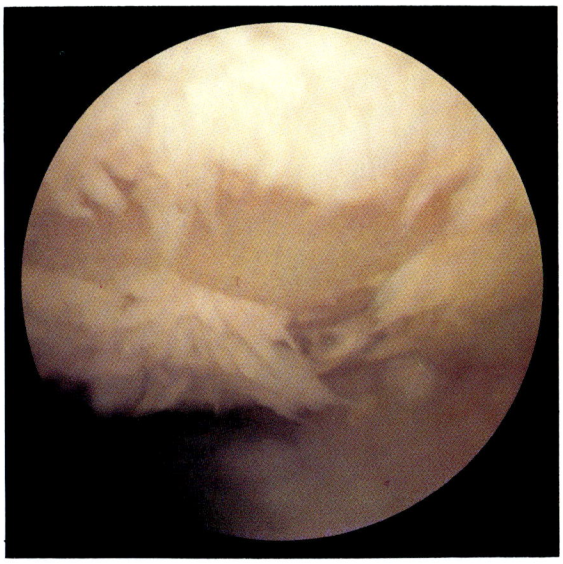

3.40

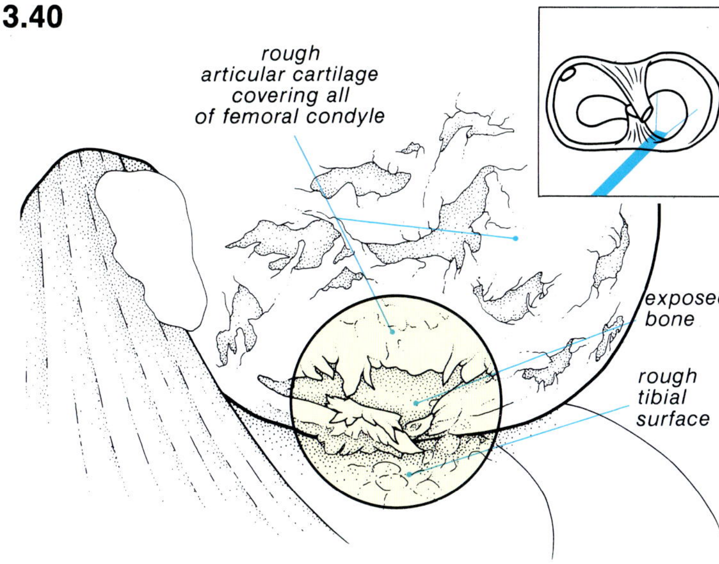

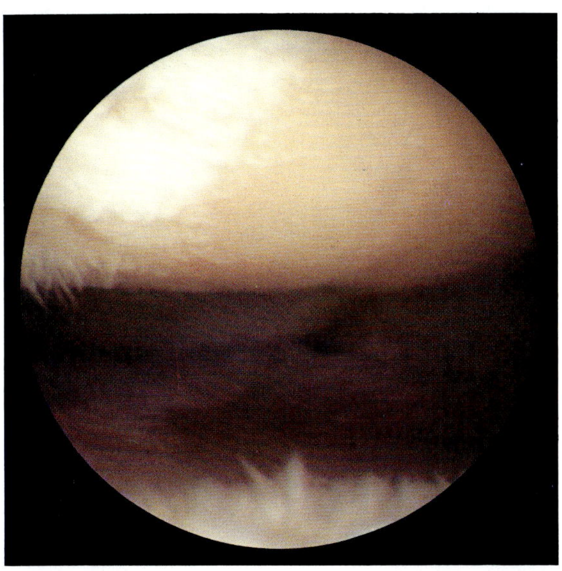

3.41

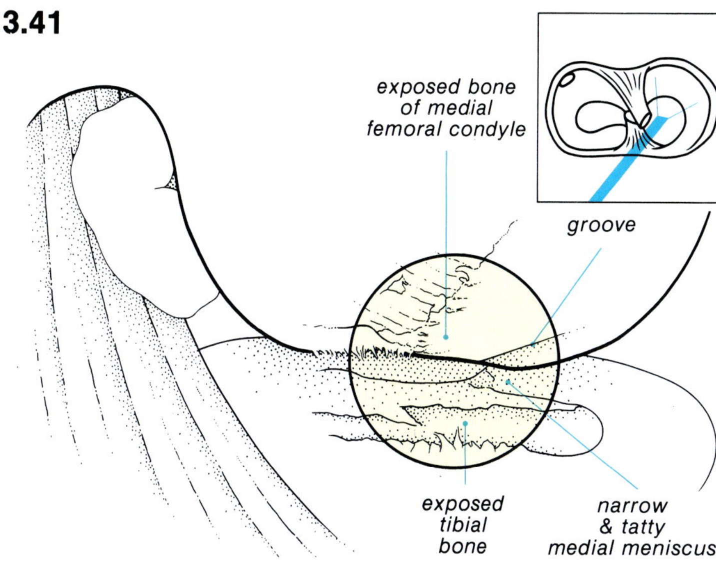

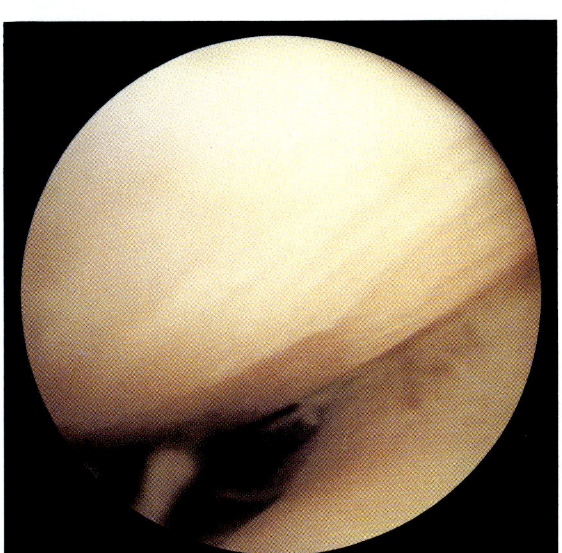

3.42

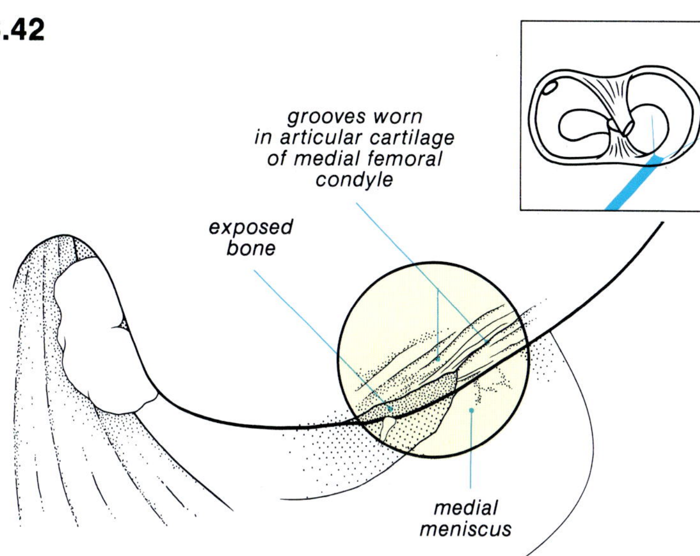

Fig.3.43 shows a later stage of osteoarthritis with eburnated grooves and ridges on the femoral and tibial surfaces. A few tiny plaques of articular cartilage persist and the bone is bleeding. It has been suggested that abrasion of osteoarthritic bone down to vascular tissue will lead to healing. In Fig.3.43, as with many patients, the natural disease process consists of abrasion down to bleeding bone, yet no evidence of healing can be seen. The concept of abrasion as a therapeutic procedure for osteoarthritis must remain questionable until long-term results are available for study.

Osteophytes, which consist of soft bone and articular cartilage, form around all joint margins but are most easily seen at the intercondylar notch. In Fig.3.44 there is

3.43

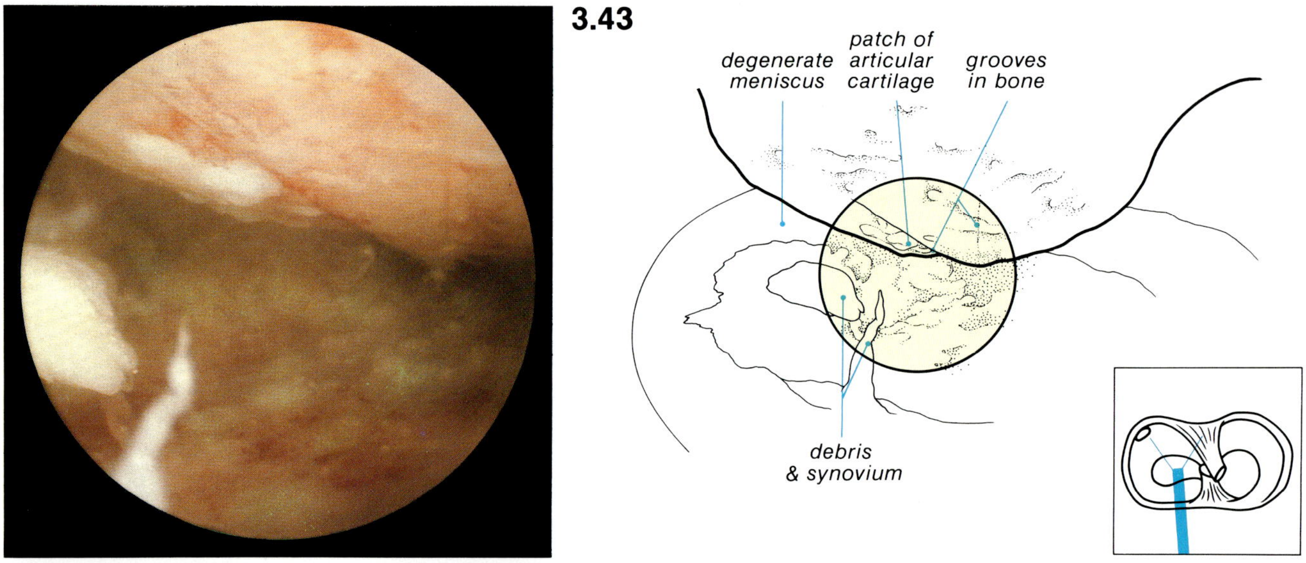

3.44

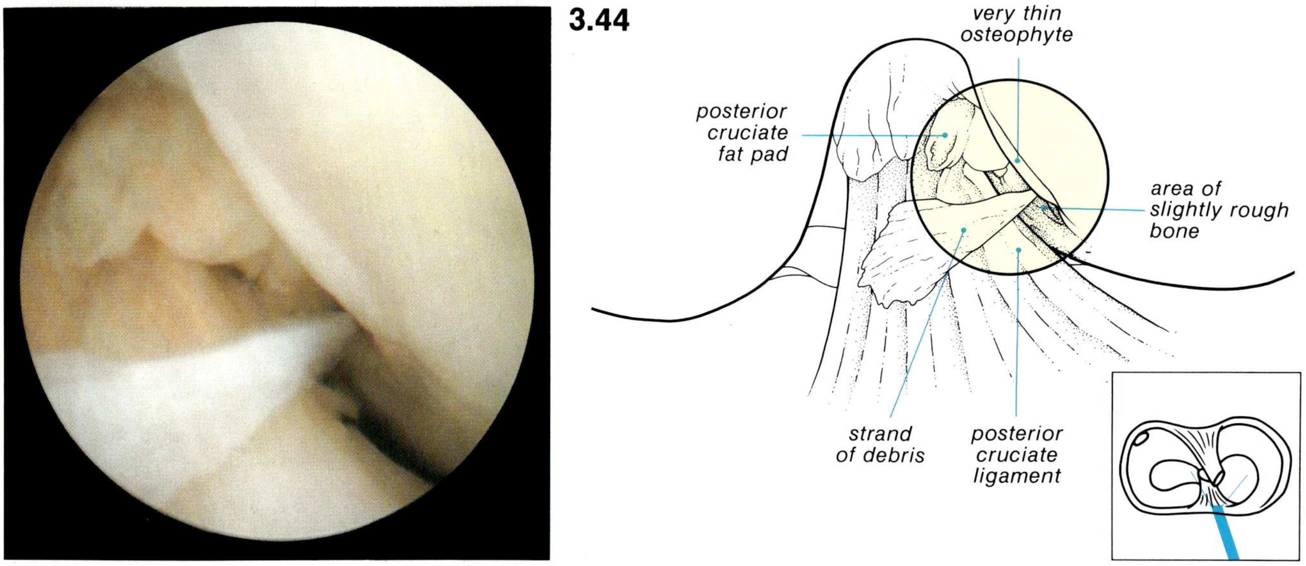

3.45

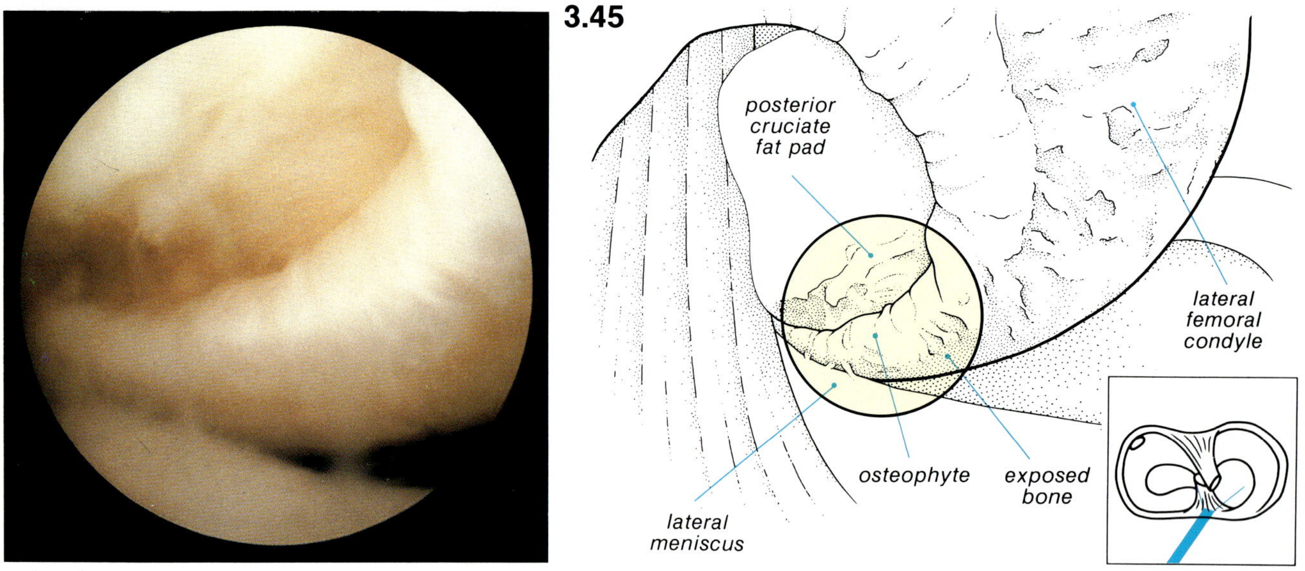

a narrow but sharp osteophyte along the margin of the medial femoral condyle but no sign of degenerative change elsewhere in the knee. Osteophytes are often seen at this site before obvious radiological or arthroscopic evidence of osteoarthritis. They are perhaps the earliest indication of articular cartilage degeneration.

As the osteoarthritis progresses, the osteophytes enlarge. Fig.3.45 shows a ridge of bone on the lateral femoral condyle extending medially to approximately 3mm from the medial edge of the condyle. Behind the osteophyte (between it and the condyle) is a narrow trough which probably serves as a trap for articular cartilage debris. Collection of debris in this situation may be the mechanism for the gradual enlargement of the central osteophyte around the intercondylar notch.

The natural termination of osteoarthritic formation at the intercondylar notch is reached when the osteophyte has completely obliterated the notch (Figs.3.46 & 3.47), leaving only a tiny defect for the infrapatellar fold of synovium. A similar appearance is seen in the hip joint, where the central osteophyte forms around the ligamentum teres.

Another osteophytic appearance is seen in Fig.3.48. The lateral meniscus had been removed many years earlier, and it is interesting to note the similarity in the shape of the osteophyte to that of the missing meniscus. It is not suggested that the body is attempting to

3.46

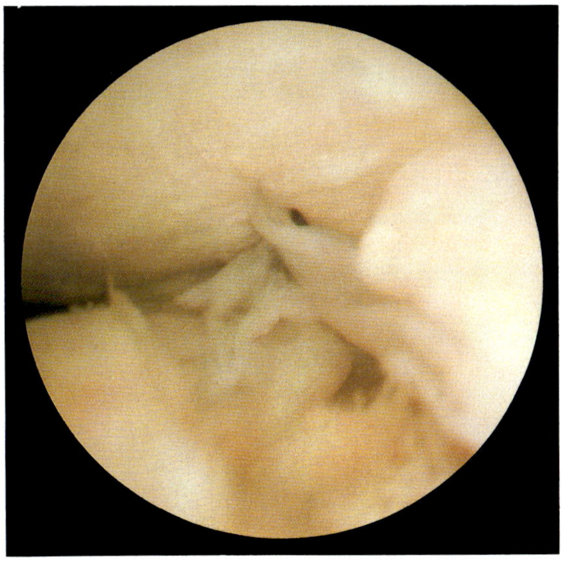

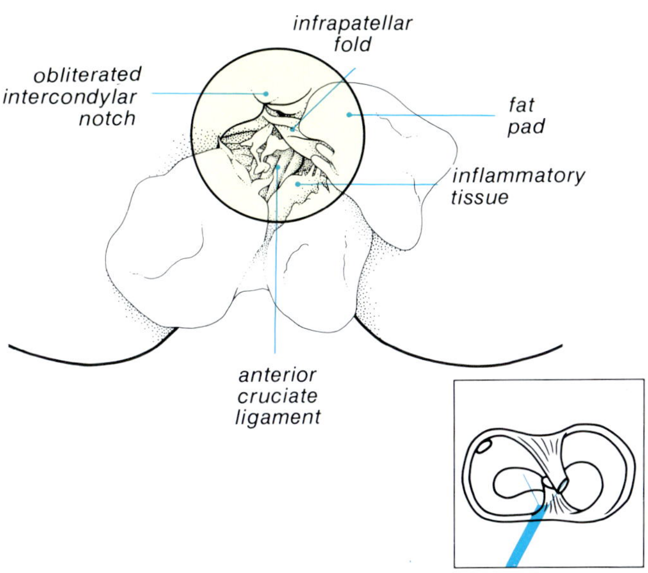

3.47

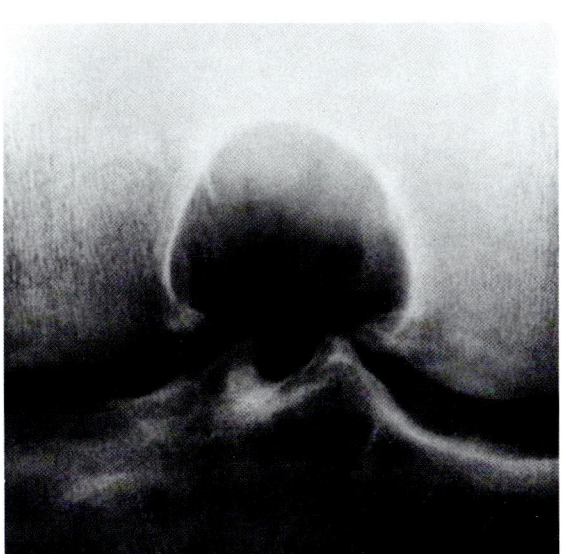

3.48

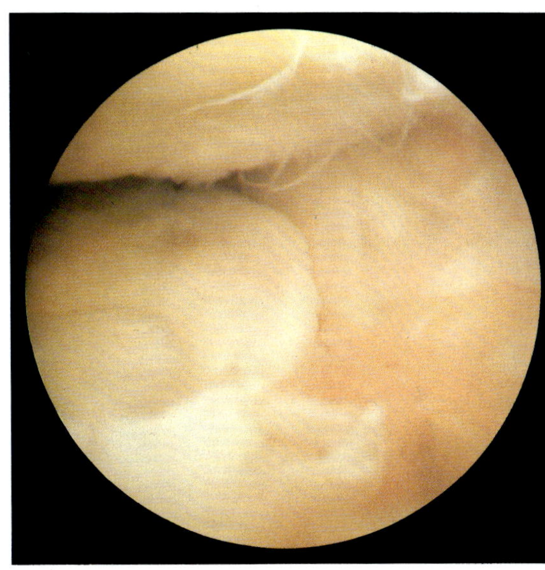

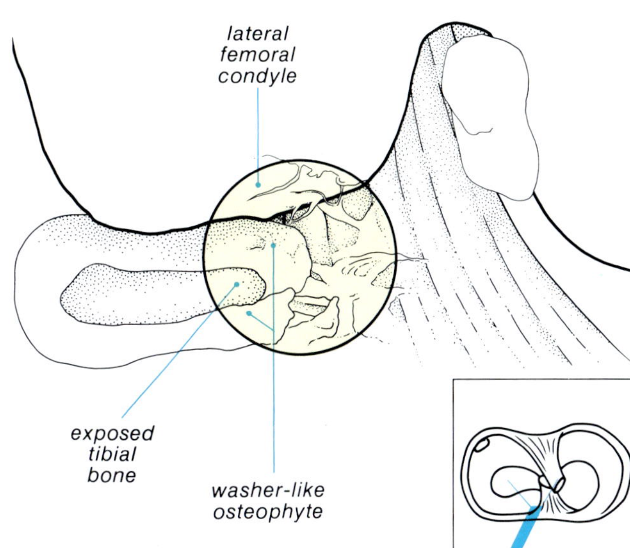

reduplicate the original meniscus; the osteophytic shape is more likely to be due to the natural tendency for wear particles to be swept to the margin of a joint surface.

In the lateral compartment, unlike the medial, osteoarthritis of the tibial plateau usually starts at its centre and not at its margin. The distribution of osteoarthritic change on the tibial plateau is probably nothing more than a reflection of the load distribution

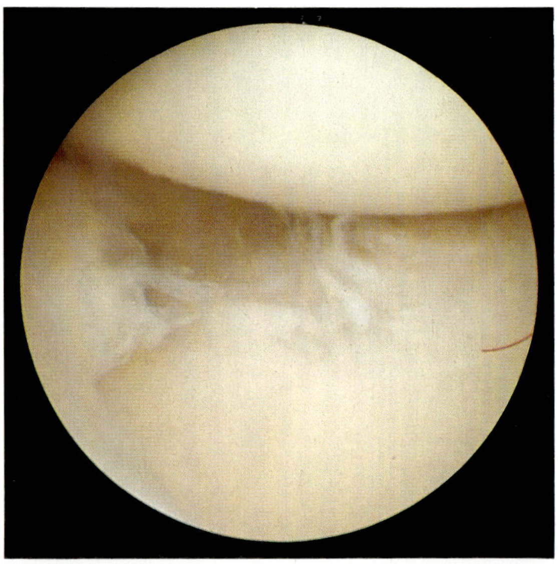

3.49

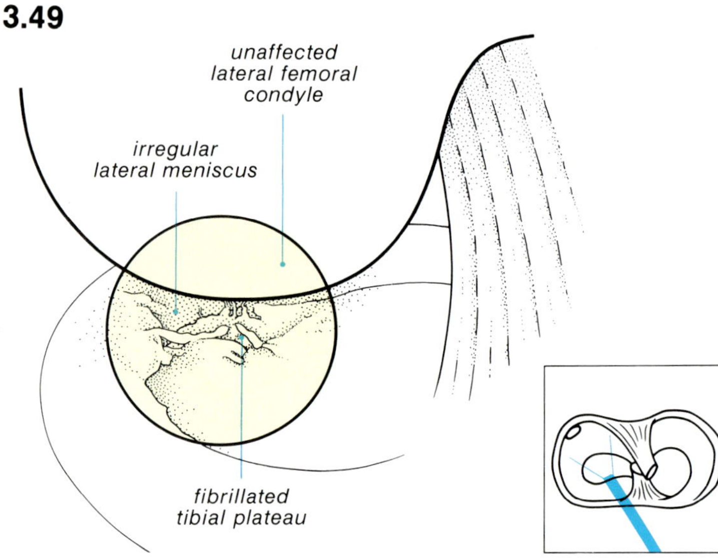

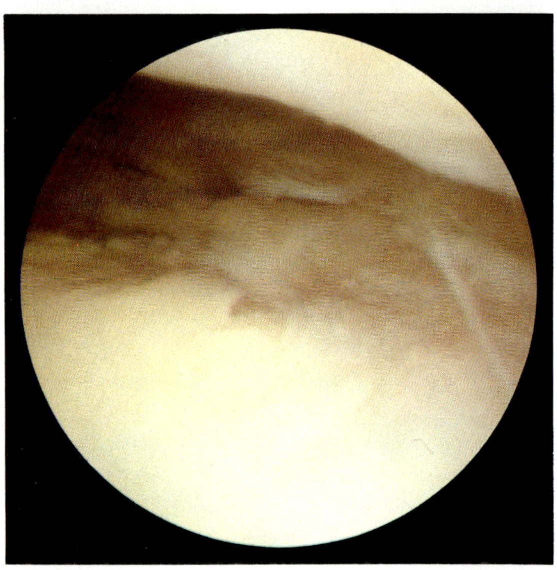

3.50

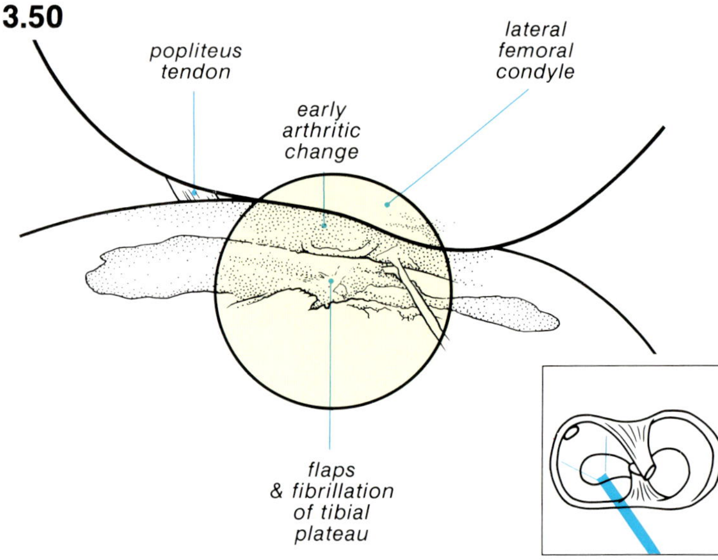

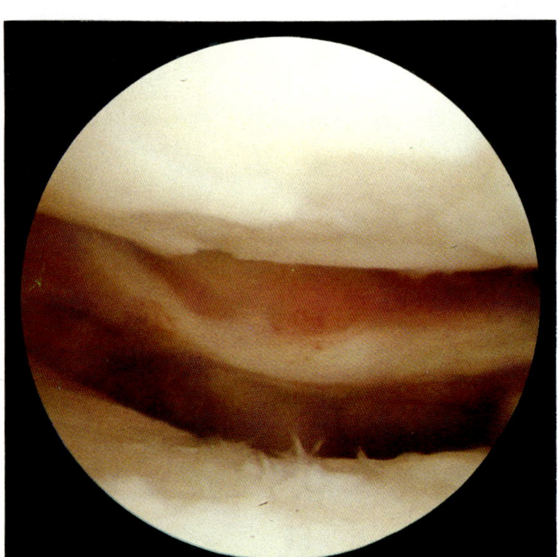

3.51

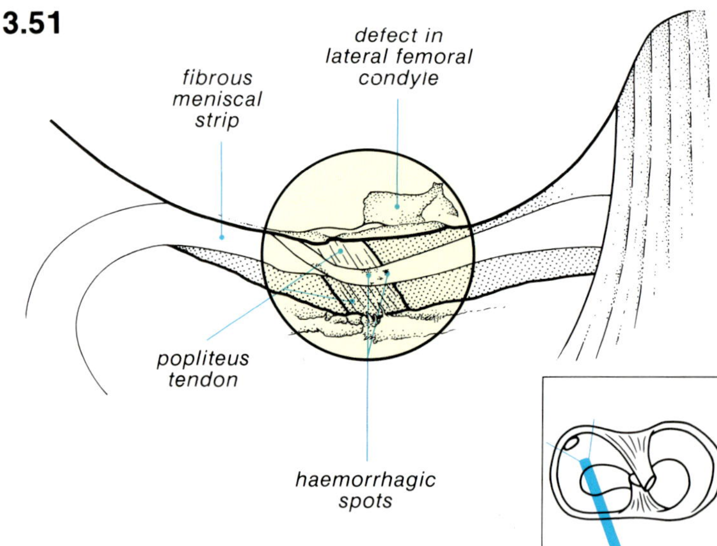

within the joint. Fig.3.49 shows a localized patch of damage to the articular cartilage at the summit of the convexity of the lateral tibial plateau. The femoral condyle is normal and the meniscus is intact, albeit with an irregular margin (Fig.3.49).

Degenerative change on the lateral tibial plateau generally spreads from the summit of the plateau and up towards the intercondylar notch and the meniscal margin. Fig.3.50 shows a more advanced degree of degeneration of the lateral tibial plateau in a patient who had previously undergone a lateral meniscectomy. Subchondral bone is exposed on the dome of the plateau, yet the rest of the compartment is in comparatively good order and the femoral condyle does not show as much degenerative change as the tibia.

Fig.3.51 is of a 22-year-old patient who had undergone a lateral meniscectomy five years previously. Although the tibial plateau is worn and irregular there is no exposed bone; but the irregular femoral condyle has a slightly recessed defect, like a sculpture in bas-relief, which is often seen on the lateral condyle.

In contrast, Fig.3.52 shows gross degenerative change in the lateral compartment ten years after a lateral meniscectomy. Exposed bone is seen over most of the tibial plateau, with a few patches of articular cartilage in the exposed area and around the edge of the plateau which, instead of having a domed centre, is slightly concave. The popliteus tendon can be clearly seen with no meniscal bridge and no sign of meniscal regeneration. Fig.3.53 shows a degenerate lateral meniscus, following a total lateral meniscectomy, with even more advanced changes than those in Fig.3.52. The concavity of the lateral tibial plateau is now more obvious and the exposed bone has spread as far as the popliteus tunnel although the femoral condyle has retained some of its articular cartilage covering.

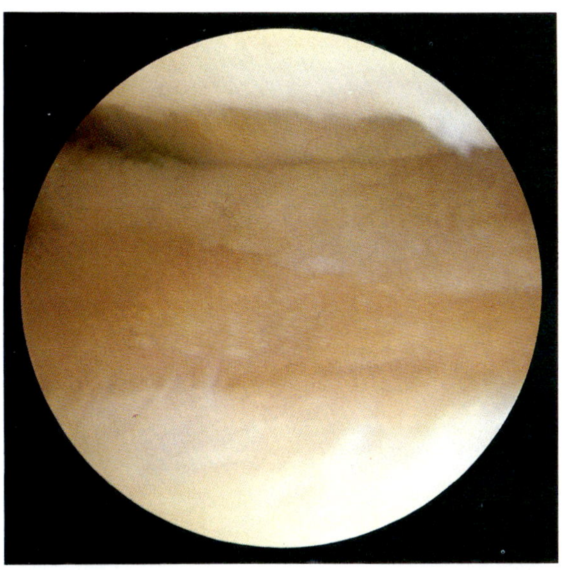

3.52

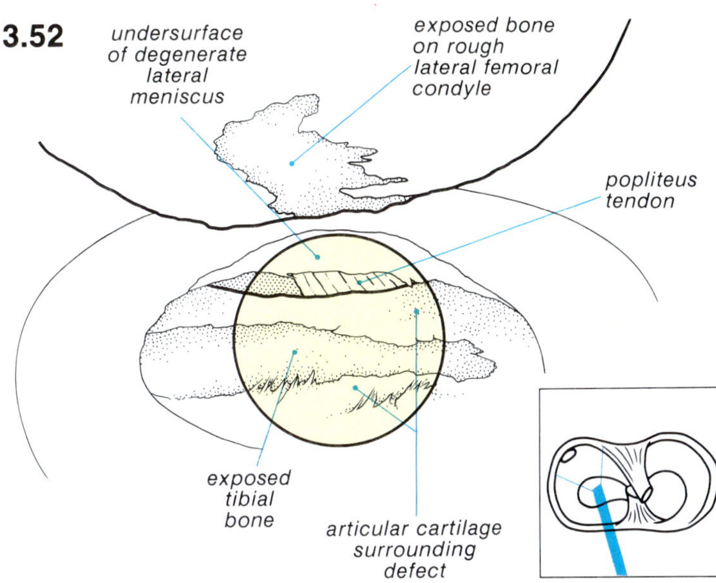

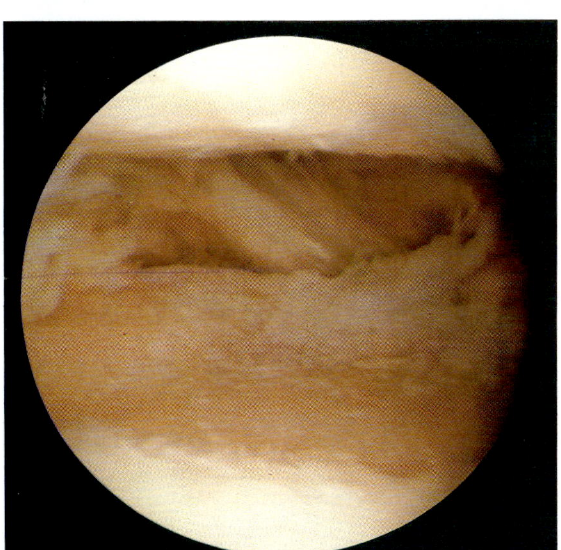

3.53

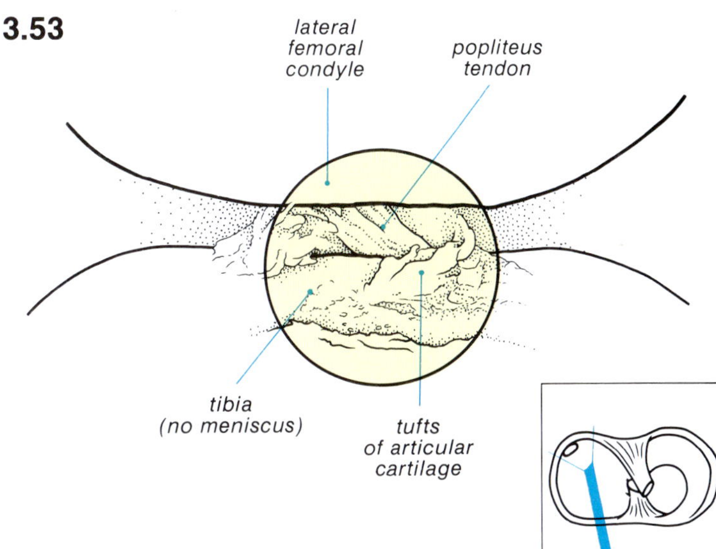

Alkaptonuria

This condition affects articular cartilage and causes damage to the menisci and synovium (see Figs.2.64 & 2.65).

In Fig.3.54 the articular surface of the femoral condyle is irregular. The open face of the lateral meniscus is encrusted with black crystals, but its surface layers and the popliteus tendon appear to have escaped crystal deposition. At a greater magnification (Fig.3.55) the palisade-like arrangement of homogentisic acid crystals is clearly seen, and a single large crystal protrudes downwards from the articular surface like a dagger.

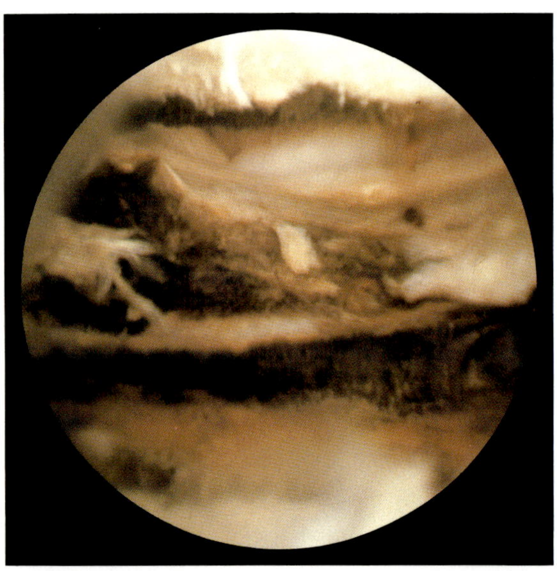

3.54

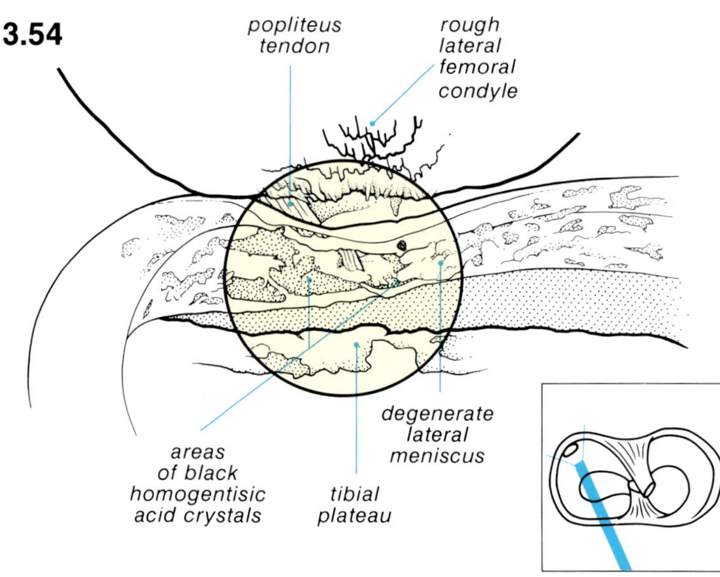

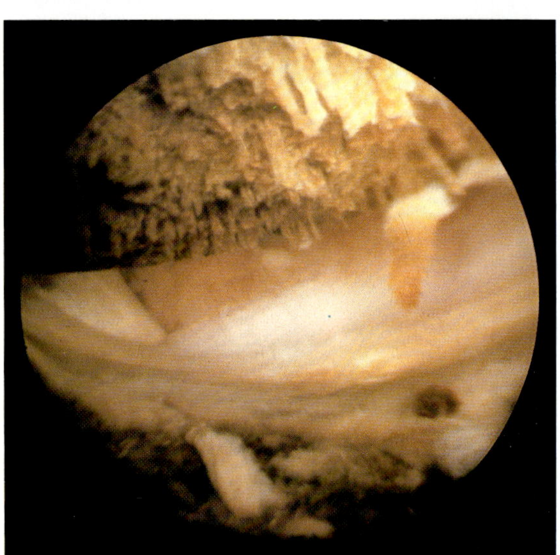

3.55

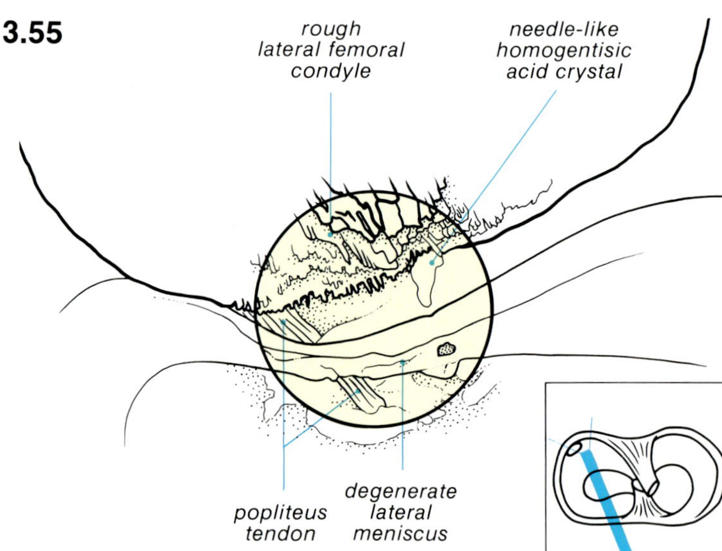

4

The Patellofemoral Joint and Loose Bodies

PATELLOFEMORAL JOINT

Chondromalacia patellae

Articular cartilage degeneration of the patellofemoral joints, and probably elsewhere, may begin as a 'blister lesion', a small pimple of softened articular cartilage on the weight-bearing surface. The lesion is probably the result of degeneration of the deep layers of the articular cartilage associated with breakdown of the long proteoglycan chains. The increase in the number of molecules in the deep layers of the articular surface will increase the osmotic pressure and lead to the imbibition of fluid. Localized swelling results. In Fig.4.1 the lesion is on the articular surface of the patella in a patient suffering from anterior knee pain. The radiographs were normal.

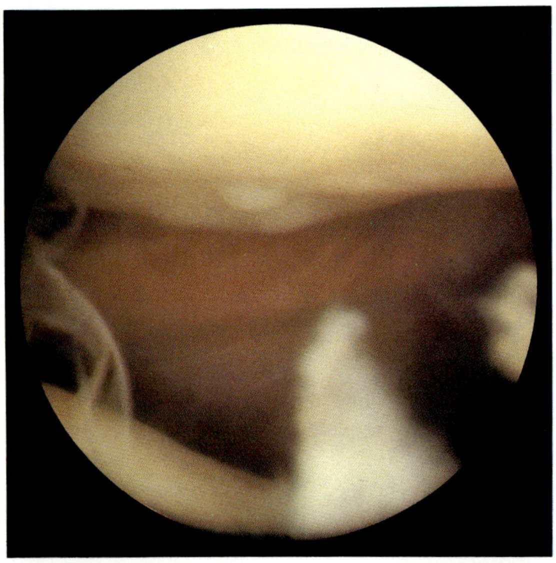

4.1

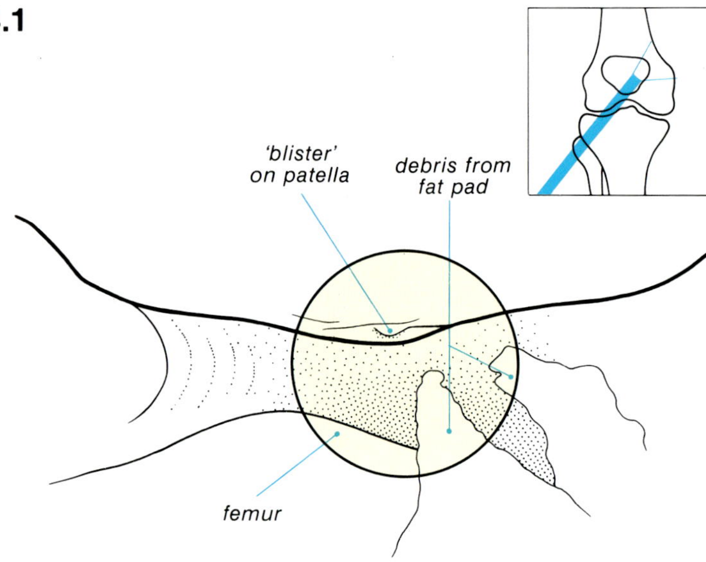

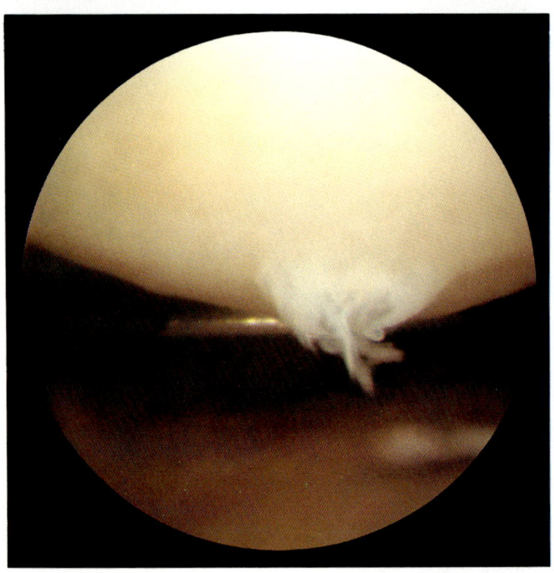

4.2

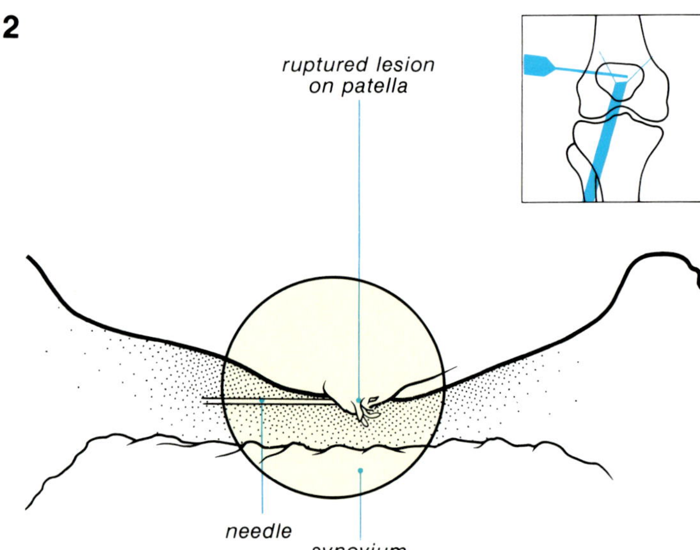

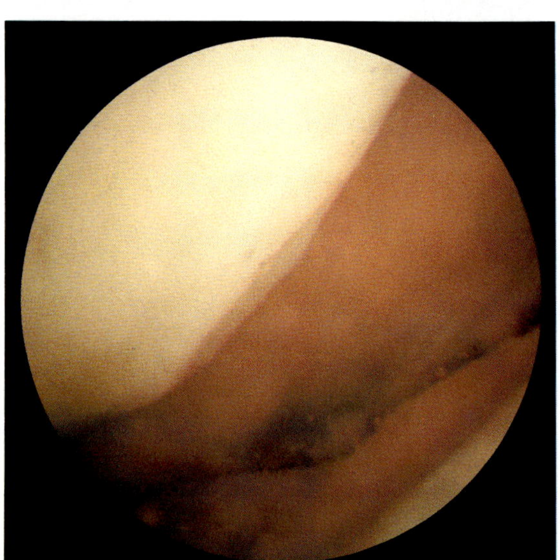

4.3

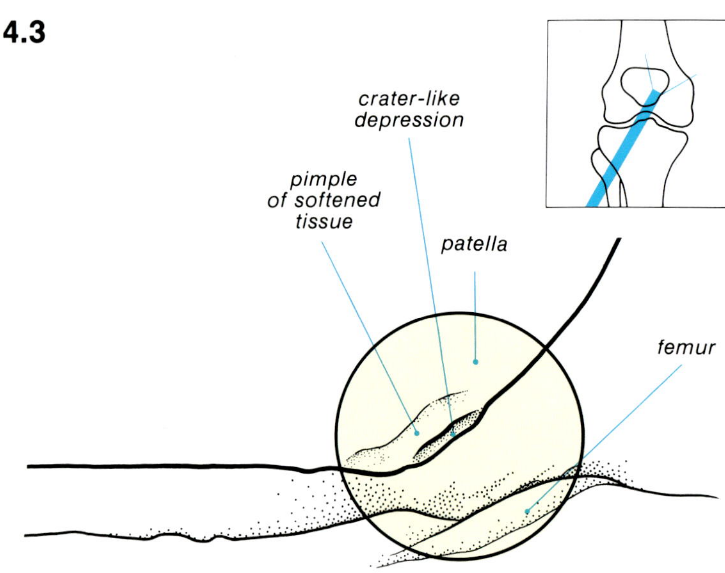

The lesion may progress to involve the superficial layers of articular cartilage and eventually rupture through the articular surface. In Fig.4.2 irregular and ruptured fibres are emerging from a small opening at the apex of the lesion as if a tiny explosion had occurred in the depths of the articular surface. The rest of the patella was normal.

The ruptured blister lesion in Fig.4.2 may proceed in one of several directions. If the centre of the lesion heals while the degenerative process in the deeper layers of the articular surface is still expanding, the result is a doughnut-like blister surrounding a central crater (Fig.4.3). The heaped-up rampart is swollen but visibly intact and its flat centre does not have the appearance of normal shiny articular cartilage.

If the lesion does not heal, the degeneration and fibrillation will spread across the patella (Fig.4.4) and may result in a large area of fine fibrillation, as if the lesion in Fig.4.2 had extended both in depth and area, or may remain as a patch of fibrillation, as in Fig.4.5 where it is localized on the medial facet. The rest of the patella was normal with no suggestion of degenerative change on the intact articular surface.

4.4

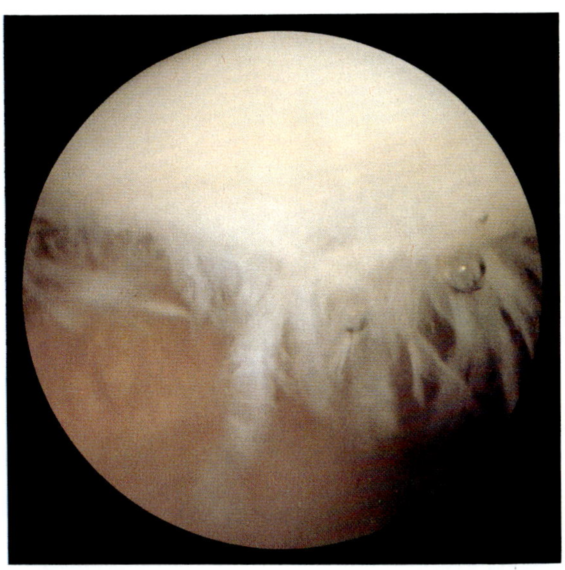

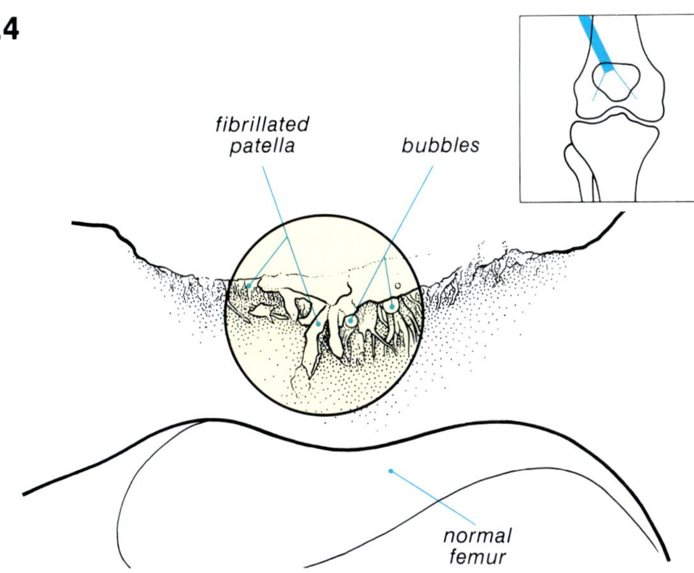

4.5

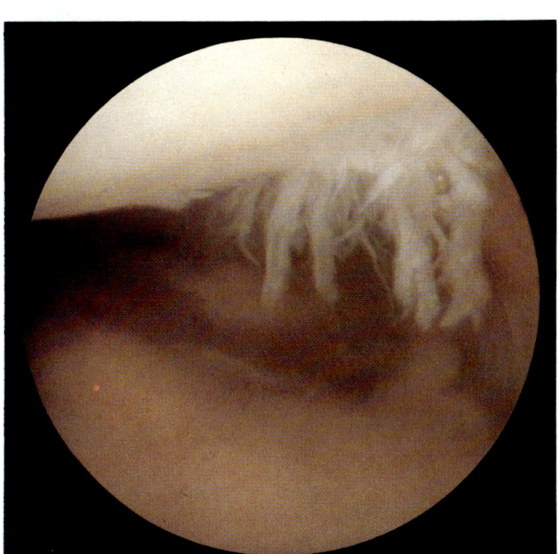

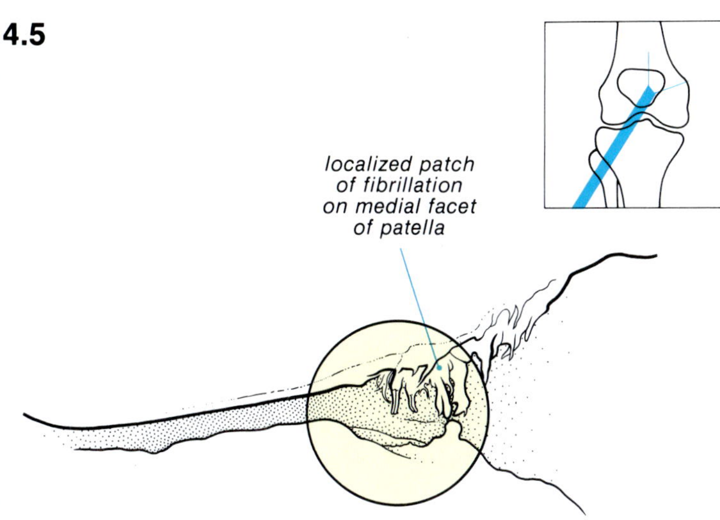

In Fig.4.6, seen from the lateral suprapatellar approach, the lower pole of the patella is affected by relatively coarse fibrillation. The fat pad lying between the femur and patella is both hyperaemic and inflamed. The articular surface was soft and podgy when examined with a probing hook, as if the blister process was occurring over a larger than normal area.

Another appearance of degenerative change on the patella is seen when the articular surface becomes softened and coarsely fibrillated but instead of the process extending into the surrounding areas, the lesion appears to be demarcated by a groove (Fig.4.7). No explanation for this 'moat' around the lesion is offered. This appearance contrasts with the umbilicated appearance in Fig.4.3.

To distinguish between idiopathic and traumatic chondromalacia is perhaps a little artificial in that the degenerative process is probably similar and differs only in the manner of its onset. Fig.4.8 shows the knee of a patient who had fallen from her bicycle, striking the front of the patella against the road. After a good early recovery, the patient was aware of crepitus and pain under the patella. The appearance of the articular cartilage under the magnification of the arthroscope was similar to that of crabmeat and localized at the point of impact. The softened material was removed and the patient made a good recovery, with relief of the crepitus, but the pain never disappeared completely. The prognosis for this patellofemoral joint must be poor.

Fig.4.9 shows the knee of a patient who, eighteen months earlier, had been involved in a motorcycle accident in which he sustained a fracture of the femur and a ruptured posterior cruciate ligament. The fracture was treated by internal fixation which, however, proceeded to non-union and was later grafted. When bony union was finally achieved and the patient was able to bear weight through his leg, he reported coarse crepitus in the patellofemoral joint although movement of the joint was painless. At arthroscopy the patella, seen from the lateral suprapatellar approach (Fig.4.9), had no

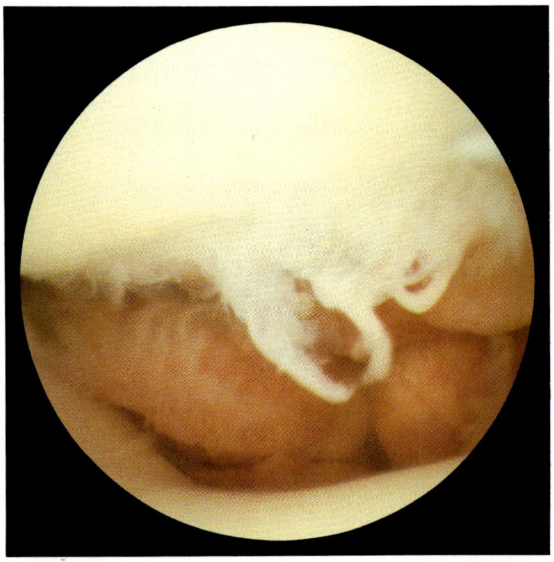

4.6

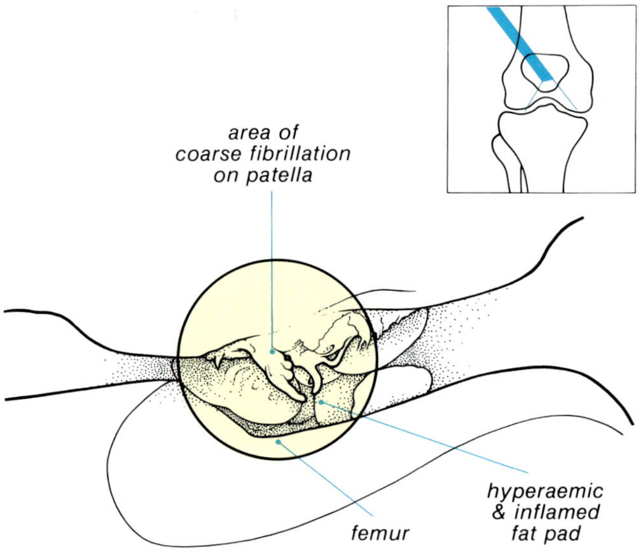

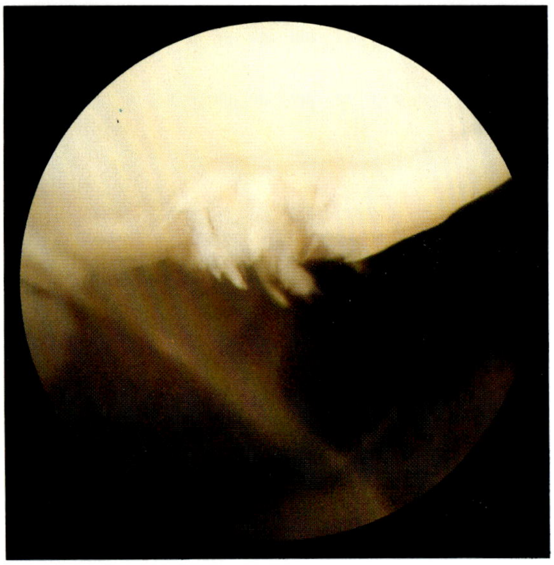

4.7

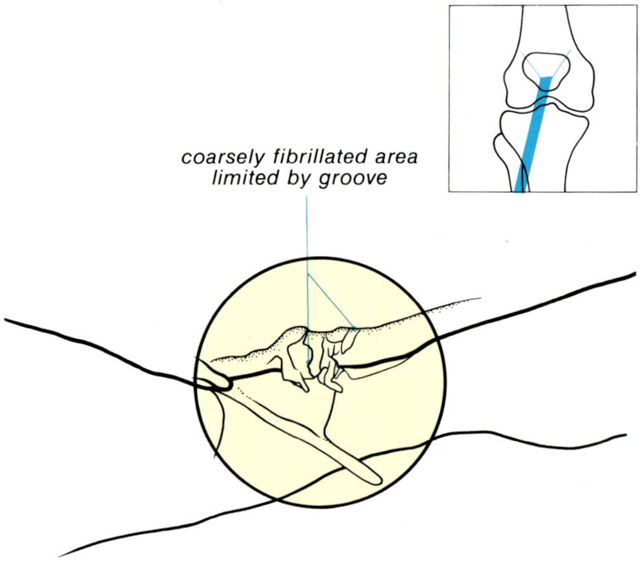

normal articular surface, the entire area being replaced by degenerate fibrillation. The femoral surface was normal, perhaps because the patellofemoral joint had not been loaded normally. The fibrillated area was shaved arthroscopically and the crepitus greatly improved.

The effects of trauma on the patellofemoral joint are not consistent. Fig.4.10 is of the patellofemoral joint of a 33-year-old woman who sustained a comminuted fracture of the patella at the age of eighteen. The fracture was treated by internal fixation, producing a good but not perfect reduction. Later, the patient experienced anterior knee pain and slight crepitus. At arthroscopy (Fig.4.10) patches of normal articular surface are

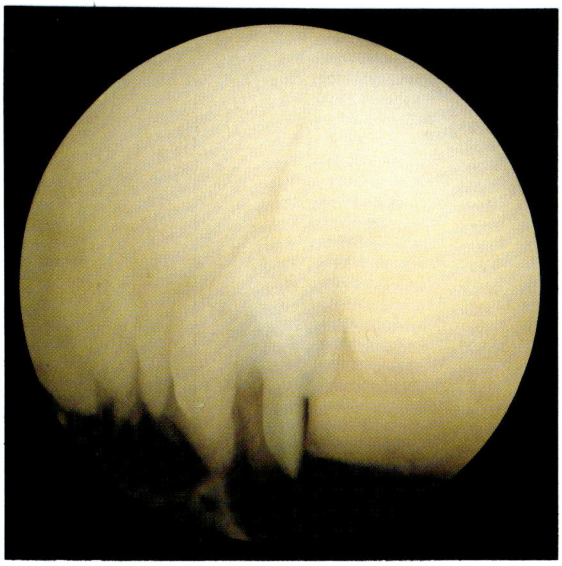

4.8

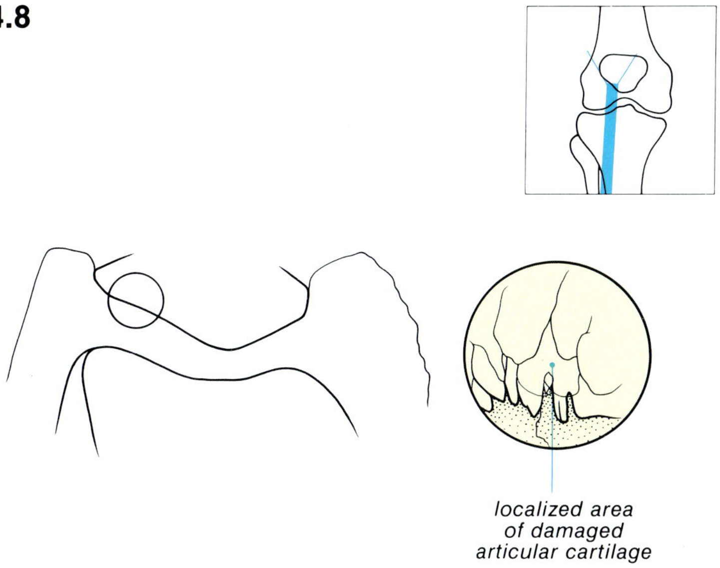

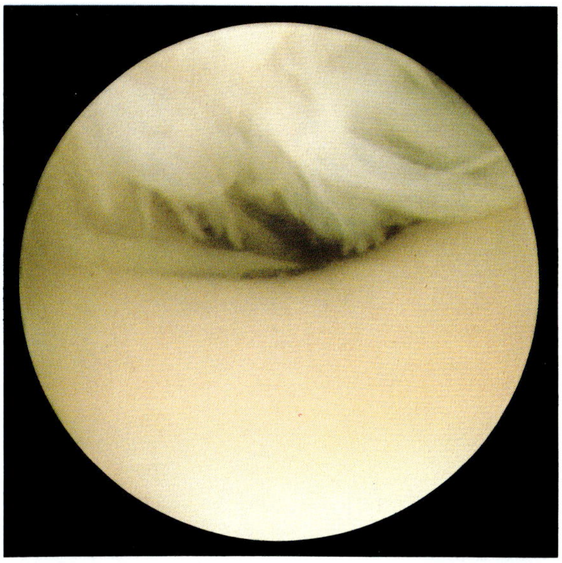

4.9

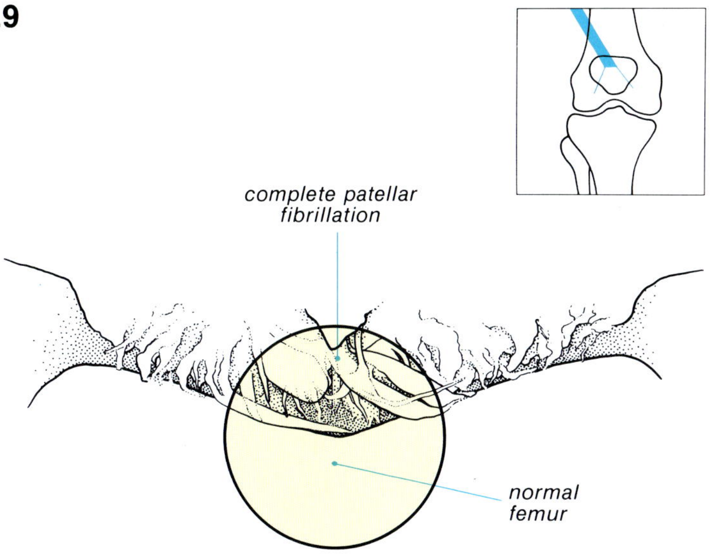

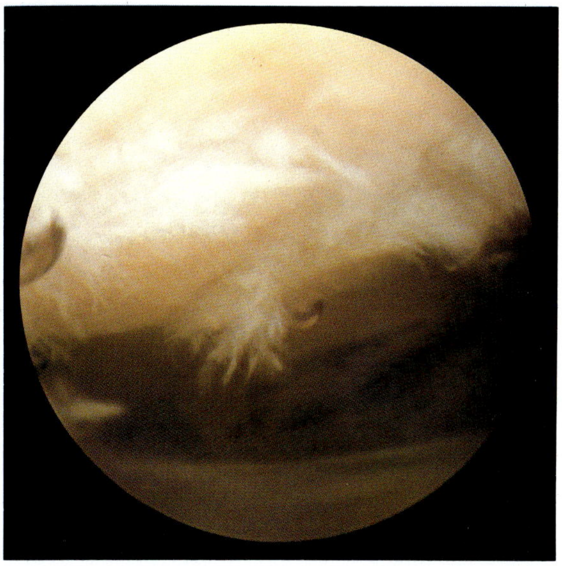

4.10

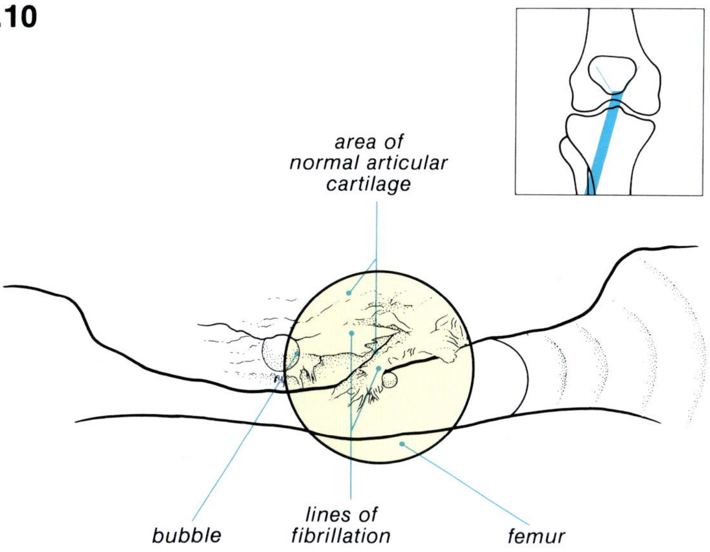

separated by lines of fibrillation curiously like grass growing between the cracks of crazy-paving. It is interesting that the fibrillation has been confined to the fracture lines and has not spread across the intervening space. The radiological appearances are shown in Figs.4.11 and 4.12.

Osteoarthritis

Gross osteoarthritis of the patellofemoral joint, as in other joints, is usually associated with irregularity of the joint surfaces and osteophyte formation around the margins. Eburnation and grooving of the joints occur much later than in the tibiofemoral joint, perhaps

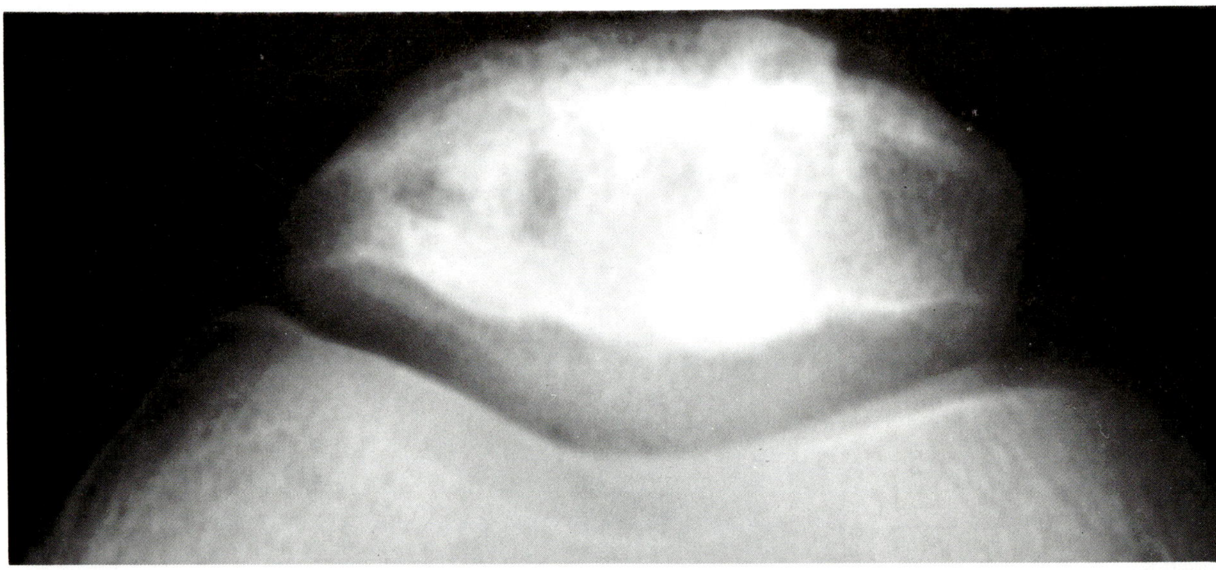

4.11

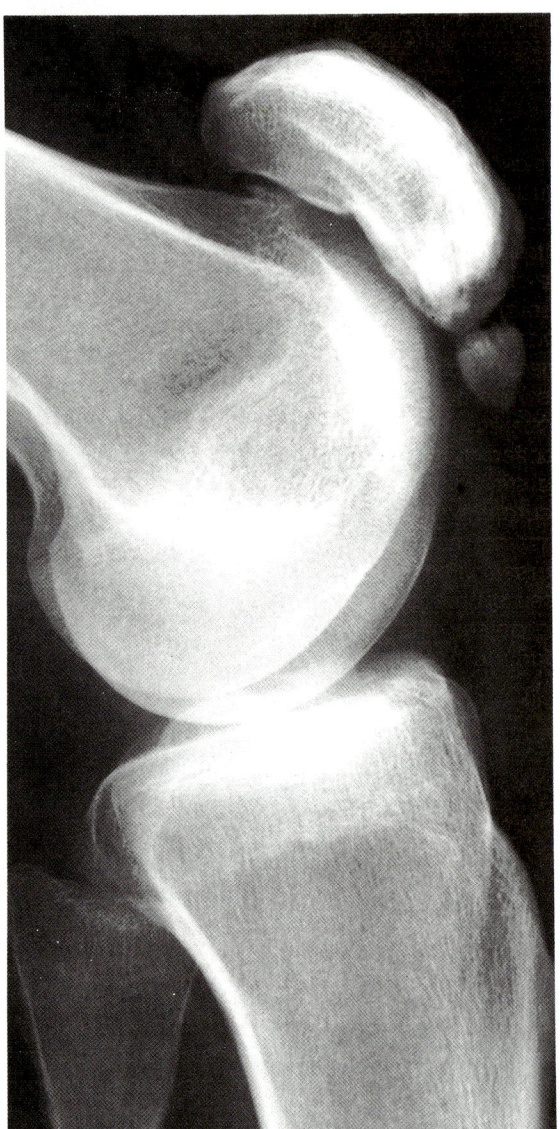

4.12

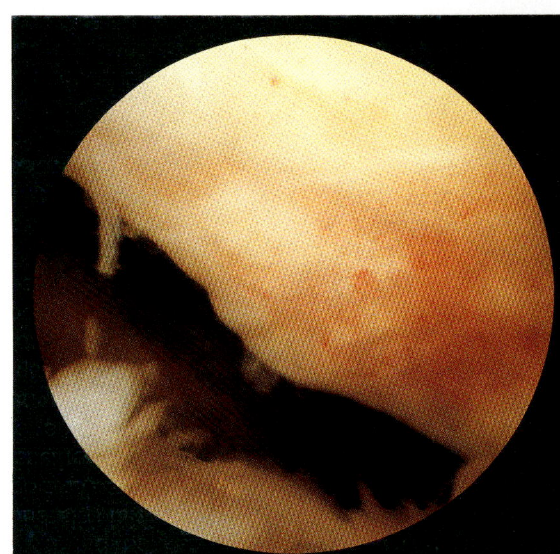

4.13

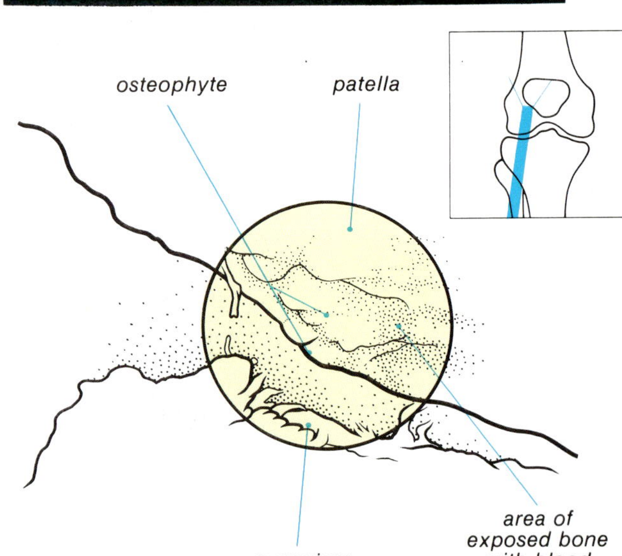

because the patient can limit the load imposed upon the patellofemoral joint by restricting flexion at the knee. In Fig.4.13 there is a small osteophyte at the margin of the patella, adjacent to an area of uneven exposed subchondral bone. The bone is blood-stained. The patient reported 'catching' and 'locking' in the knee. The irregularity and the osteophyte were probably responsible for these symptoms, which are not uncommon in patients with patellofemoral osteoarthritis.

In Fig.4.14 a large ridged osteophyte lies transversely at the upper margin of the patella, coming into contact with an equally large osteophyte at the upper end of the articular surface of the femur during flexion of the knee and producing a true mechanical locking of the knee that was eased only by manipulation of the patella itself. True mechanical locking of the patella in full extension is a rare phenomenon. Arthroscopic removal of the osteophyte abolished the catching mechanism but the patellofemoral arthritis continued to be troublesome.

Fig.4.15 shows a particularly large irregular osteophyte at the superomedial corner of the patella. The patient's knee flexion was grossly restricted by osteoarthritis of the tibiofemoral joints so that the osteophyte was not involved in mechanical action of the joint. It may be that the absence of movement over the femur enabled the osteophyte to grow to such an unusual size.

Osteophytic formation around the patellar margin is a leading feature of osteoarthritis of the patellofemoral joint. Eburnation of subchondral bone also occurs,

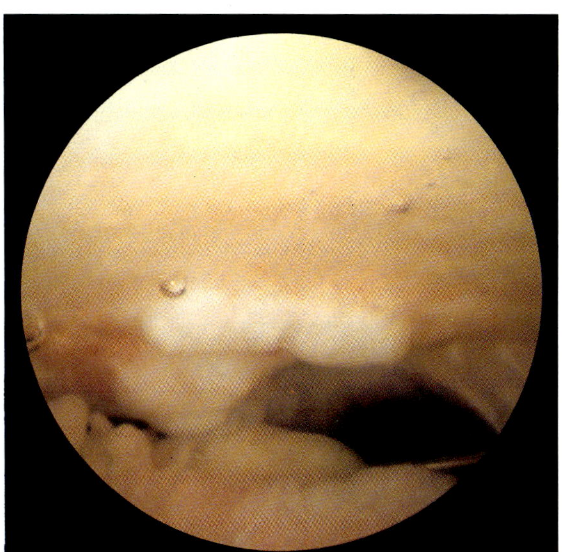

4.14

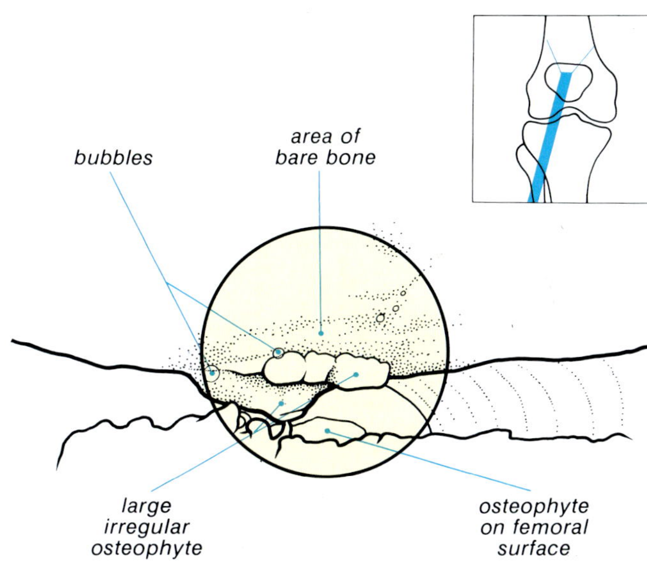

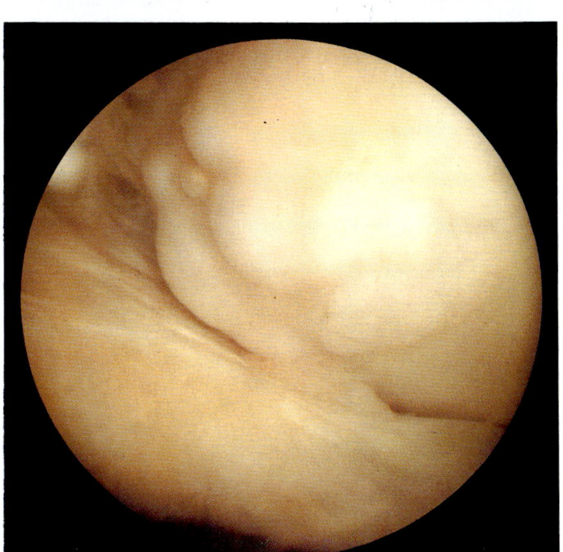

4.15

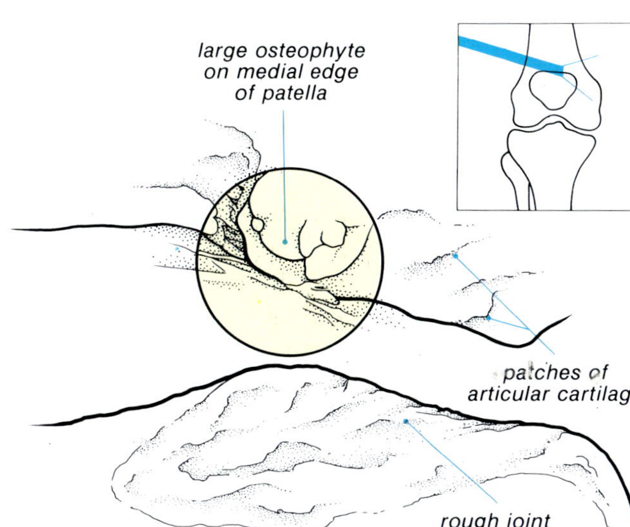

though less often, and in Fig.4.16 is seen on the lateral facet of the patella. No osteophytes were found and there was no history of injury. When degenerative change is localized to the lateral facet it is often the natural end result of the excessive lateral pressure syndrome, in which abnormal tracking of the patella places excessive load on the lateral facet, resulting in its early and rapid degeneration.

Osteochondritis dissecans

Osteochondritis dissecans of the patella, despite its obvious radiological abnormality, is not usually accompanied by a corresponding arthroscopic lesion. Fig.4.17 shows the articular surface of a patella from the lateral suprapatellar approach in a boy with vague anterior knee pain. The radiograph (Fig.4.18) shows a definite patellar defect, yet careful arthroscopic search of

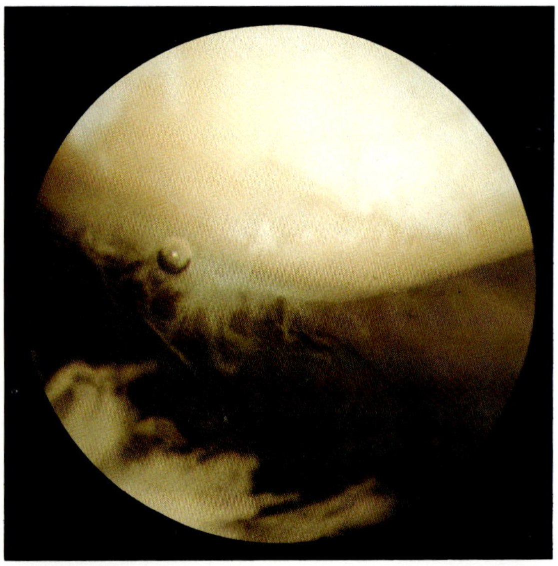

4.16

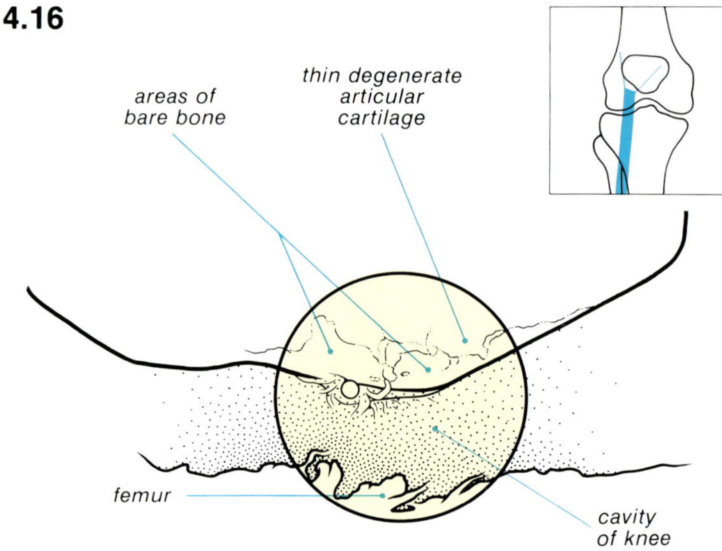

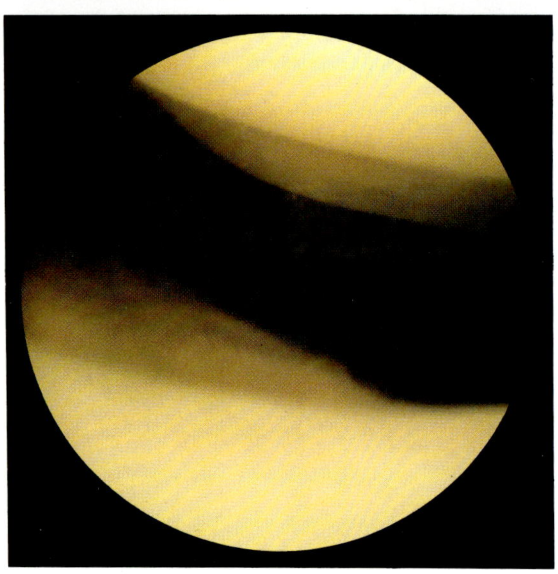

4.17

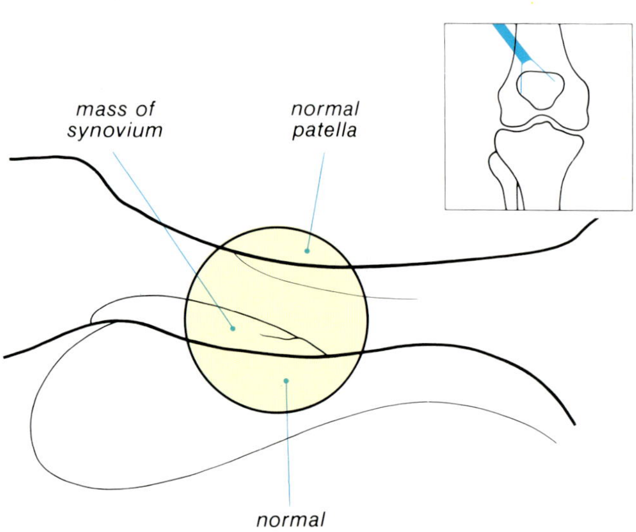

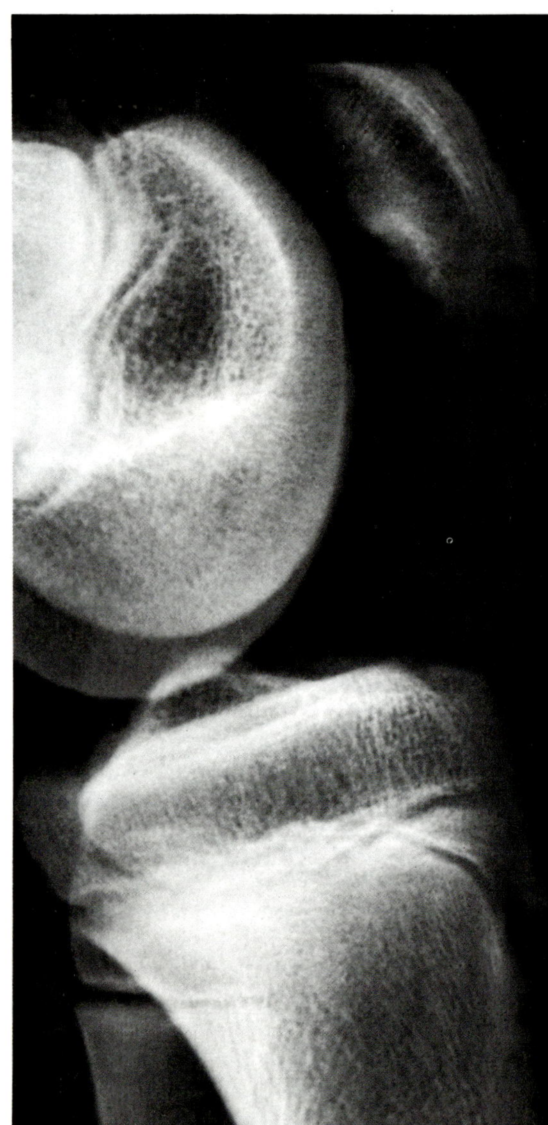

4.18

the patellar surface revealed no cracks, splits, fissures, softening or other abnormality, suggesting that the changes of osteochondritis dissecans of the patella are deep and do not involve the articular surface.

Chondral separation

Localized lesions of articular cartilage, including osteochondritis dissecans, chondral separation and osteochondral fractures, can occur in the patellofemoral joint just as they do in the tibiofemoral joint. Fig.4.19 shows a large chondral flap on the lateral margin of the patella. The patient was a semi-professional tennis player who felt sudden pain and a click in the knee while serving. He was able to continue the game but later developed an effusion of fluid in the knee. He was aware of a click when the knee was bent and pain on the lateral side of the joint. A torn lateral meniscus was suspected. The lesion proved to be a partial separation of the articular surface, involving just over half its thickness, and was comparable to the chondral flap of the femoral condyle seen in Fig.3.22. The catching and clicking were relieved by removal of the flap.

A slightly different lesion is seen in Fig.4.20 which shows the superior pole of the patella from the lateral suprapatellar approach. There is a well-defined area of chondral separation which bears a great resemblance to the femoral lesion seen in Fig.3.21. The patient's symptoms were pain and clicking on flexion of the knee but there was no history of injury. The loose articular cartilage around the margin of the lesion was removed and the symptoms were relieved.

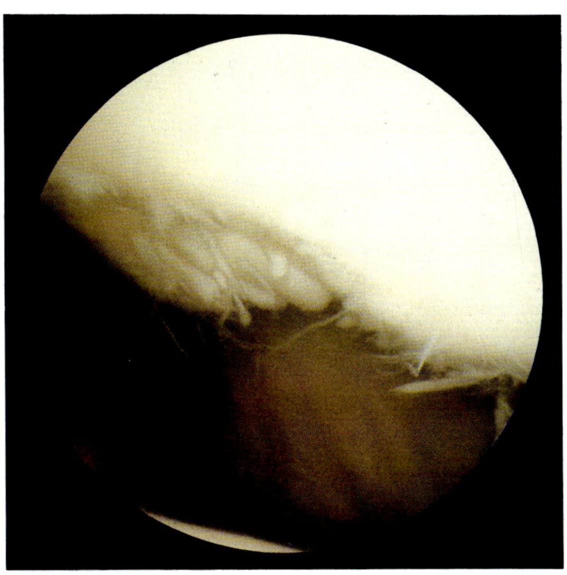

4.19

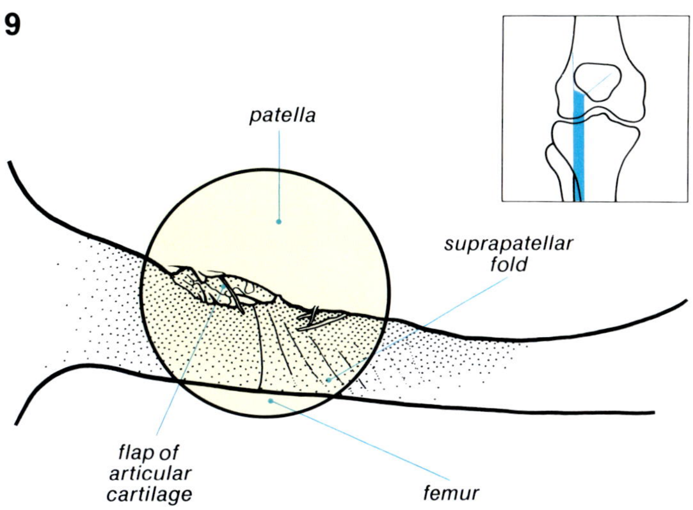

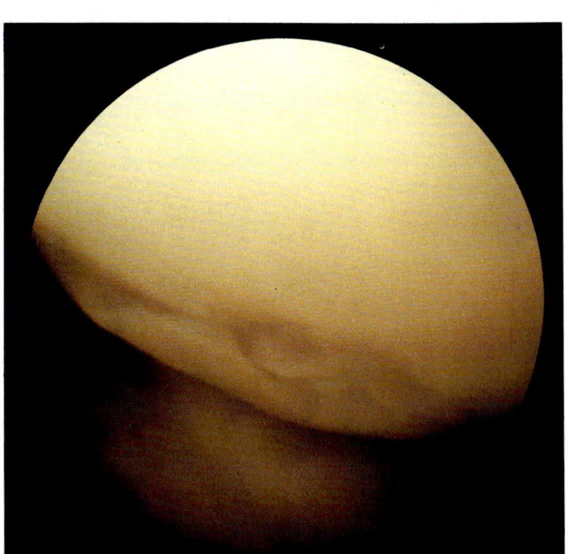

4.20

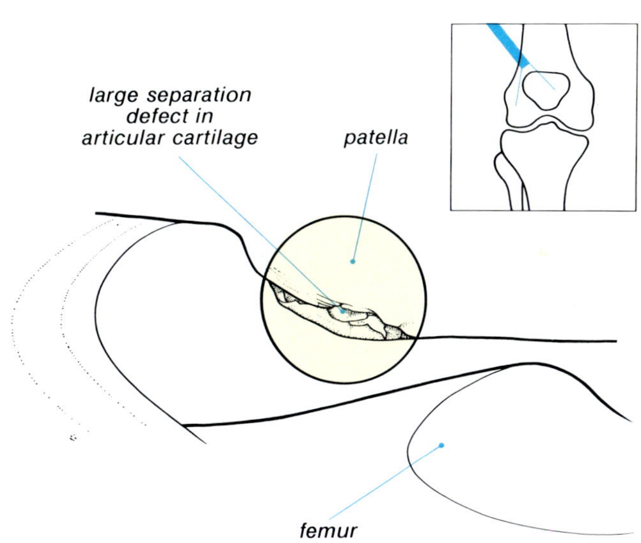

Osteochondral fractures

Figs.4.21, 4.22 and 4.23 show the patellofemoral joint of a patient who sustained an osteochondral fracture of the patella during karate practice. The patient had flicked his right foot smartly through the air in the direction of his opponent's head but failed to make contact. During this manoeuvre there was sudden and severe pain around the anterior aspect of the knee and he could not continue. A haemarthrosis developed and the patient was later referred to hospital with a loose body in the knee. The largest fragment to arise from this lesion had separated and was removed as a loose body, but part of the articular surface remained attached by one edge to the blood-stained bed of the lesion (Fig.4.21). Fig.4.22 shows the same lesion, the blood-stained base and the clean articular cartilage margin.

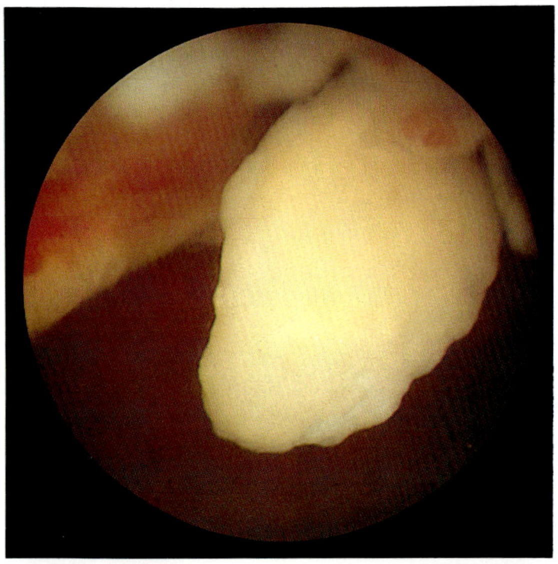

4.21

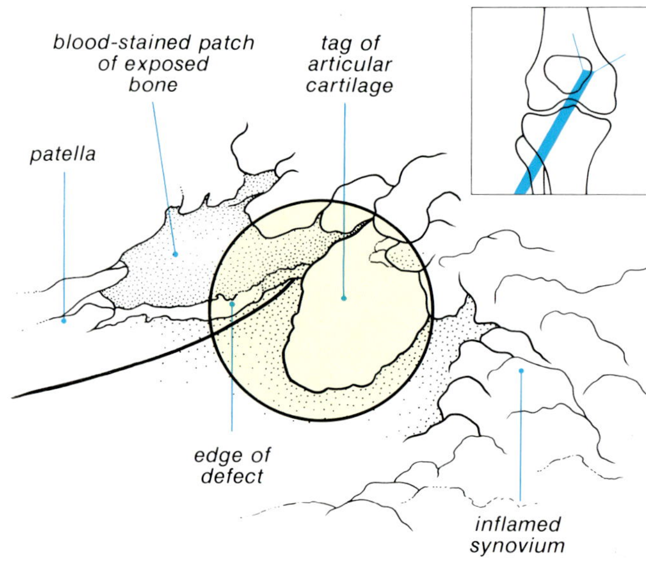

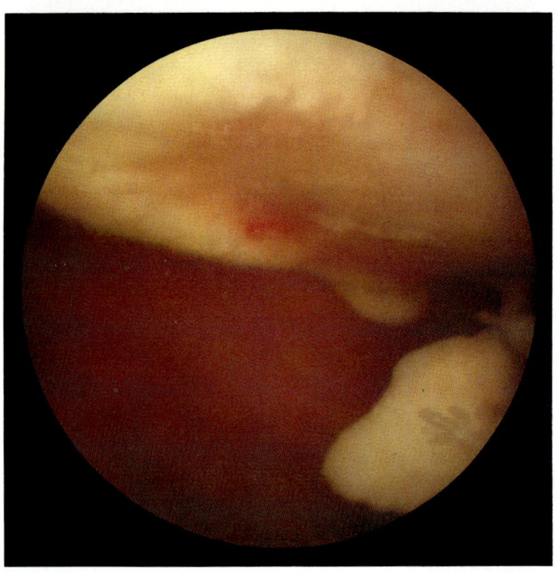

4.22

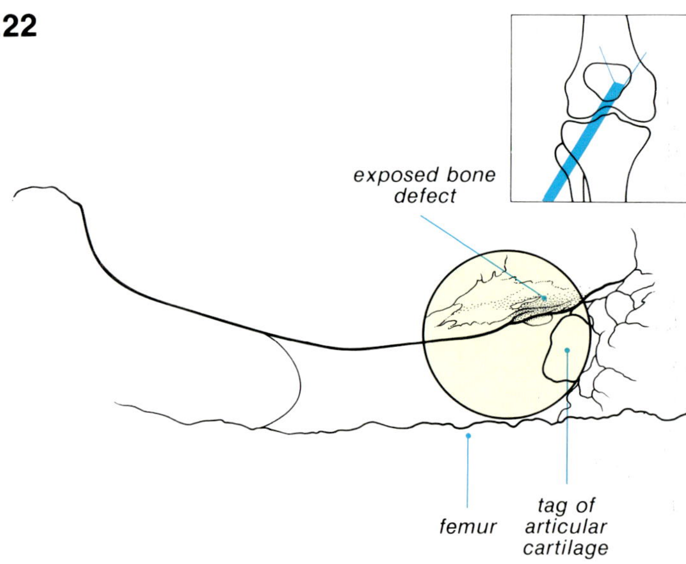

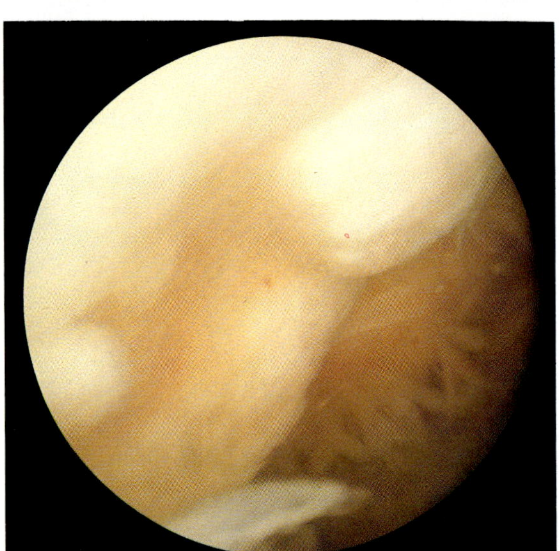

4.23

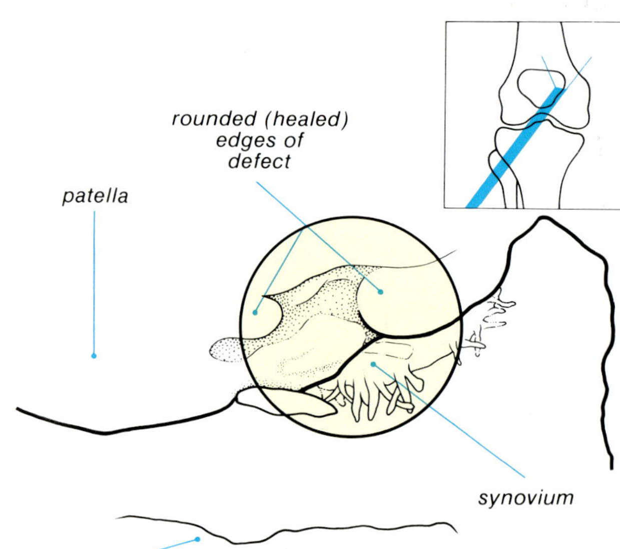

Four years later the patient sustained another injury to the same knee, giving the opportunity to inspect the site of the original lesion. At the time of this second examination (Fig.4.23) the base of the original defect had filled in substantially and the edges had become well rounded. There was no sign of degenerative change at any point on the patella, which suggests that excision of defective articular cartilage and the underlying cortical bone is a rational treatment for articular cartilage lesions.

Fig.4.24 shows an un-united fracture of the patella, a condition that must be distinguished from a bipartite patella. The patient recalled clearly the moment of fracture. The fracture line did not involve the superolateral corner of the patella but extended vertically down its medial half and could be clearly seen at arthroscopy. The fracture line could be opened with an irrigation needle. In patients with a bipartite patella, the patellar surface is usually normal although a little fibrillation is sometimes seen on the undersurface of the fragment.

Patellar dislocation

The relative positions of the patella and femur are variable, but in full extension there is usually an overhang of between one-quarter and one-third of the patellar width. In patients with dislocation of the patella the overhang may be more than one-half of the patellar width. In those with permanent dislocation of the patella, almost the entire width may be seen extending beyond the lateral edge of the femoral condyle. Fig.4.25 shows a normal patella overhang of just over one-third of its diameter in a sixteen-year-old female athlete who was troubled by persistent pain on the lateral side of the patella and was considered to have the excessive lateral pressure syndrome. After conservative management had failed, a lateral release of the extensor mechanism was performed arthroscopically which relieved the symptoms. Although there are no specific arthroscopic features in Fig.4.25 to distinguish this knee from others, some factor may one day be found which will

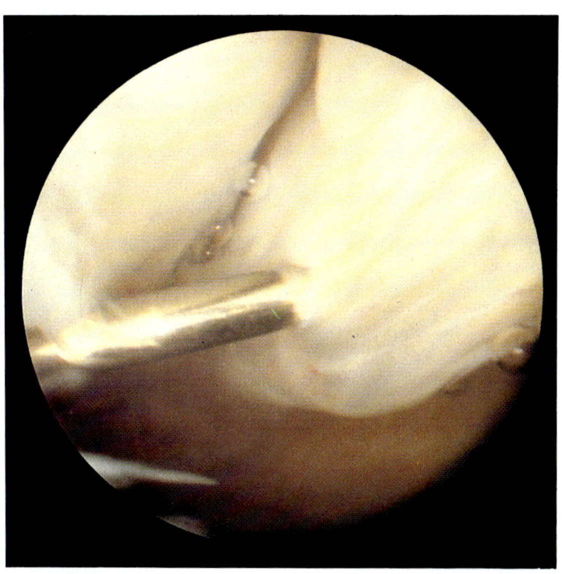

4.24

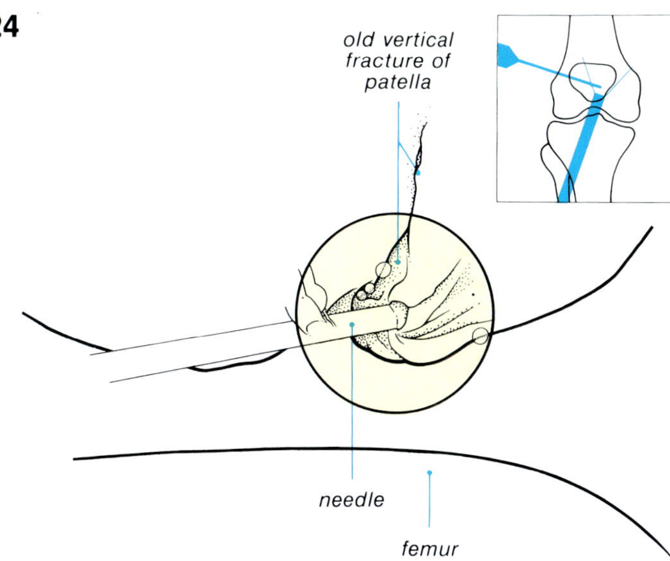

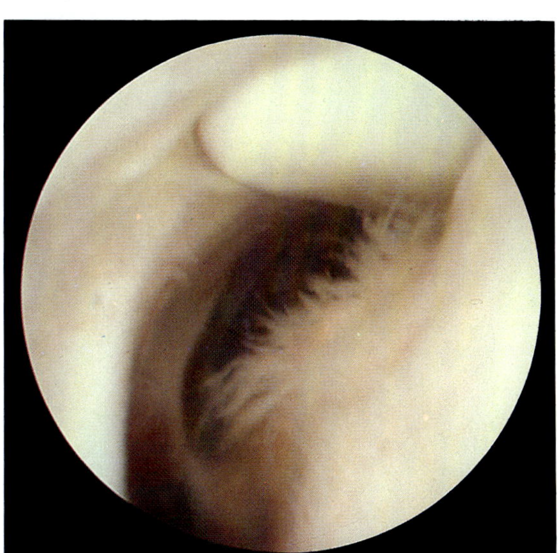

4.25

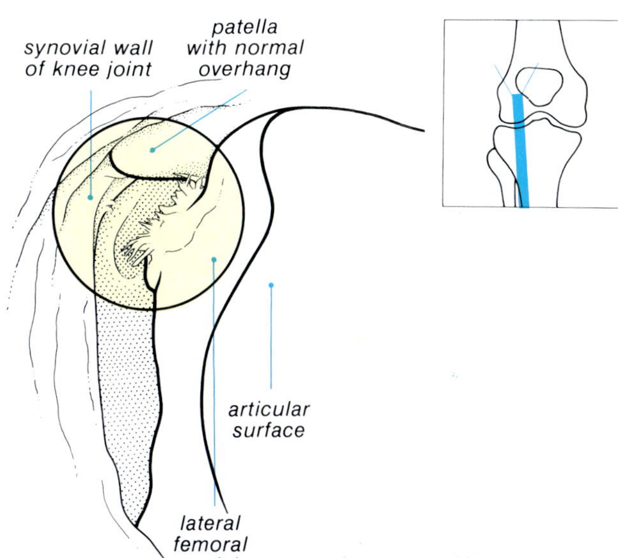

discriminate between those patients who will gain from a lateral release and those who will not. Until such a criterion is determined, the clinician must rely on radiographs, the distribution of patellar tenderness and the characteristics of the patient's symptoms as a basis for deciding whether operation is necessary.

Acute dislocation of the patella is associated with subsynovial haemorrhage on the medial side of the knee (Fig.4.26). The patient was a keen sportsman, with a previous history of one episode of dislocation, who had twisted his knee sharply while playing football. The patient had generalized ligamentous laxity. When

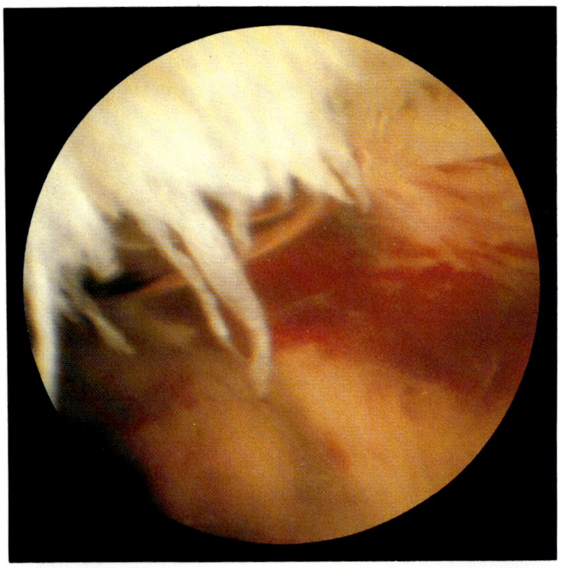

4.26

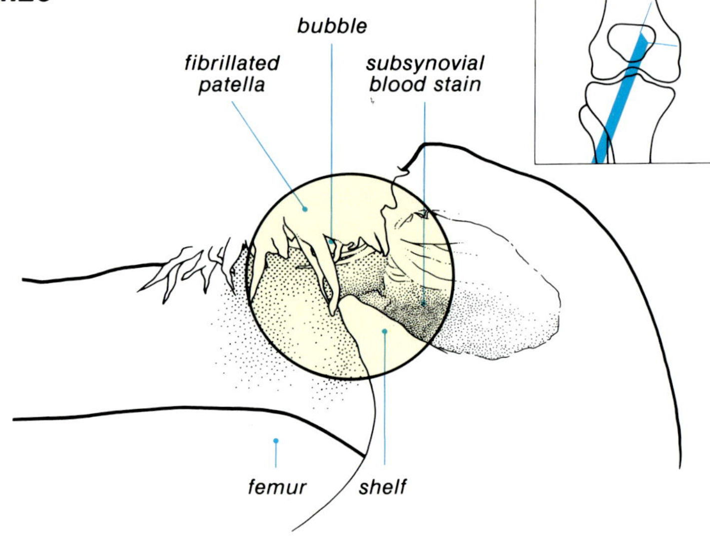

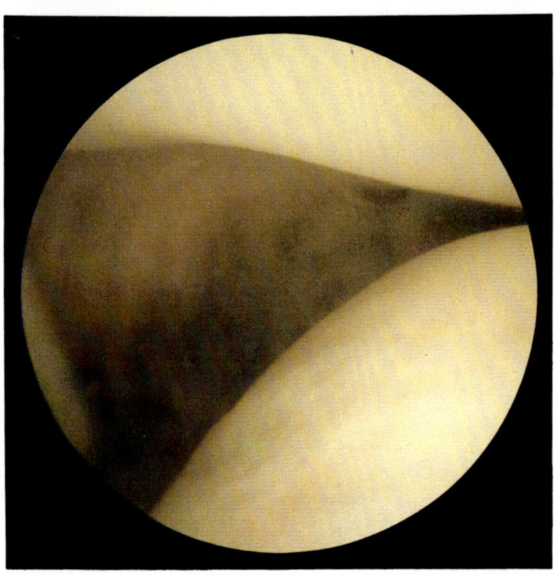

4.27

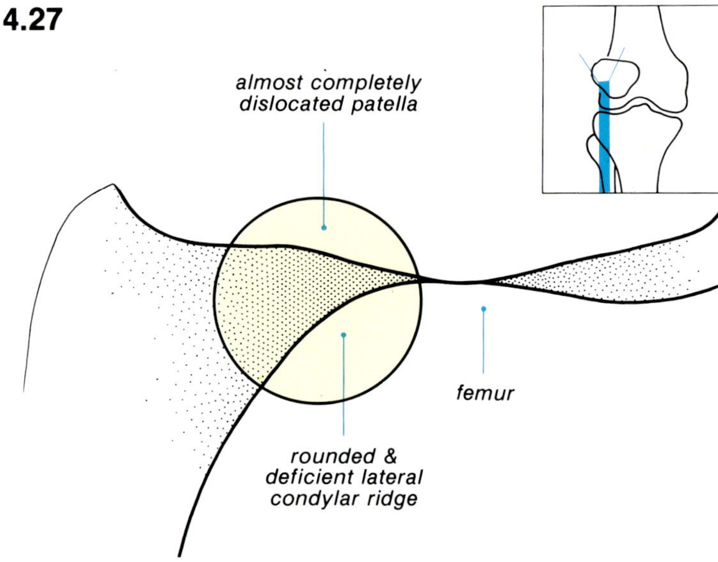

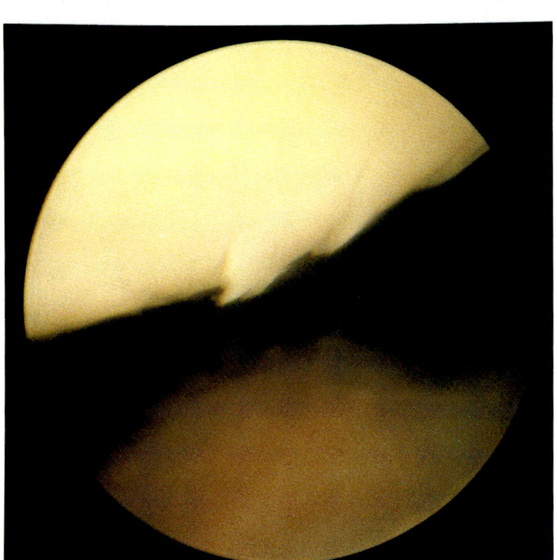

4.28

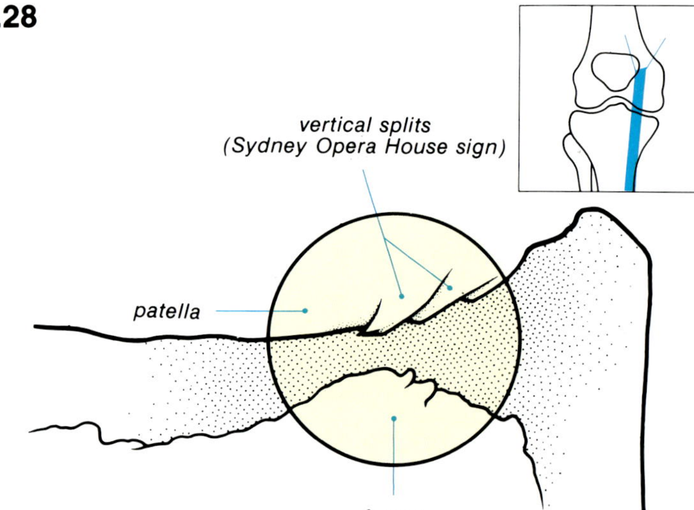

examined three days after the injury, it was possible to push the patella almost completely beyond the lateral edge of the femoral condyle, a manoeuvre accompanied by pain and discomfort. The medial parapatellar structures seen in Fig.4.26 were tender and at arthroscopy the synovial staining was noted.

Fig.4.27 shows the patella of a boy with habitual dislocation associated with nail-patella syndrome. The patella was found lying in a position of almost complete dislocation in full extension. The lateral edge of the femoral condyle was poorly developed but the patellar surface was normal. Fig.4.27 was taken with the knee in full extension; the patella dislocated completely at thirty degrees of flexion.

Repeated subluxation of the patella can produce changes in the articular cartilage. In Fig.4.28, vertical splits are seen on the medial patellar facet. The appearance, with its alternately vertical and sloping surfaces, is a common finding in adolescents with recurrent subluxation or dislocation of the patella and has not been observed in any other condition. Because its appearance of interlocking curved shells resembles the Sydney Opera House, it is sometimes known as the Sydney Opera House sign.

LOOSE BODIES

Loose bodies within the knee vary greatly in size and the smallest may cause no symptoms whatsoever. Fig.4.29 shows an accumulation of fragments of articular cartilage debris in the posteromedial compartment. There was a chondral separation on the femoral condyle and the mechanical action of the joint acting on the fragment from the defect had probably produced the fine granular debris. The patient's symptoms arose from the chondral separation and not from the tiny fragments of articular cartilage, which were too small to cause any noticeable mechanical symptoms. Despite this, the irritation from the fragments must have contributed to the inflammation of the synovium.

Articular cartilage fragments arising from defects in the joint surface may be milled into particulate debris or they may adhere to the synovium, forming cartilaginous plaques. Such a plaque of articular cartilage (Fig.4.30), lying in the posteromedial compartment adherent to the synovium overlying the posterior capsule, has thickened synovial ridges radiating from the fragment. The ridges are perhaps an indication of the inflammatory response of the synovium to the articular cartilage.

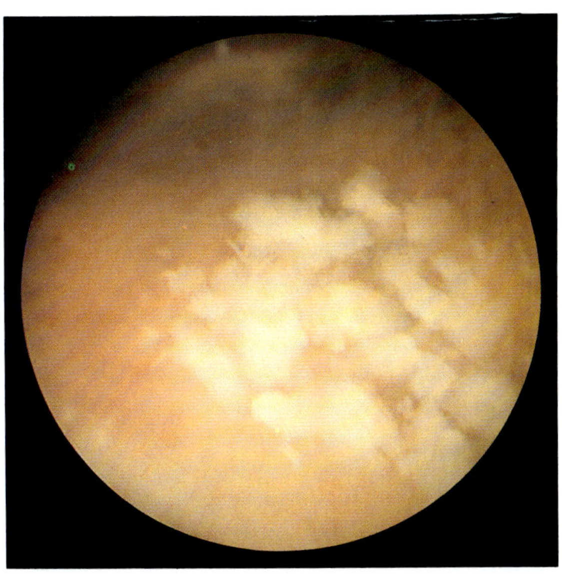

4.29

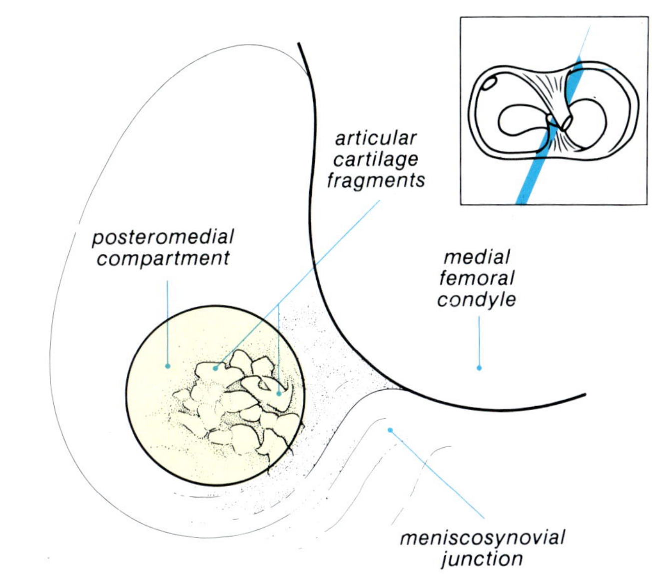

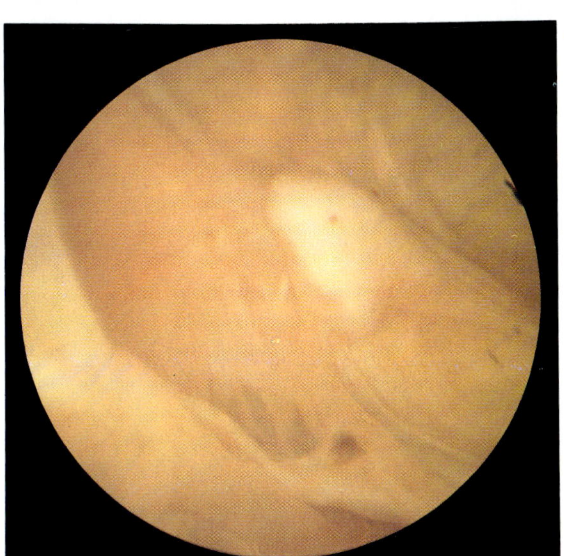

4.30

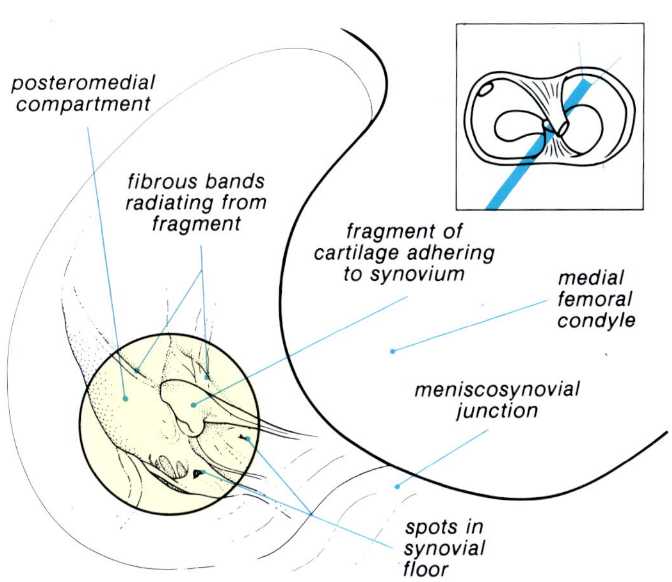

In Fig.4.31 an articular cartilage fragment lying in the lateral gutter of the knee was firmly adherent to the synovium at the lowermost point of the gutter. Its upper portion, however, remained free and could be manipulated with a percutaneous needle (Fig.4.31). The fragment was not visible radiologically.

A more substantial loose body is seen in Fig.4.32 lying adjacent to the medial meniscus. Although appearing to be quite large in the illustration, its vertical height was only 3mm at its greatest. However, it was not visible radiologically because it consisted of soft tissue only.

The conventional idea of a loose body is a calcified ovoid object surrounded by a smooth cartilaginous covering and is mobile and elusive. Calcified loose bodies are denser than saline or gas and therefore sink to the bottom of the knee and tend to accumulate in the posteromedial or posterolateral compartment where they may be concealed from the surgeon.

Fig. 4.33 shows a typical loose body in the posteromedial compartment of the knee, behind the femoral condyle and above the posterior third of the medial meniscus. The loose body was removed from the posteromedial approach. Small loose bodies can reach the posteromedial compartment through the intercondylar notch, but larger loose bodies, such as in Fig.4.33, are more likely to reach the compartment by slipping down the medial gutter into the posteromedial corner of the knee when the knee is flexed.

Although the posterolateral compartment is smaller than the posteromedial and therefore less likely to accumulate loose bodies, they can still find their way into the posterolateral compartment. Fig.4.34 shows a fragment of bone with a cartilaginous covering lying between the posterior horn of the lateral meniscus and the lateral femoral condyle. Its flat and rounded contour made it particularly elusive, but it was successfully

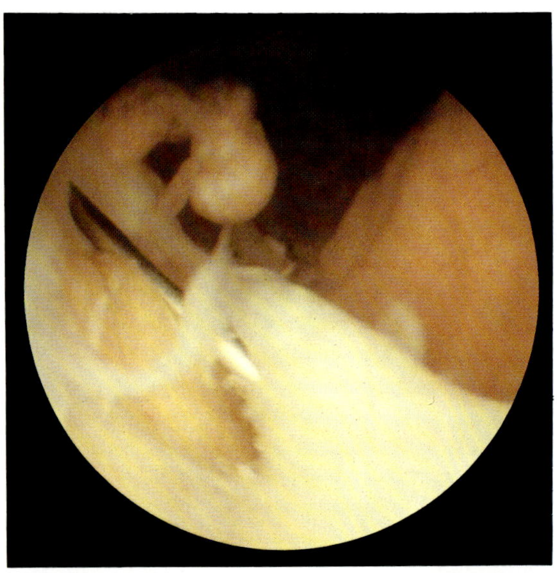

4.31

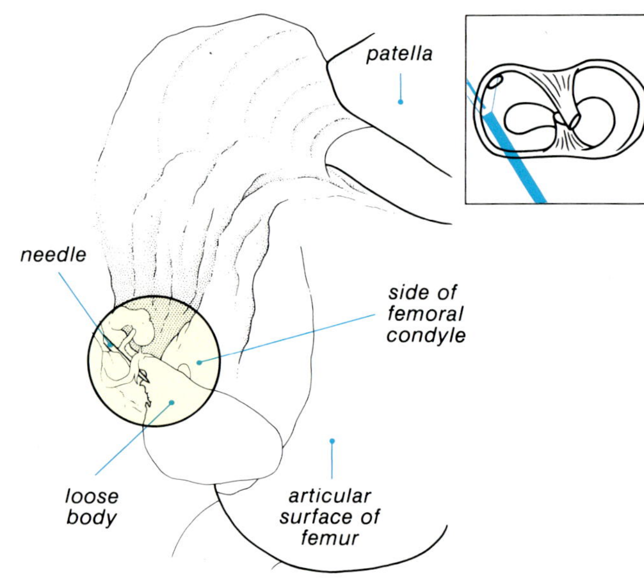

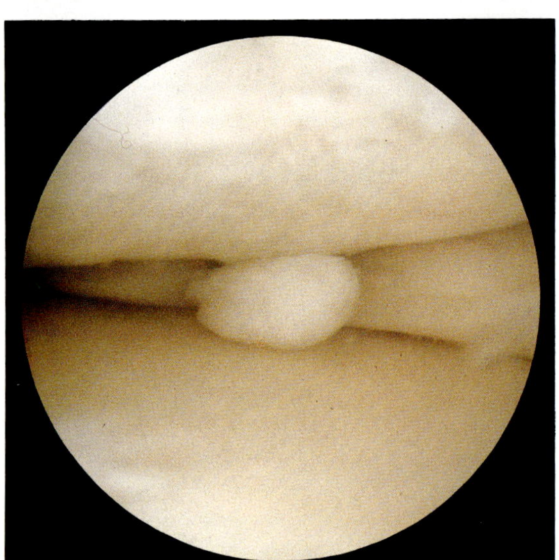

4.32

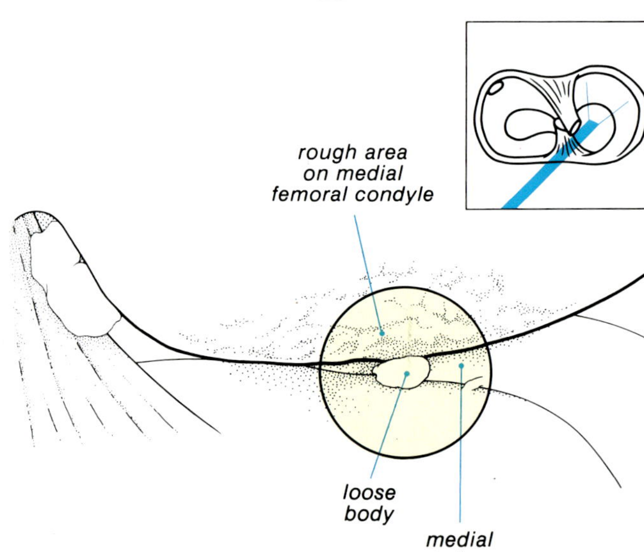

removed with grasping forceps inserted from the posterolateral approach.

There are many other places in the knee where loose bodies may settle and escape detection. One such refuge is the space beneath the lateral meniscus, between the inferior meniscosynovial junction and the lateral femoral condyle. This space is surprisingly large and can accommodate a loose body almost 1cm in diameter (Fig.4.35).

4.33

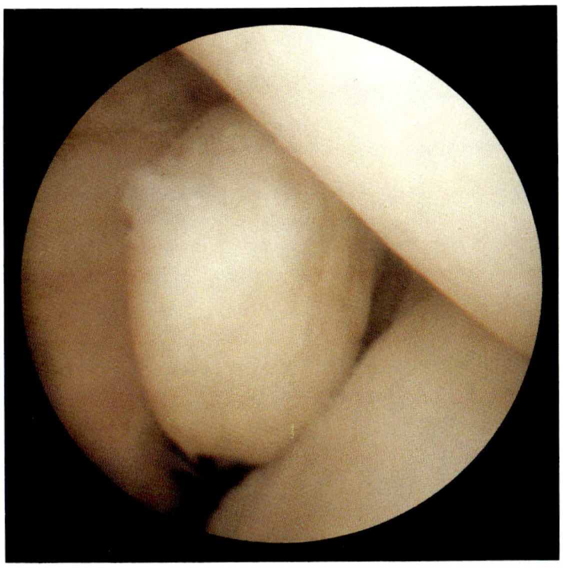

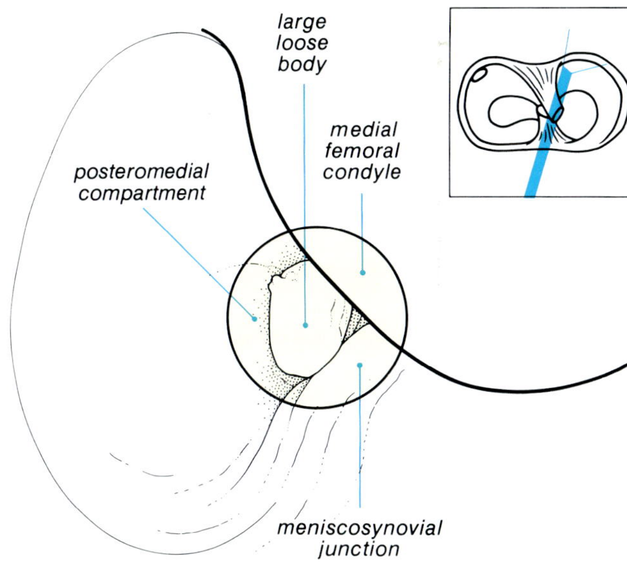

4.34

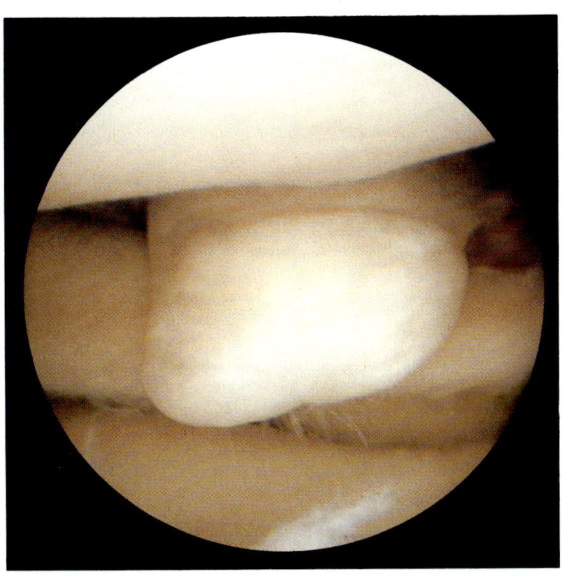

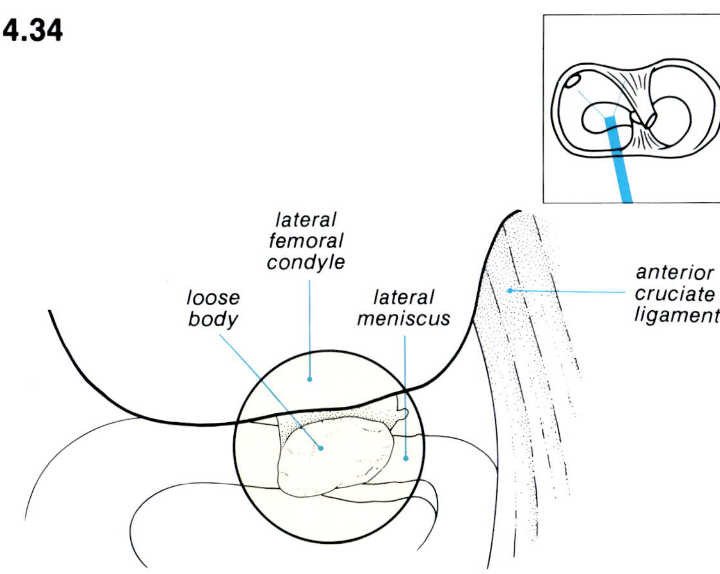

4.35

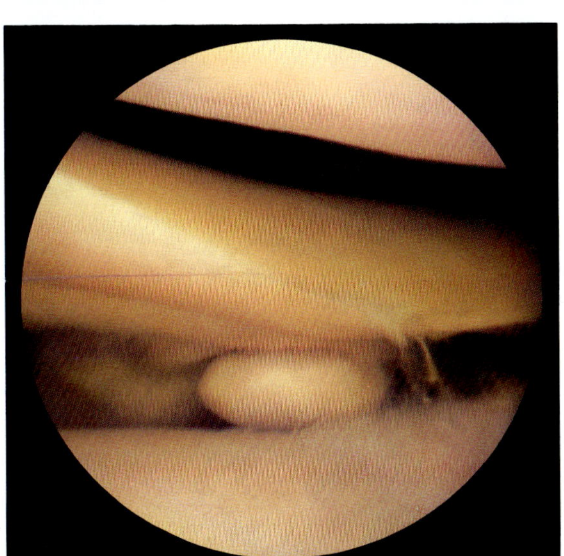

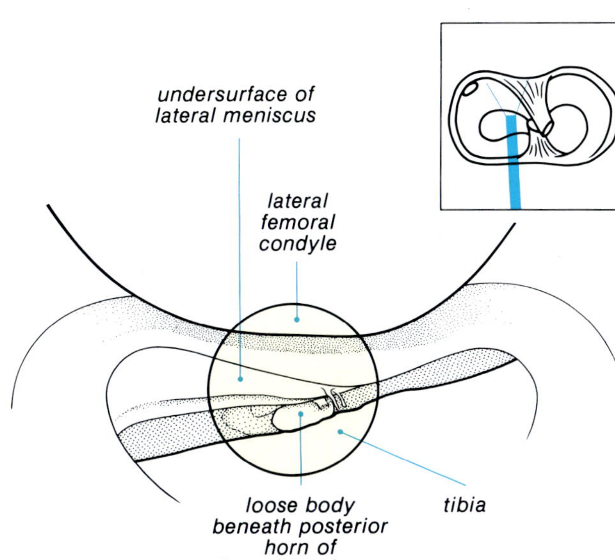

Fig.4.36 shows a glass fragment approximately 8 x 5 x 5mm which had entered the front of the knee when the patient slipped and landed on a bottle. The fragment (Fig.4.36) is lying in front of the inferior meniscosynovial junction near the posterior horn of the lateral meniscus and was found by placing the arthroscope under the posterior horn of the meniscus.

In the suprapatellar pouch, 'loose' bodies are sometimes seen attached to the margin of the patella by a soft tissue stalk (see Figs.4.21 & 4.22). Fig.4.37 shows a large pedunculated loose body, measuring 2 x 1 x 1cm, tethered by a vascular pedicle 5mm in thickness which had to be divided before the fragment could be removed. The fragment had arisen from an osteochondral fracture of the patella and had increased in size by gradual accretion until it was larger than its bed.

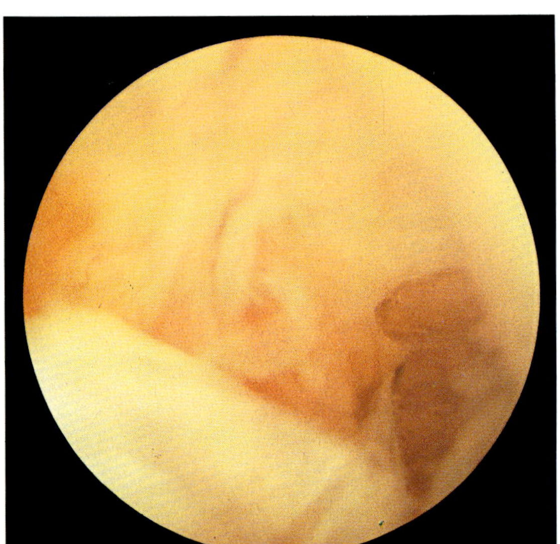

4.36

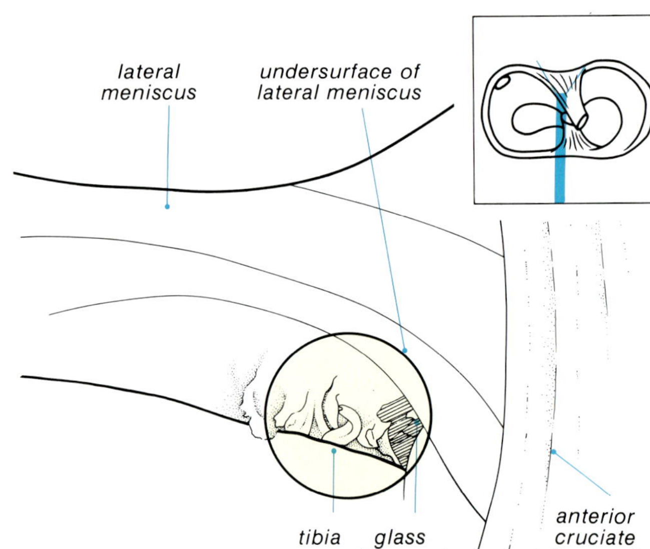

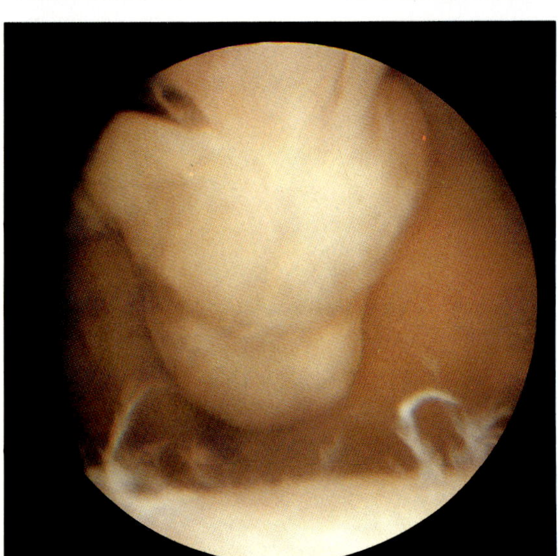

4.37

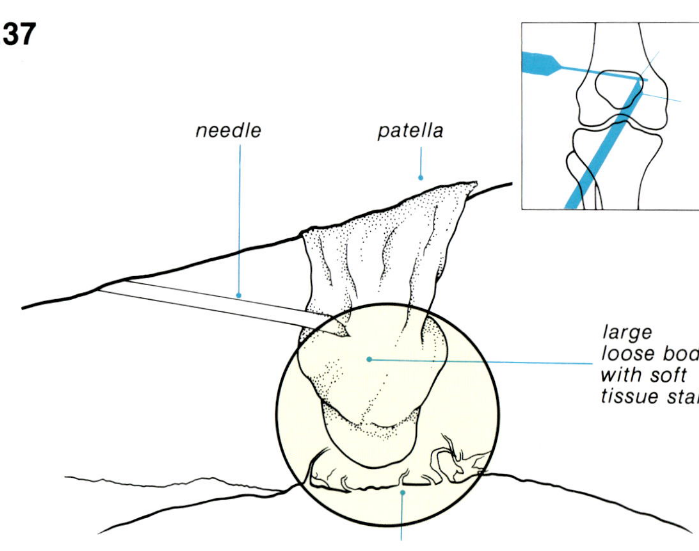

5
Lesions of Ligaments

ANTERIOR CRUCIATE LIGAMENT

The anterior cruciate ligament is not a simple band of fibrous tissue but is twisted upon itself in such a way that it is functionally divided into posterolateral and anteromedial bands. The posterolateral band runs from the posterior part of the femoral insertion to the lateral side of the tibial insertion and twists round the anteromedial band as it does so. Though the two components are usually fused, they sometimes appear quite distinct from each other, almost as two separate ligaments (Fig.5.1). The posterolateral band is taut when the knee is in full extension and the anteromedial is taut

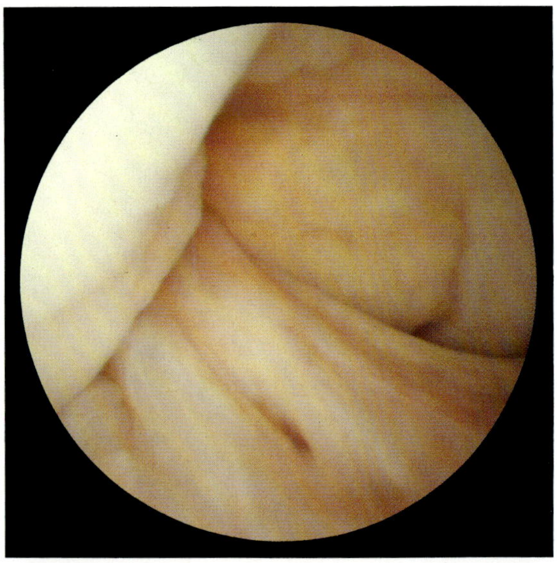

5.1

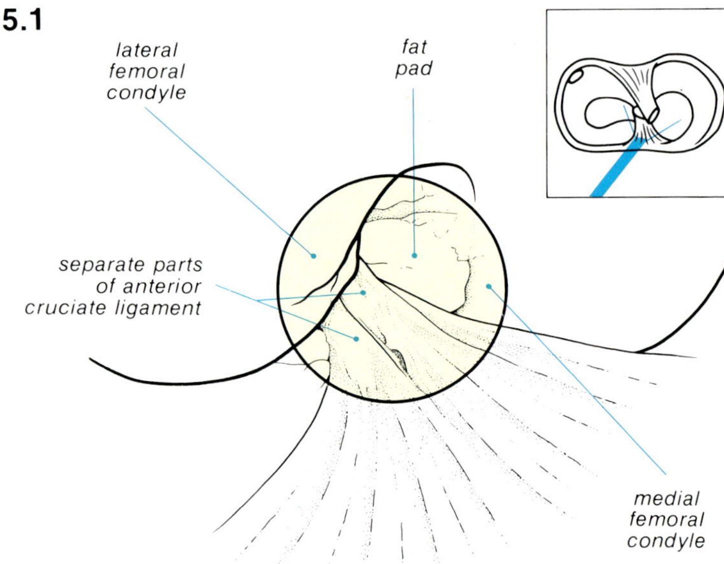

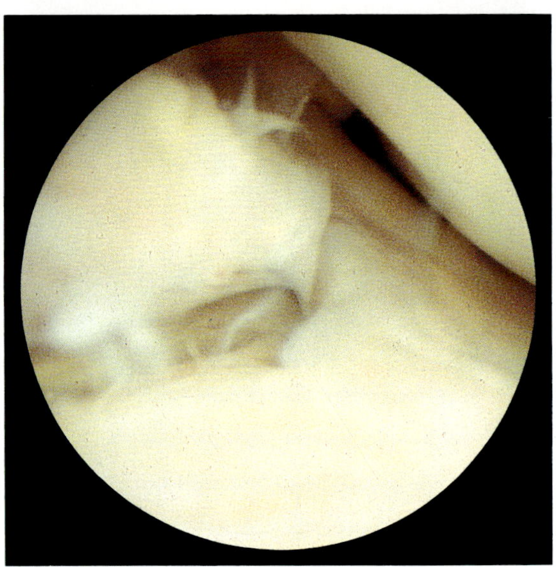

5.2

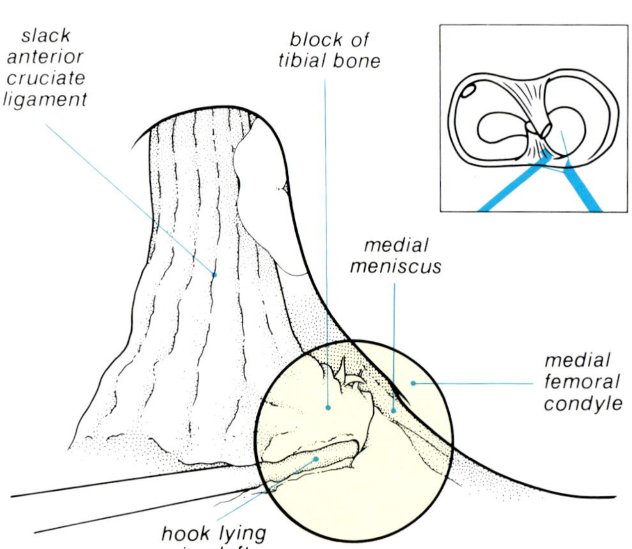

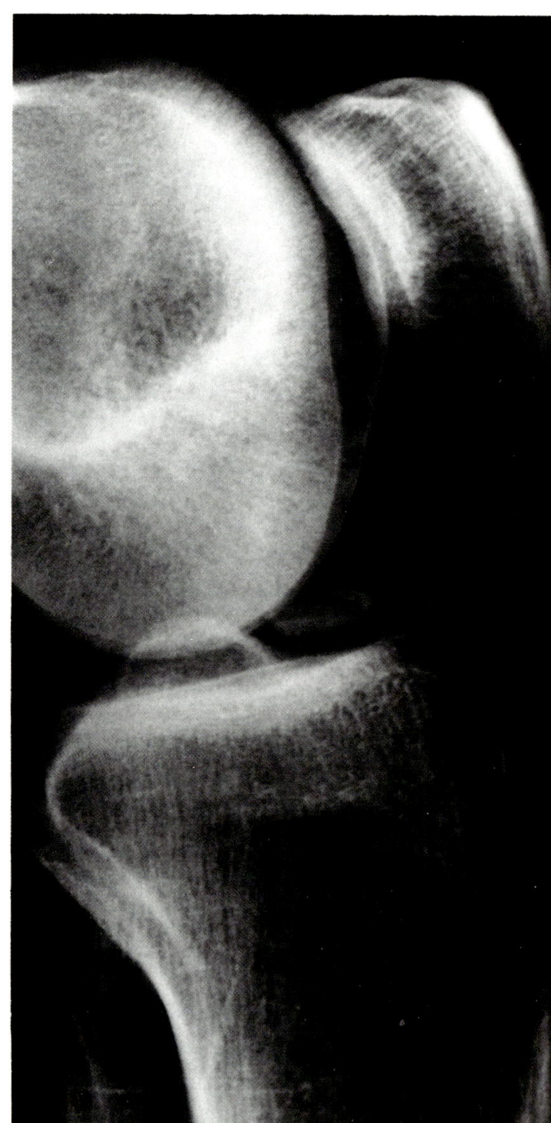

5.3

during flexion. Rupture of the posterolateral band is associated with a positive Lachman sign and positive shift or jerk test, but the anterior draw sign will be negative unless the anteromedial band is also ruptured. Isolated rupture of the anteromedial portion alone is associated with the opposite clinical features: a positive anterior draw sign, but negative Lachman, pivot shift and jerk signs.

The anterior cruciate ligament can be ruptured at any of several points. Its tibial insertion can be avulsed along with a block of bone, an injury most commonly seen before skeletal maturity. Fig.5.2, however, shows the tibial insertion avulsed with a piece of tibia in a 28-year-old man. A probing hook lies in the cleft between the fragment and the tibia. The lesion was eight months old at arthroscopy, and the fragment had failed to unite with its bed after conservative management (Fig.5.3).

More proximally, the ligament can rupture immediately above its tibial attachment, leaving a short fringe of ruptured fibres. In Fig.5.4 there is a short fringe of fibres and no soft tissue mass large enough to hold suture material.

The most common site for anterior cruciate rupture is the middle third of the ligament. If the ligament ruptures in the central part, it will not heal. The ends contract into rounded stubs of tissue at the base of each insertion (Fig.5.5). As in Fig.5.4, the remnants of the ligament fibres are not substantial enough for suturing.

5.4

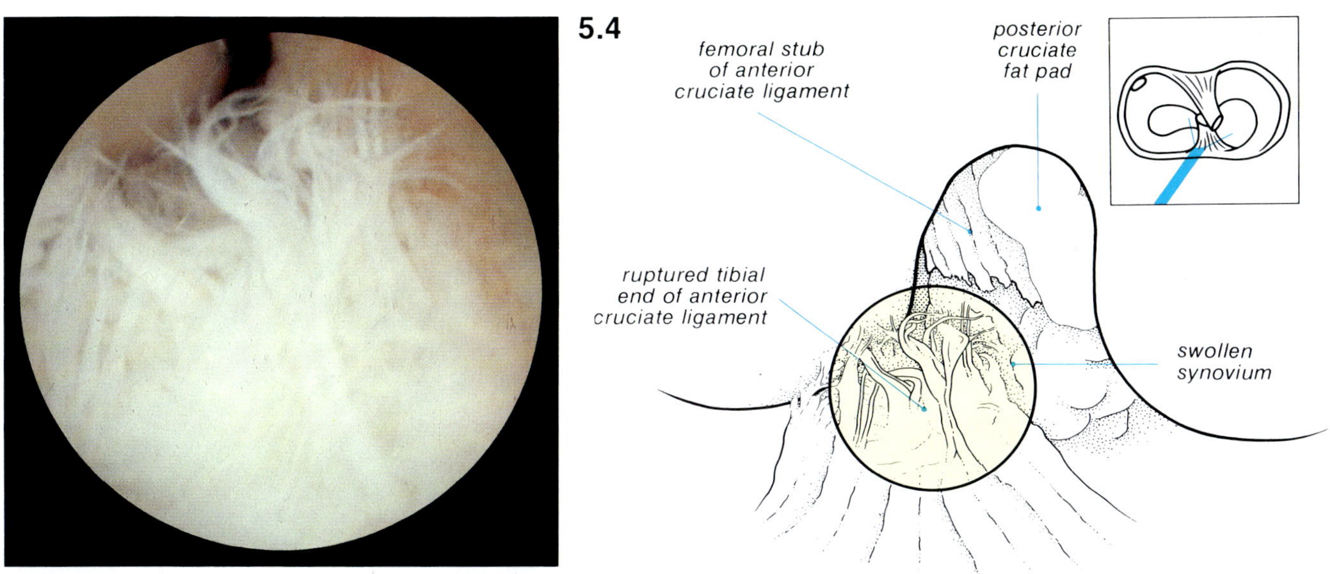

5.5

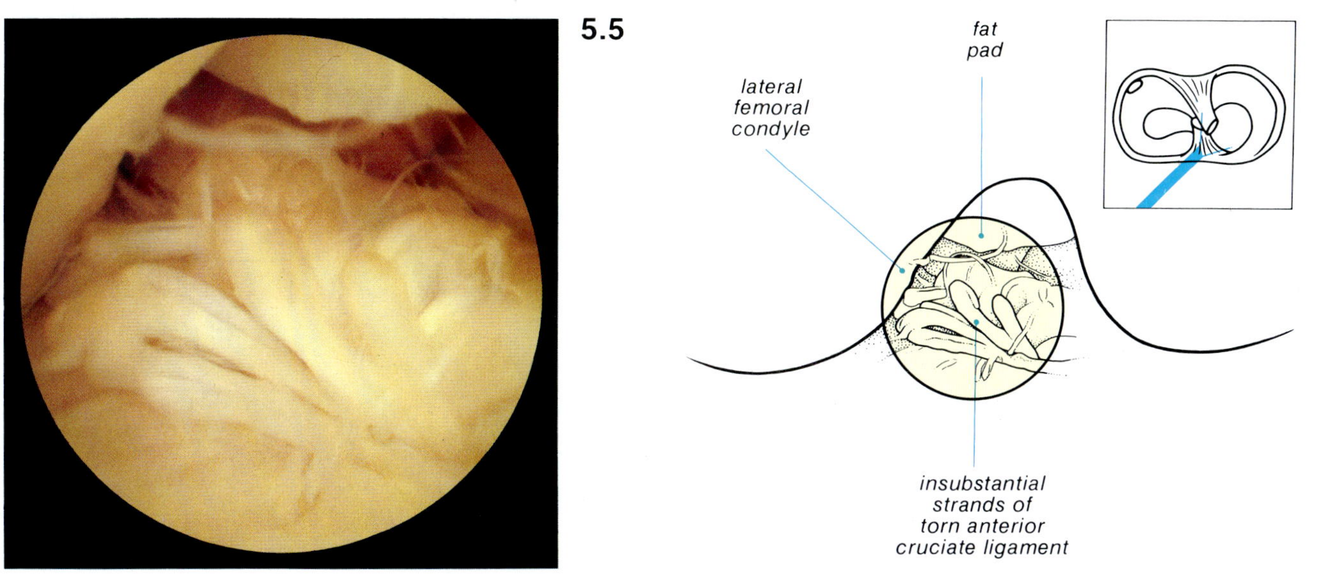

Fig.5.6 shows another rupture of the midportion of the anterior cruciate. The lesion is four weeks old. The stub is contracted and appears swollen and oedematous with its surface covered with blood. It is large enough to obstruct extension of the knee. This type of stub is often associated with a painless block to extension but restoration of full extension as soon as the patient is anaesthetized. This painless block to knee extension may be due to involvement of the profuse supply of proprioceptive fibres in the anterior cruciate ligament which may be responsible for reflex inhibition of extension.

Until recently, the concept of an isolated rupture of the anterior cruciate ligament was the subject of controversy. Although it is now generally agreed that the anterior cruciate can be completely ruptured in the absence of damage to other structures in the knee, the idea of a partial rupture of the anterior cruciate is not so widely accepted. In Fig.5.7, only the posterolateral band of the anterior cruciate ligament has ruptured. The ruptured fibres protrude through the synovial sheath covering the ligament, but the synovium covering the anteromedial portion remains intact. The patient had a negative anterior draw sign but the Lachman and pivot shift signs were positive.

Fig.5.8 shows a ruptured posterolateral band of the anterior cruciate ligament which has undergone cystic degeneration so that the tip of its stub is now a bulbous three-lobed ganglionic cyst, being pulled forward with a hook in the illustration, which blocked extension of the knee. Before arthroscopy the patient complained of intermittent episodes of internal derangement as well as the classical high-speed instability associated with rupture of the anterior cruciate ligament. After removal of the stub under arthroscopic control the mechanical symptoms were abolished.

Fig.5.9 shows another partial rupture of the anterior cruciate ligament. The round white object in Fig.5.9 which would appear, at first sight, to be a loose body is, in fact, the rounded stub of the posterolateral band of the anterior cruciate ligament which has come to lie in a position similar to the lesion in Fig.5.8. The intact anteromedial band can seen running through the intercondylar notch in the normal position but without its normal synovial covering.

The torn end of a ruptured anterior cruciate ligament is not always easily seen. If the rupture occurs within the synovial sheath, the ligament may appear to the casual or uncritical observer to be intact though 'attenuated'. The concept of the attenuated anterior cruciate ligament

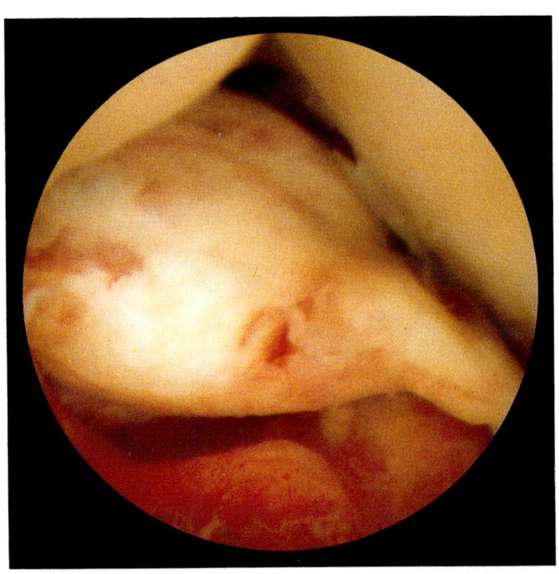

5.6

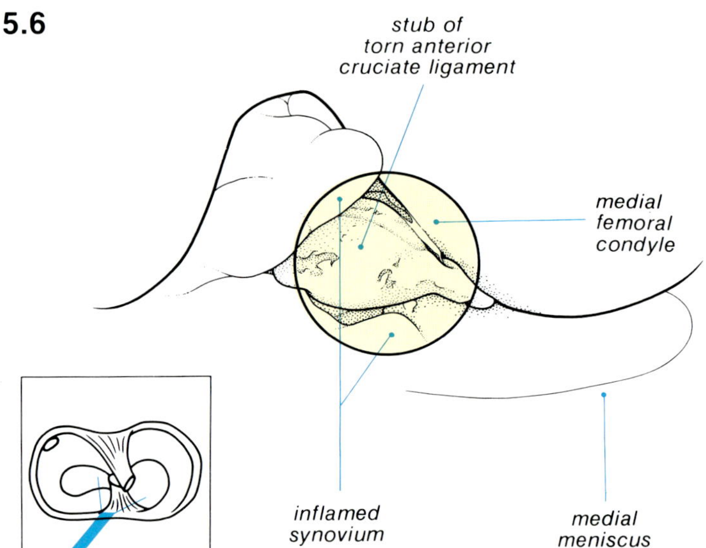

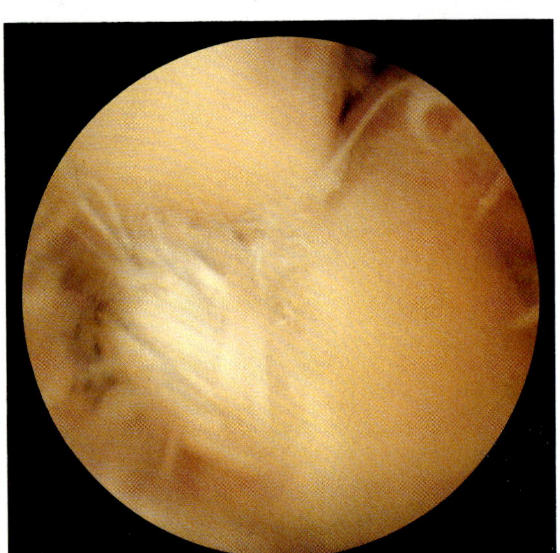

5.7

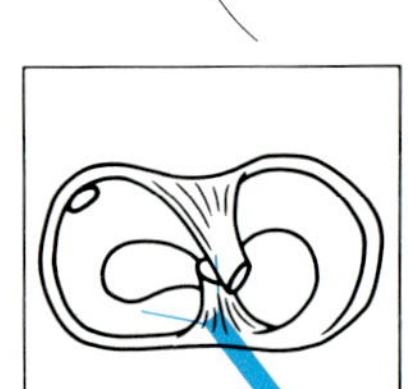

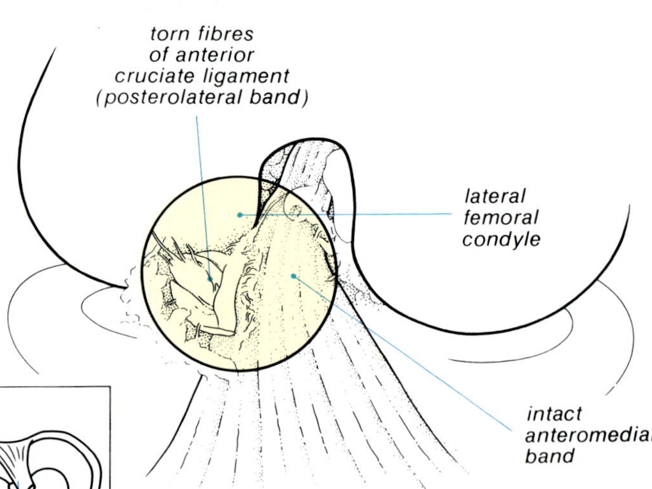

probably accounts for some of the many anterior cruciate ligament ruptures that have escaped diagnosis in the past.

Fig.5.10 shows an irregular anterior cruciate ligament; its proximal portion is narrower and its blood vessels more obvious than in the distal portion. The explanation for this appearance is that the cruciate ligament has ruptured within its sheath and become adherent to the posterior cruciate ligament. The proximal part of the sheath is empty while distally it contains a swollen mass of ligamentous tissue. If this ligament were to be incised, its torn fibres would protrude, giving an appearance similar to that of Fig.5.7.

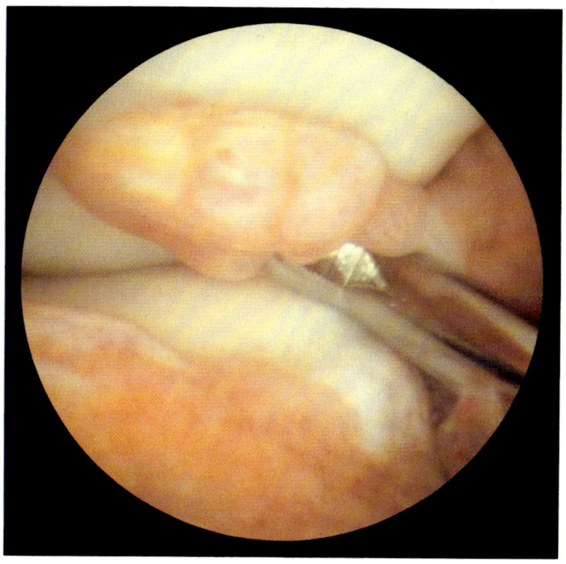

5.8

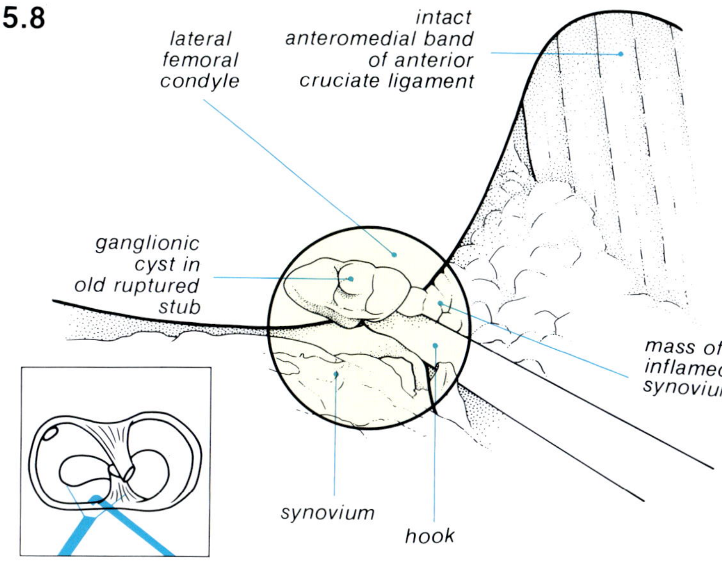

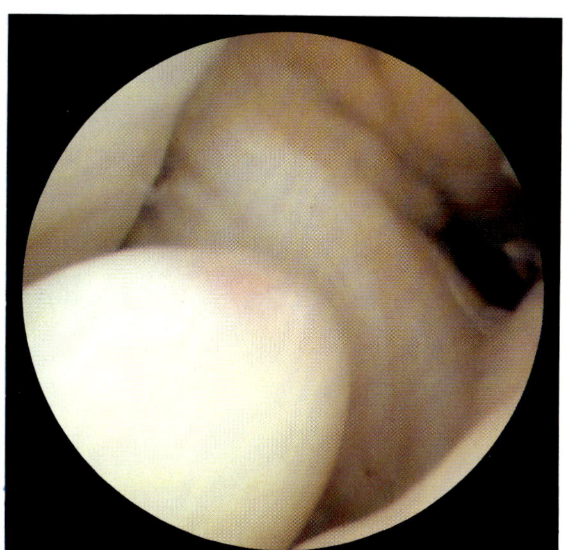

5.9

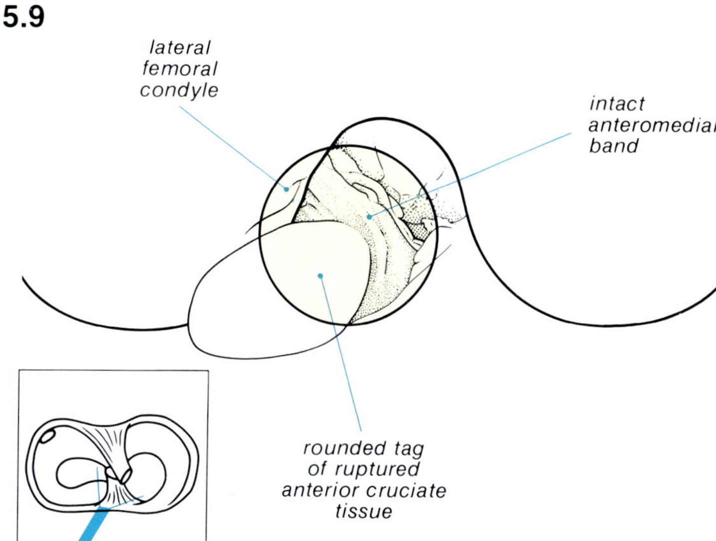

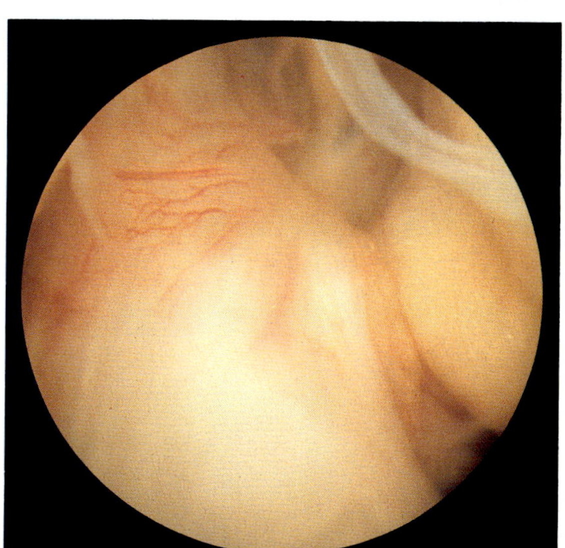

5.10

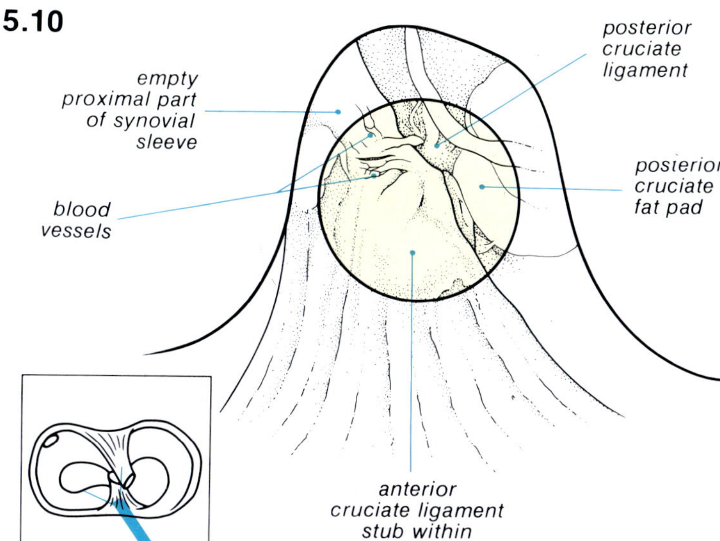

Fig.5.11 shows the anterior cruciate ligament of a fifteen-year-old boy. The anteromedial band appears to have a swelling, suggesting a rupture within the sheath similar to that in Fig.5.10. On clincial examination the knee was normal, with negative anterior draw, pivot shift and Lachman signs. The arthroscopic appearances, however, strongly suggest an intrasynovial lesion of the anteromedial band. It may be that a partial rupture of the ligament has occurred and that, because the ends of the ligament are held in close apposition by the remaining intact ligament and synovial sleeve, healing has taken place spontaneously. The temptation to incise the

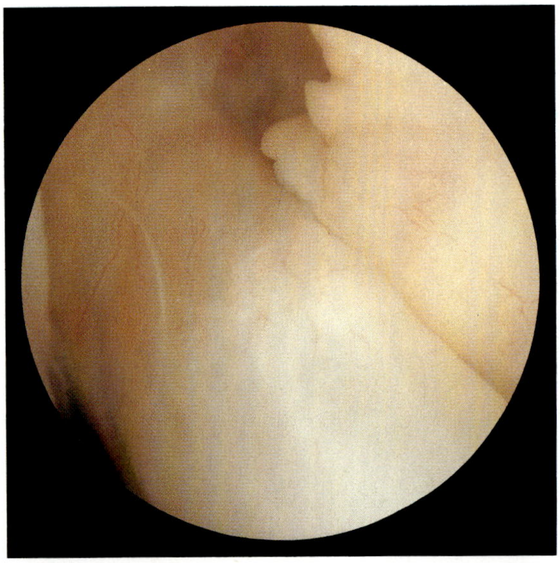

5.11

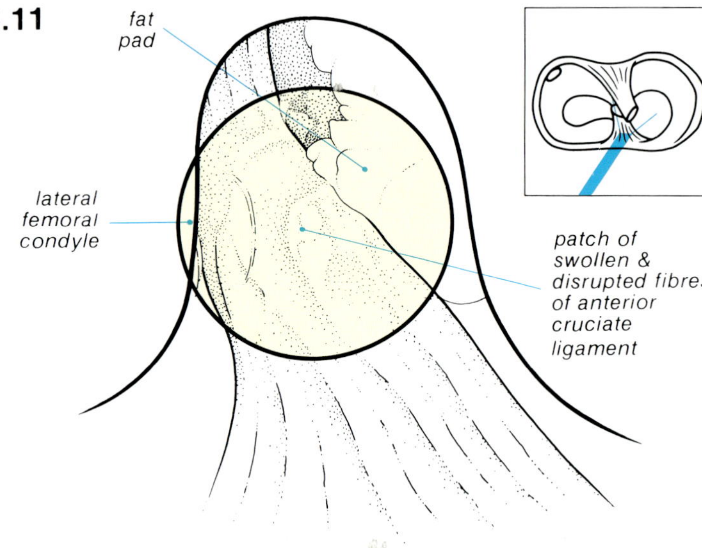

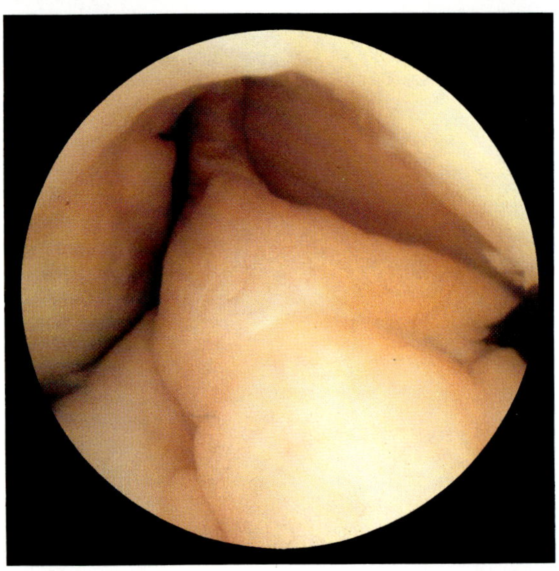

5.12

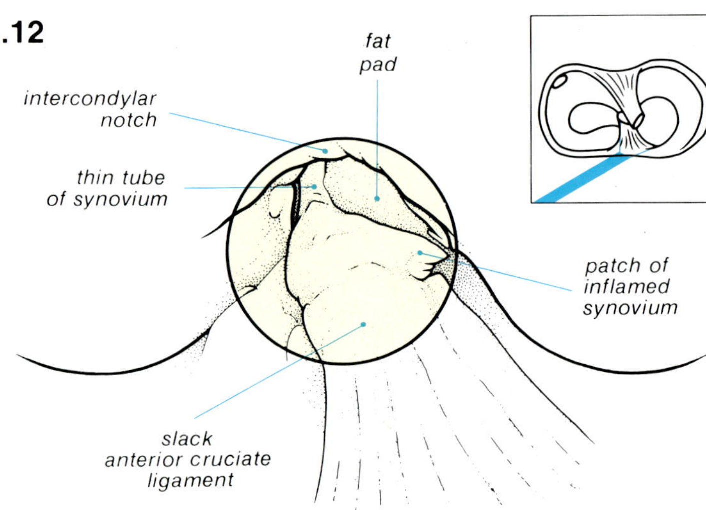

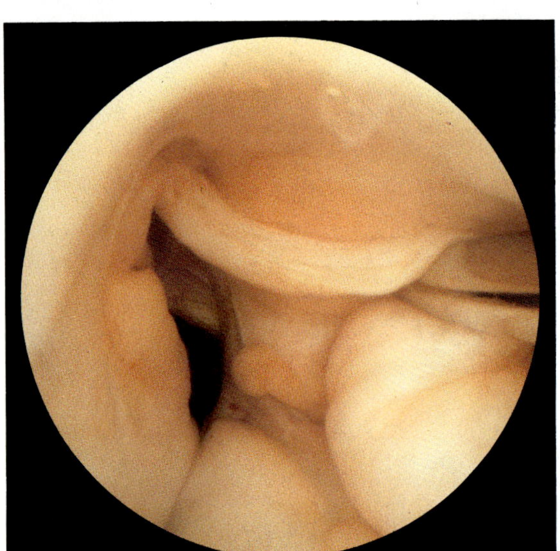

5.13

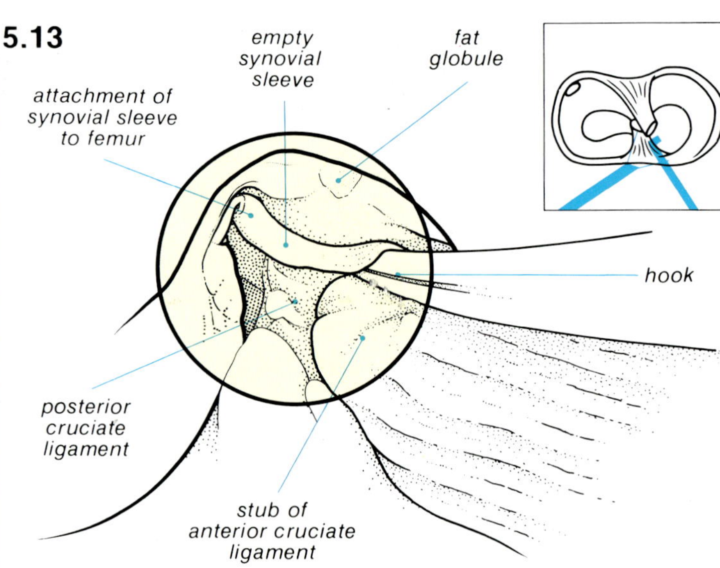

synovial covering of the lesion and inspect the tissue within was resisted.

Fig 5.12 shows another example of an 'attenuated' anterior cruciate ligament which at first sight appears to be slack but intact. Although the ligament is not as tense or taut as normal, no ruptured fibres are seen. When retracted with a probing hook (Fig.5.13), it becomes clear that the appearance of continuity depends solely upon a narrow sleeve of synovium which runs from the tip of the ligament to its femoral insertion. This appearance is consistent with the suggestion that the ligament has ruptured within its synovial sheath and contracted to form a swollen functionless stub based on the tibial insertion, leaving an empty synovial tube running upwards to the femoral insertion.

Late ruptures of the anterior cruciate are also found in which the infrapatellar fold remains intact while the notch itself is empty (Fig.5.14). It is possible that the casual observer might consider these strands to represent the so-called attenuated anterior cruciate ligament, but careful observation will show that they run from the front of the intercondylar notch into the infrapatellar fat pad, which is not the course of the anterior cruciate ligament. If the arthroscope is passed beyond the strands of tissue, a space at the former site of the anterior cruciate ligament will be seen (Fig.5.15). The posterior cruciate ligament can be seen deep within the intercondylar notch, running from the fat pad that covers its femoral insertion to the tibial insertion below. The ligament does not have a normal synovial covering.

Avulsion of the anterior cruciate from the tibia, ruptures at its tibial insertion, midportion ruptures and ruptures within the synovial sheath have been discussed. The final site of anterior cruciate detachment is at its attachment to the femur, which is side-to-side rather than end-to-end as on the tibia. The femoral attachment is therefore less easily seen than that of the tibia.

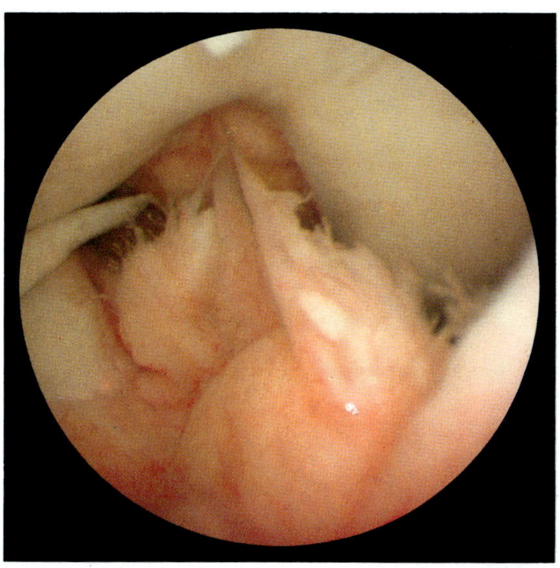

5.14

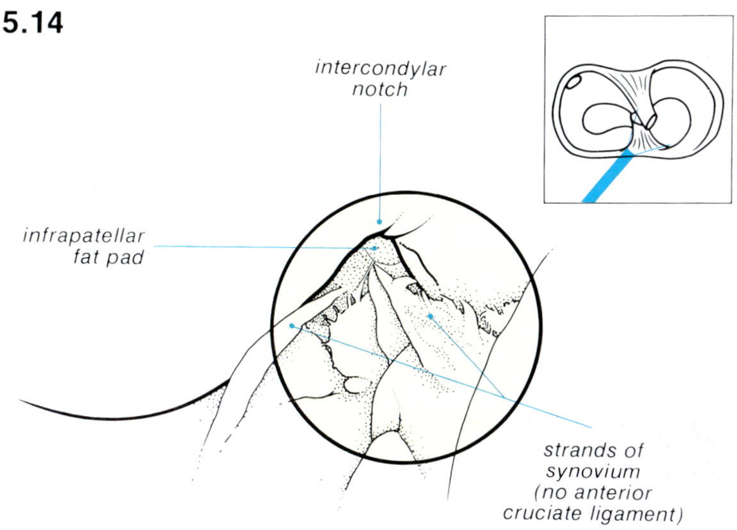

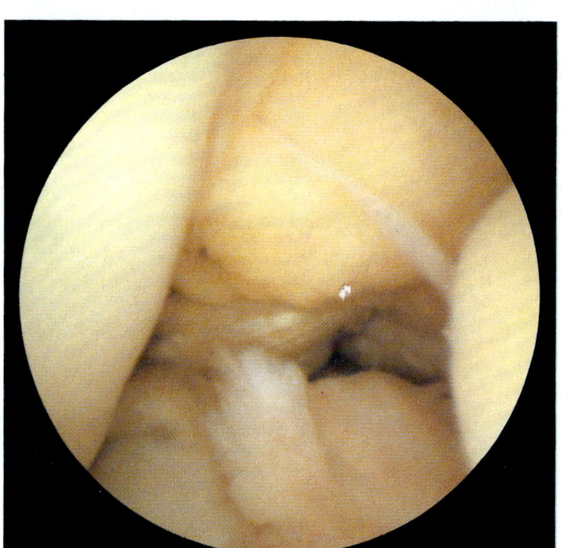

5.15

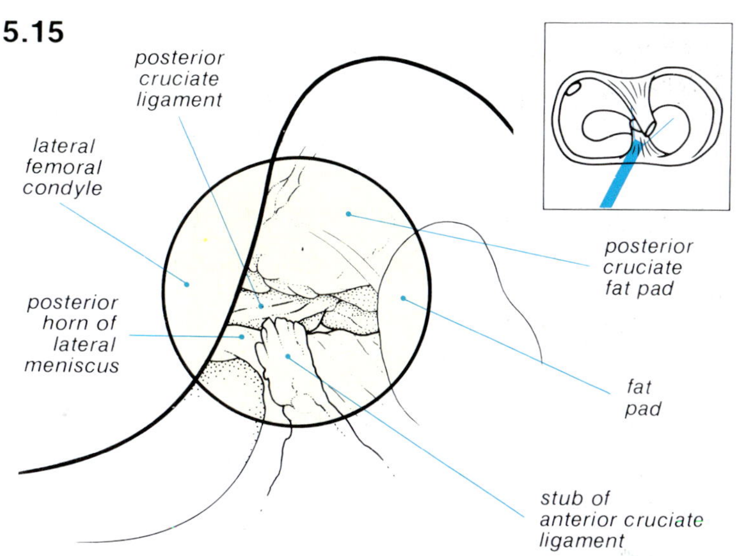

Moreover, detachment at this point is accompanied by haemorrhage and swelling which further obscure the view in an already tight part of the knee. In Fig.5.16, subsynovial bleeding, a torn synovial edge and swelling indicate the site of avulsion of the anterior cruciate ligament from the femur (compare with the normal appearance in Fig.1.56).

Anterior cruciate reconstruction

The anterior cruciate ligament can be replaced with fascia, patellar ligament, tendon, or prosthetic material such as carbon fibre or polyester. At arthroscopy the appearances of the substitute may be misleading in that they give no indication of its strength or of its contribution to the functional stability of the knee. If the ligament substitute is clearly disrupted, however, it can be concluded that the procedure has failed. Fig.5.17 shows a strip of fascia taken from the iliotibial tract, passed through the intercondylar notch and attached to the femur and tibia at the anatomical point of insertion eleven months previously. The new 'ligament' appears sound, smooth and in a good position, but no judgement can be made about its strength or vascularity since no vascular markings can be seen.

A similar ligament substitute (Figs.5.18 & 5.19), inserted by the same surgeon using the same technique approximately seven months earlier, ruptured (Fig.5.18), leaving the tibial stump of the graft in the intercondylar notch. It is interesting to note that vessels are apparent on the fascial stump, perhaps indicating revascularization. The graft itself was identified with little difficulty (Fig.5.19), lying free in the intercondylar notch and bearing a strong resemblance to a bucket handle tear of the medial meniscus. The fragment was removed.

Filamentous carbon fibre has been used as an anterior cruciate substitute on the supposition that it will provide a scaffolding for ingrowth of new fibroblasts that will eventually reconstitute a ligament which will closely resemble the original structure. Personal experience with this material has suggested that fibroblastic ingrowth does not occur in the synovial cavity of the knee. One opportunity to examine a carbon fibre ligament substitute fifteen months after insertion (Fig.5.20) arose when the patient sustained a lateral

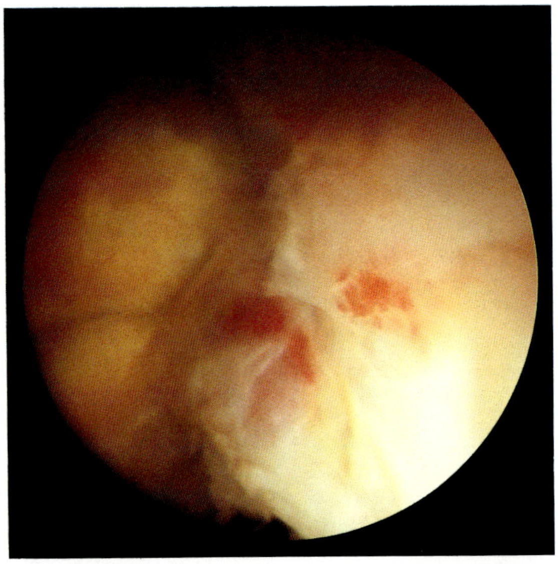

5.16

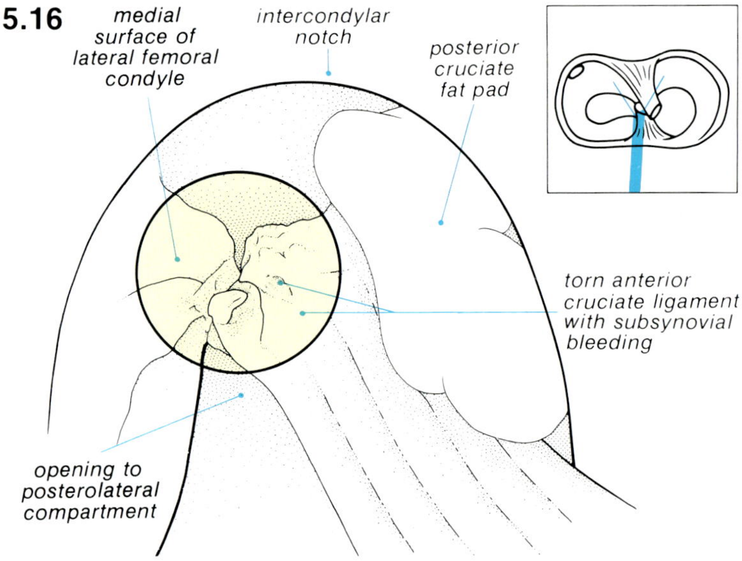

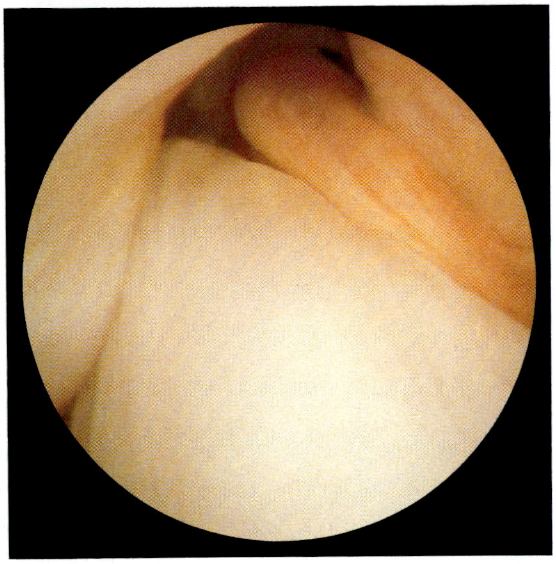

5.17

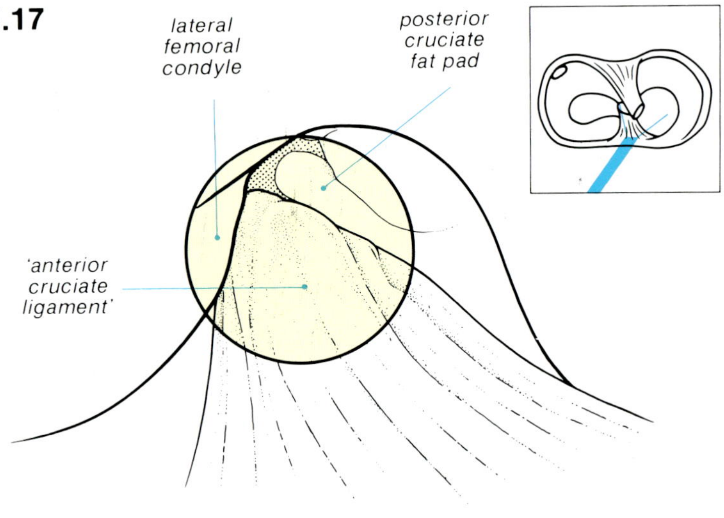

meniscus injury in the same knee and required an arthroscopic meniscectomy. The carbon fibre 'ligament', seen running through the intercondylar notch, was covered with a filmy layer of fibrous tissue that resembled synovium histologically. The underlying carbon fibre, however, was unchanged with no sign of fibrous ingrowth beyond the superficial layer. The fact that the 'ligament' has remained intact suggests that it is probably performing a mechanical function, but its appearance is essentially that of a prosthesis and not of a regenerated ligament.

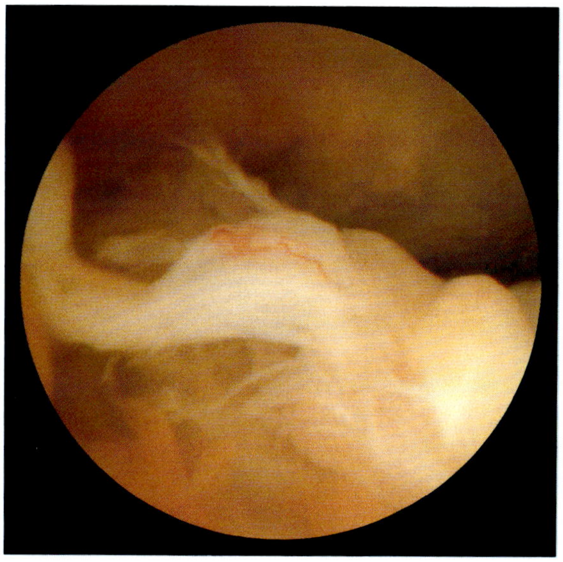

5.18

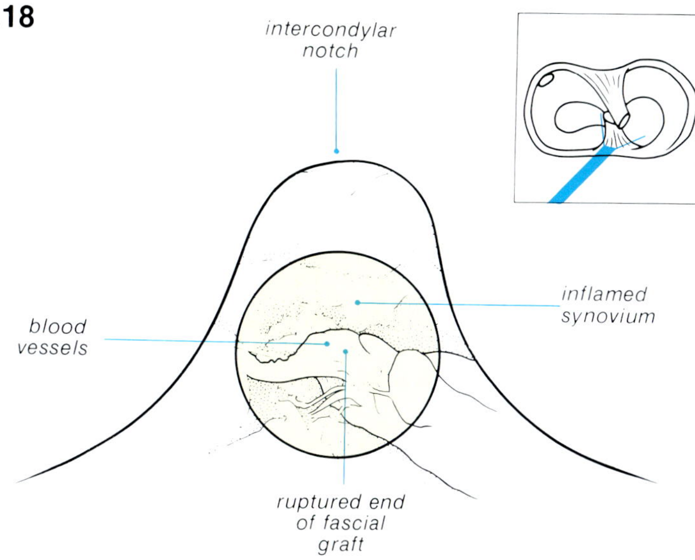

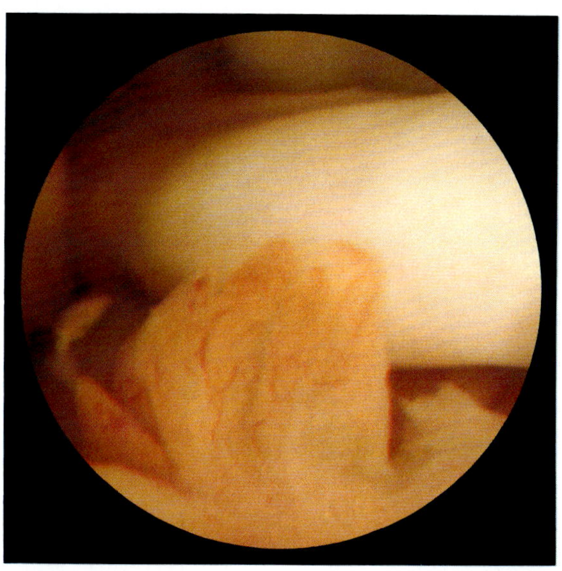

5.19

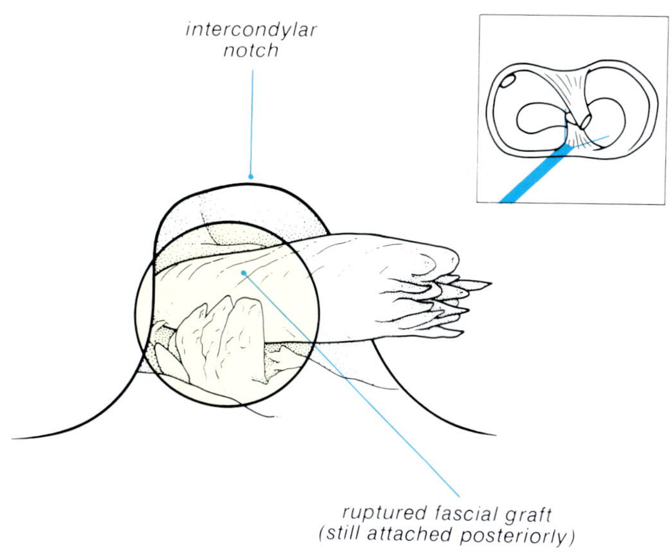

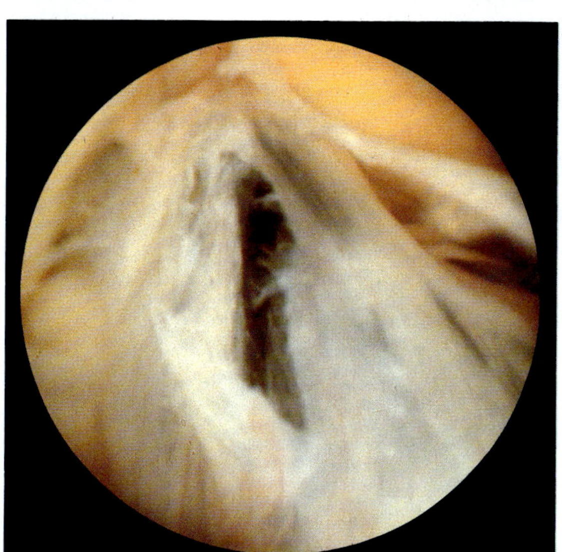

5.20

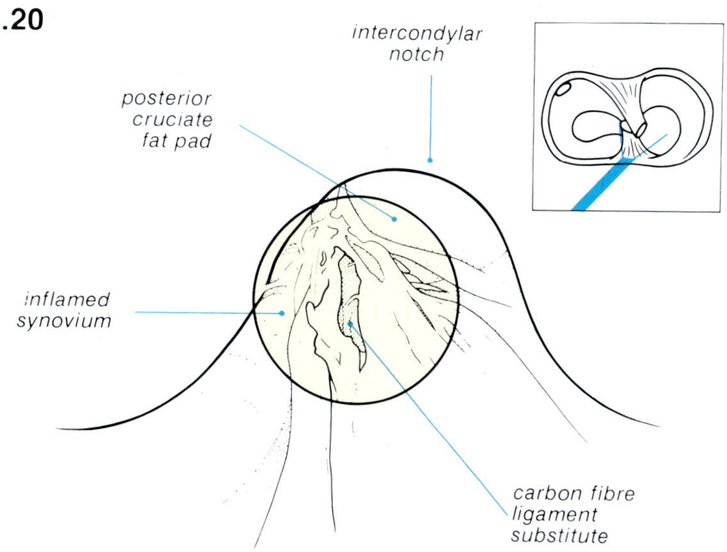

Fig.5.21 shows the intercondylar notch of a patient whose knee was affected by continuing synovitis two years after substitution. The carbon fibre is no longer intact but is replaced by a strip of fibrous tissue similar in appearance to an 'attenuated' anterior cruciate ligament. The surrounding synovium appears black because of the accumulation of carbon fibre particles. Carbon fibre pigmentation was also seen on the articular surface and at the meniscosynovial junction.

Staining of the synovium with carbon fibre particles is a common finding after the insertion of a prosthetic carbon fibre ligament and may be seen throughout the knee. Fig.5.22 shows such staining immediately above the medial synovial shelf in a knee that was examined arthroscopically because of persistent synovitis. The fragments in the synovium lie parallel to one another and to the shelf. The reason for this orientation is not clear but perhaps represents alignment with either lymphatic or blood vessels.

POSTERIOR CRUCIATE LIGAMENT

Because the posterior cruciate ligament lies behind the anterior cruciate, it is less easily seen at arthroscopy from the anterior approaches and often requires a posteromedial approach. Acute tears of the posterior cruciate ligament are particularly difficult to assess because of the inevitable haemorrhage and synovial swelling. Fig.5.23 shows an acute rupture of the posterior cruciate ligament seen from the posteromedial approach using the thirty degree arthroscope. The haemorrhagic stub of the ligament is lying above the tibia with a patch of exposed posterior capsule behind it. The space between the ligament and the posterior capsule is not found in a normal knee and in this case permits an arthroscope to be passed into the posterolateral compartment from the posteromedial approach, a manoeuvre that is normally obstructed by the posterior cruciate ligament and its surrounding synovial folds. In Fig.5.24, obtained by passing the seventy degree arthroscope through the intercondylar notch and directing its angle of vision

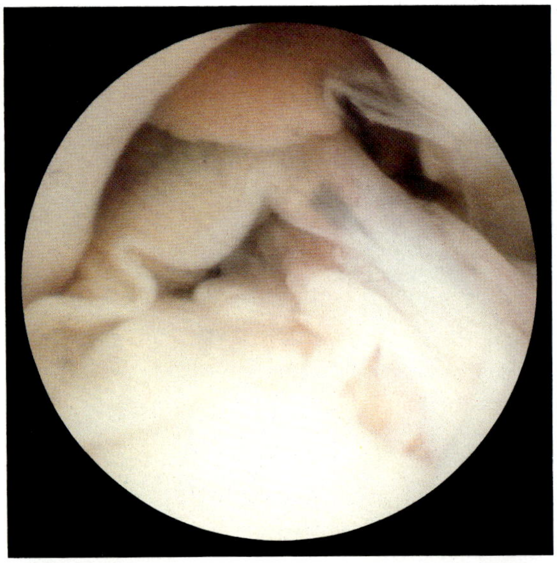

5.21

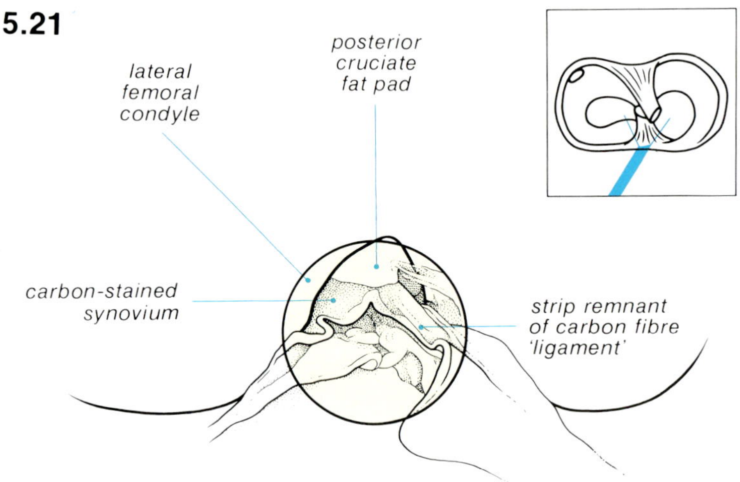

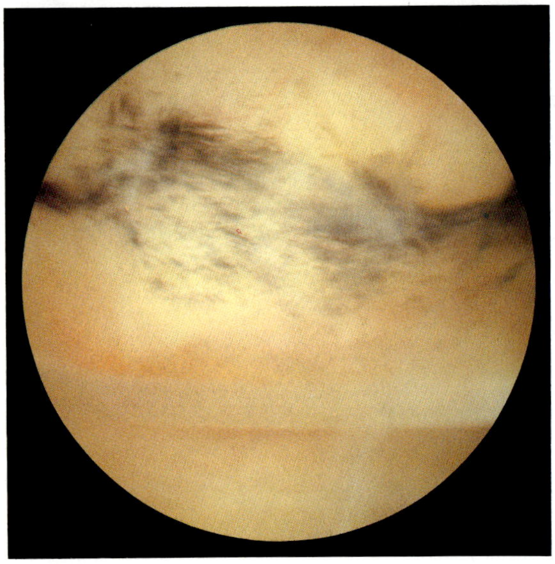

5.22

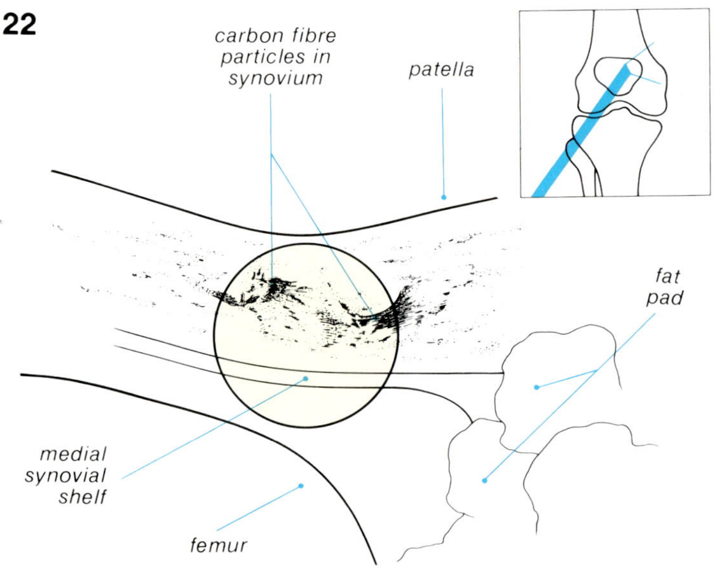

medially, the posteromedial insertion used in Fig.5.23 can clearly be seen with blood-stained fibrinous debris floating above it.

The posterior cruciate ligament can be seen from the anteromedial or anterolateral approach by passing the arthroscope through the intercondylar notch. Fig.5.25 shows a posterior cruciate ligament ruptured in its mid-portion, seen with a seventy degree telescope passed through the intercondylar notch and with the tibia pushed well back in relation to the femur to take full advantage of the telescope's capacity to look backwards towards the eyepiece at the proximal extremity of its field of vision. The ruptured fibres of the ligament are contracted and present an appearance similar to a rupture of the anterior cruciate ligament. It is difficult to imagine such an irregular ligament stub being successfully sutured.

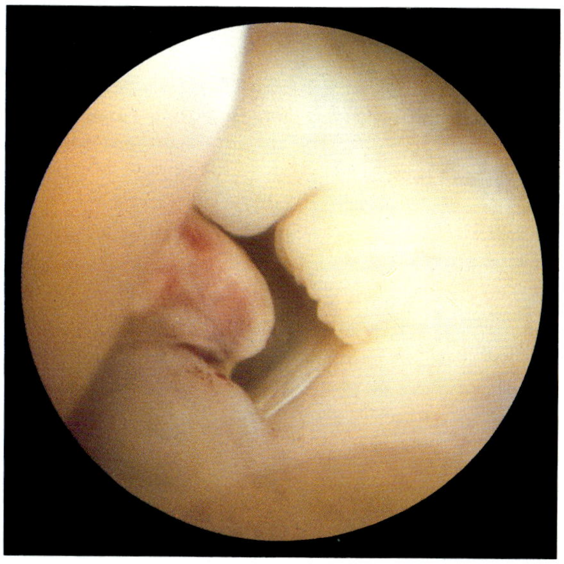

5.23

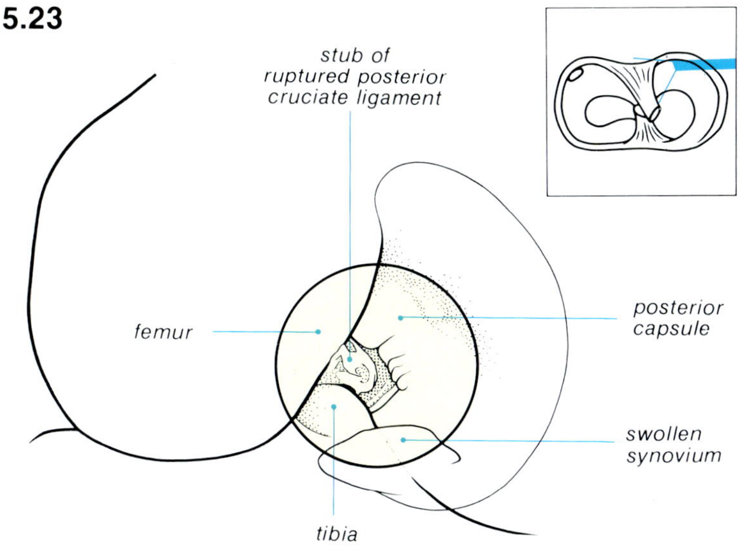

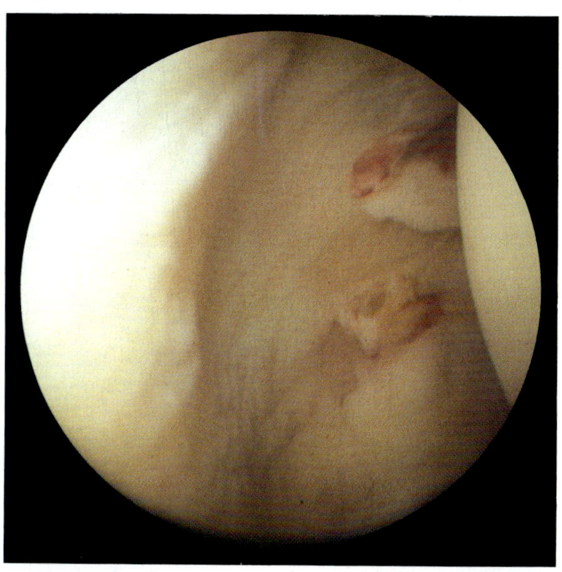

5.24

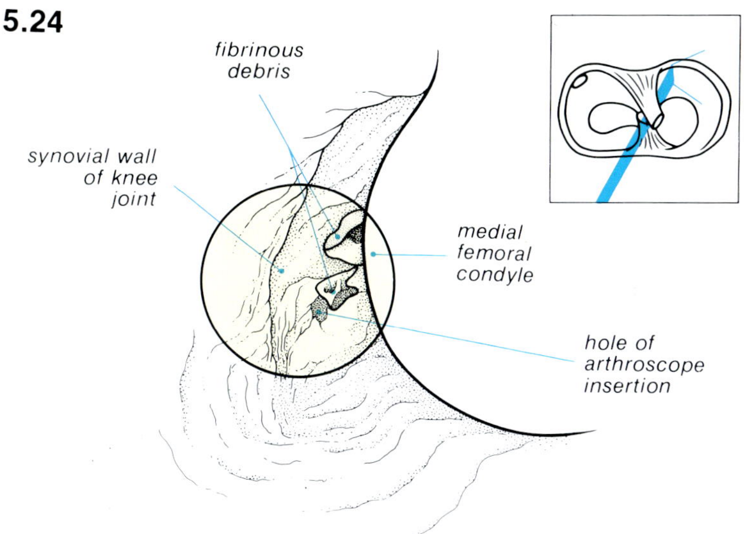

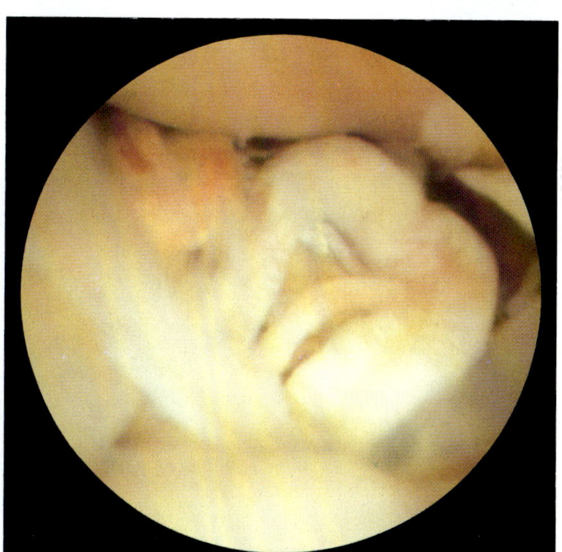

5.25

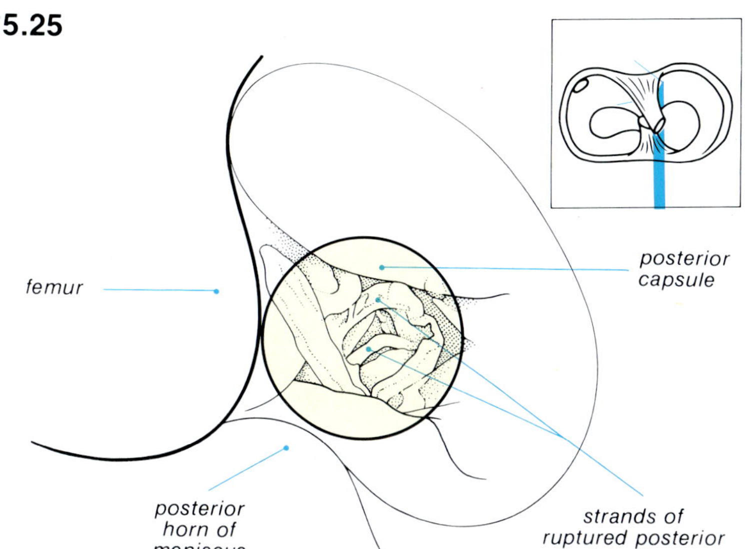

A less recent rupture of the posterior cruciate ligament is seen in Fig.5.26 where the point of rupture lies in the posterior cruciate tunnel, between the posterior horn of the medial meniscus and the tibia. The swollen and haemorrhagic appearance of the stub, lying just above the posterior horn of the medial meniscus, and the fact that it has been withdrawn from its synovial tunnel make it unlikely that these lesions will heal soundly if treated conservatively. On the other hand, replacing the distal stub of the ligament in its tunnel and reattaching it to the tibia present formidable technical problems and it is doubtful if accurate surgical reposition could be achieved.

Fig.5.27 shows a posterior cruciate ligament ruptured at its midportion, seen from the same approach as in Fig.5.26. Instead of the normal stout posterior cruciate ligament (see Fig.1.55), the tunnel is filled with irregular debris (compare with the anterior cruciate stub in Fig.5.5). The intact part of the ligament (seen in the upper part of the picture) is probably held in position by the synovial sleeve surrounding the ligament.

One result of rupture of the posterior cruciate ligament is abnormal posterior mobility of the tibia on the femur. In Fig.5.28, with the knee flexed to ninety degrees, the femur, tibia and the posterior cruciate ligament in the background are in their normal positions. When the tibia is pushed backwards in relation to the femur and allowed to sag posteriorly, a small defect is seen in front of the posterior cruciate ligament (Fig.5.29) through which the arthroscope could just be passed. Although no frank rupture with free fibres is seen, the ligament lacks the normal firm appearance and is undoubtedly incompetent. The explanation for such incompetence in the absence of a frank rupture is probably that the ligament is ruptured within its synovial sheath.

Rupture of the posterior cruciate ligament within its synovial sheath (Fig.5.30) has a similar appearance to rupture of the anterior cruciate (see Figs.5.10 & 5.11). Seen from the posteromedial approach with a

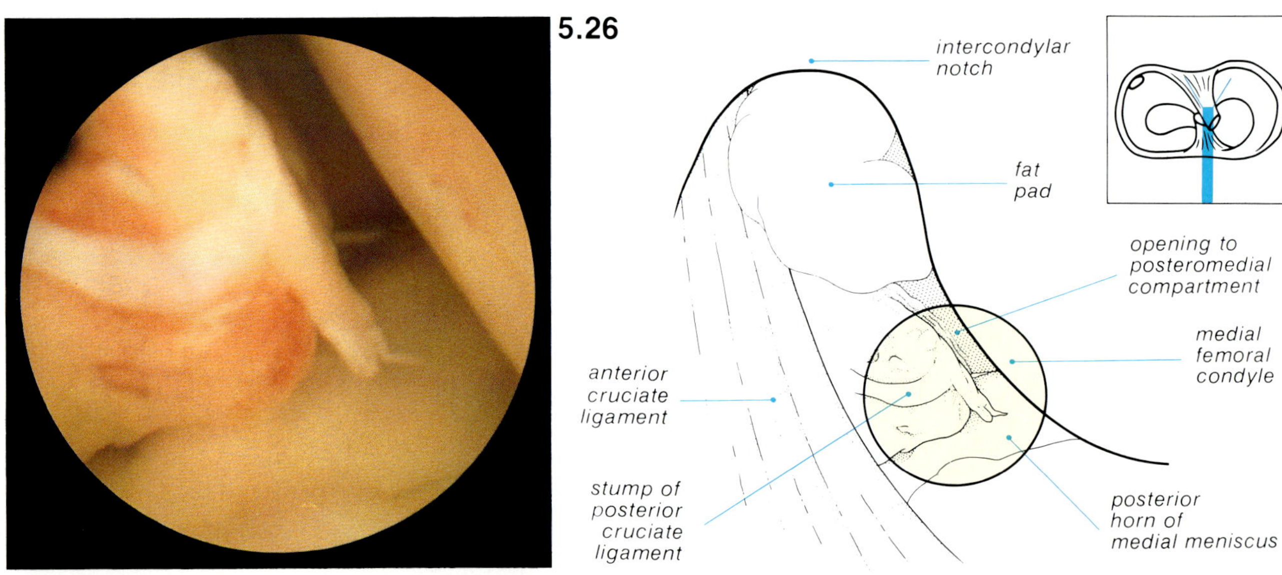

5.26

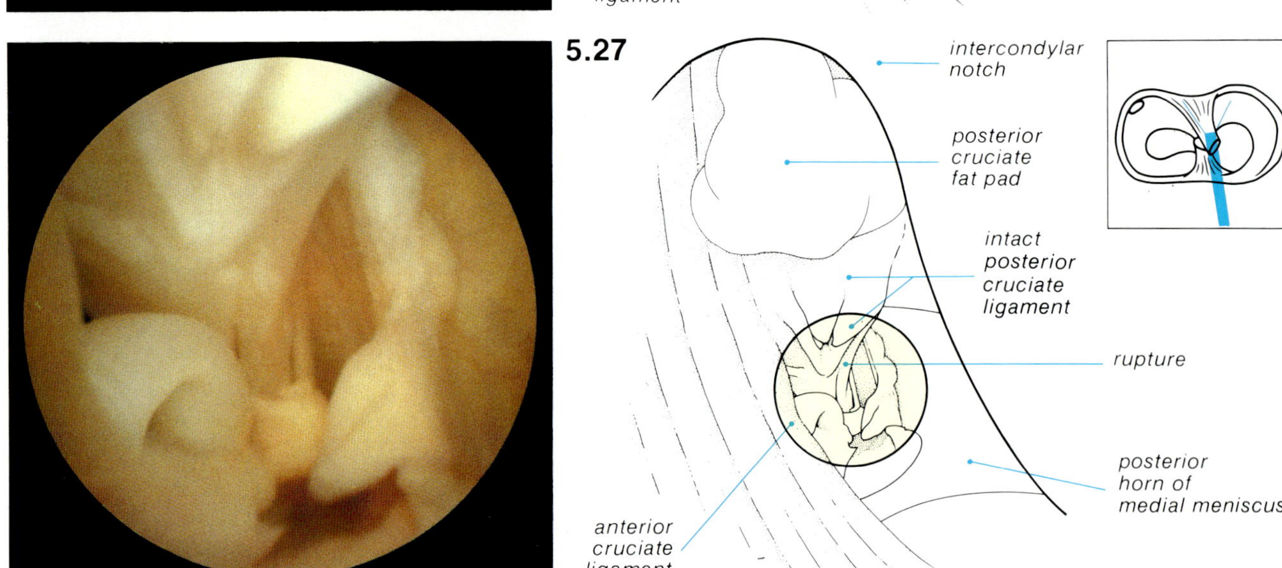

5.27

backward force applied to the tibia, the posterior cruciate shown in Fig.5.30 is covered by synovium but comes to a rounded stub in its midportion. The ligament is present distally but proximally has contracted, failing to reach its insertion in the intercondylar notch. Although there was a defect in front of the damaged ligament, it did not allow passage of the arthroscope into the posterolateral compartment.

Ruptures of the posterior cruciate ligament can be inferred from other arthroscopic findings even if the ligament itself cannot be seen. If the popliteus tendon is visible in the posterolateral compartment when the arthroscope is passed through the intercondylar notch as in Fig.1.74, there is abnormal backward mobility of

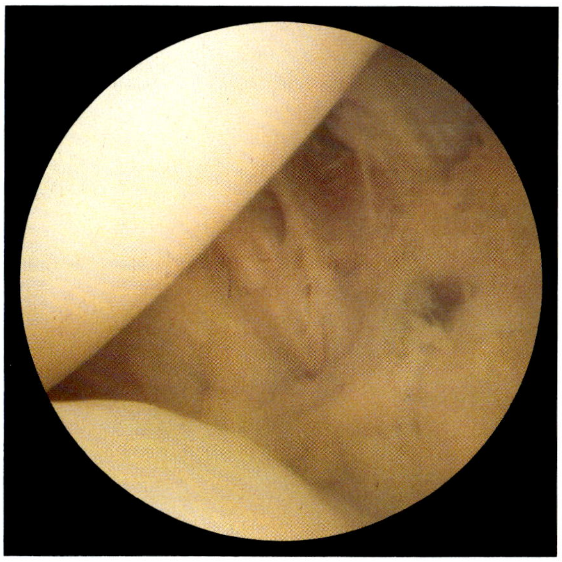

5.28

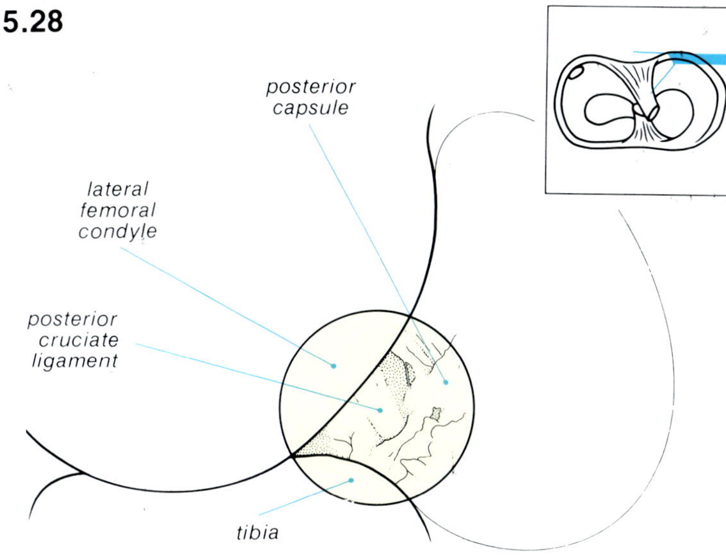

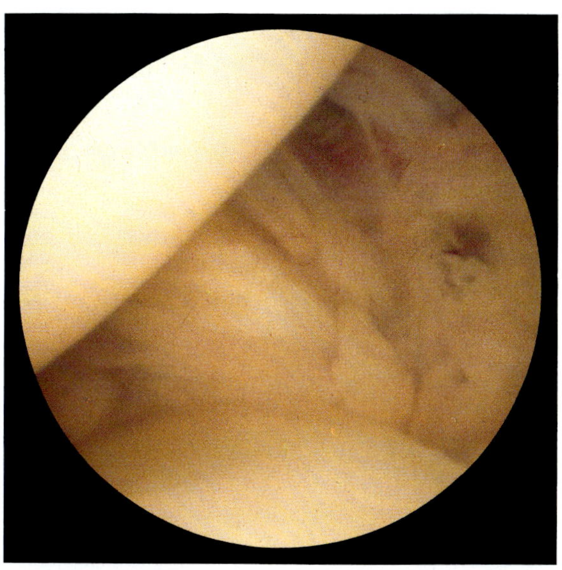

5.29

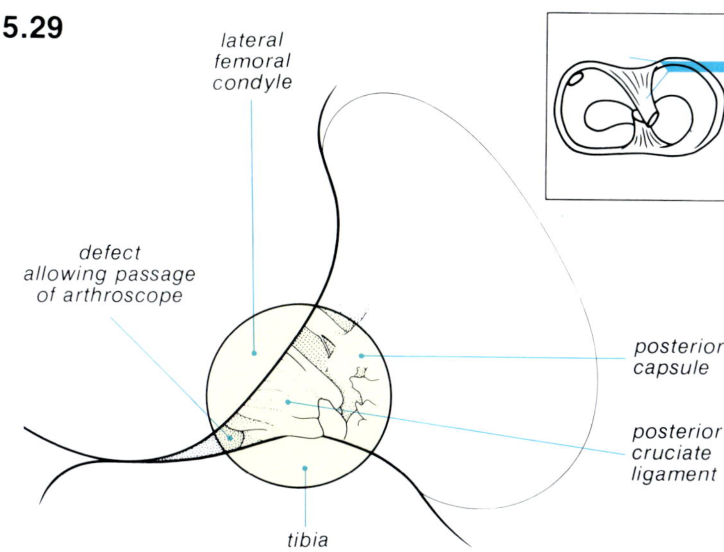

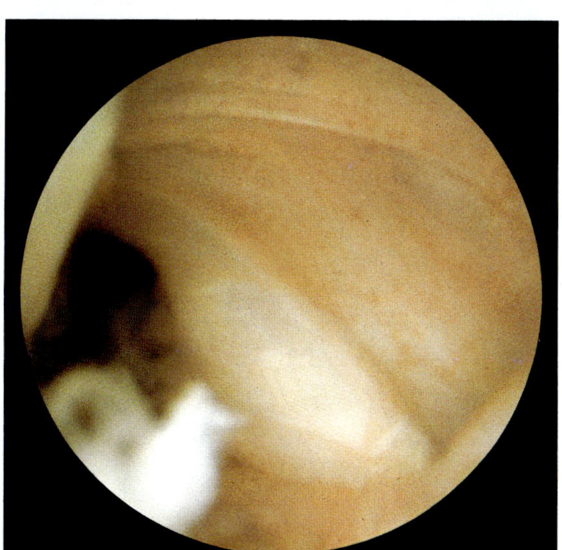

5.30

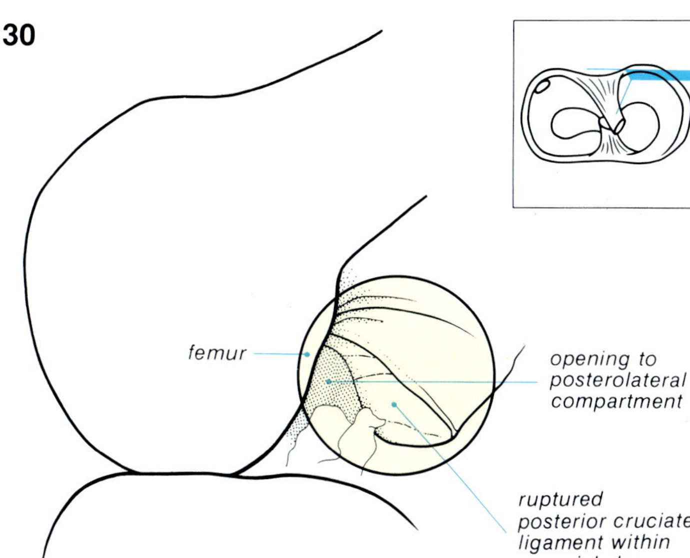

the tibia on the femur. Another indirect indication of posterior cruciate rupture is abnormal laxity of the anterior cruciate ligament. In Fig.5.31 the anterior cruciate ligament is lying in front of the posterior cruciate but has a crumpled appearance, indicating that it is not held at its normal tension. The kink in the anterior cruciate disappeared when the tibia was held in its normal position but became obvious when the unsupported tibia was allowed to fall backwards. Such a crumpled anterior cruciate ligament should alert the surgeon to the possibility of a posterior cruciate rupture if this has not already been suspected on the basis of clinical examination and examination under anaesthetic.

Ganglionic degeneration can occur in the posterior cruciate ligament as in the anterior cruciate (see Fig.5.8). In Fig.5.32 a ganglion overlying the tibial stub of a ruptured posterior cruciate ligament is seen medial to the posterior horn of the lateral meniscus. The stub is swollen with several loculi and differs from the cluster of posterior horn ganglia in Fig.2.51.

MEDIAL LIGAMENT

The medial ligament lies outside the synovial cavity and cannot be seen from within unless the overlying synovium is torn. Assessment of the integrity of the medial ligament must therefore depend on clinical examination and on the appearance of intra-articular structures related to the medial ligament rather than on the appearance of the ligament itself. If the medial ligament is lax, the medial meniscus, which normally is closely applied to the tibial plateau, will appear to float above the medial tibial plateau (Fig.5.33). This appearance is seen only in knees with abnormal laxity of the medial ligament, either as part of a generalized ligamentous disorder or as the result of trauma. In Fig.5.33, the patient had a long-standing rupture of the medial collateral ligament. In the normal knee, the superior meniscosynovial junction may be lax and mobile when probed with a hook, but the inferior meniscosynovial junction is tighter. In Fig.5.34 the meniscus has been lifted with a hook and the arthroscope passed beneath the meniscus to reveal a

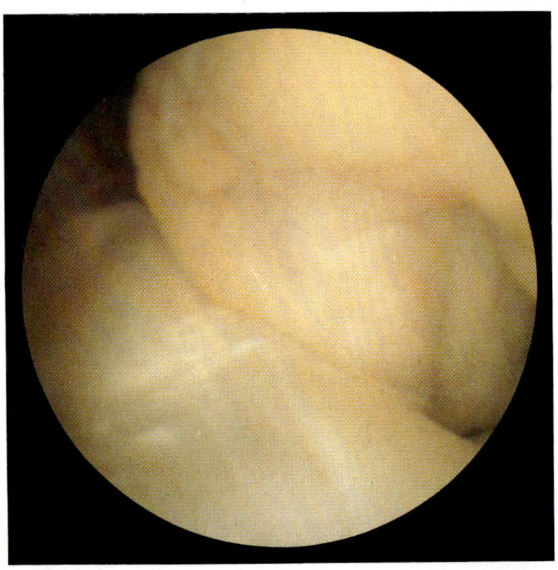

5.31

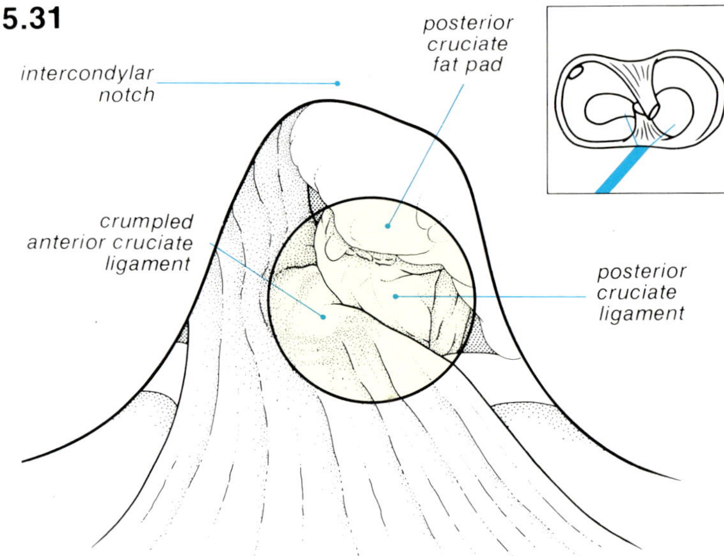

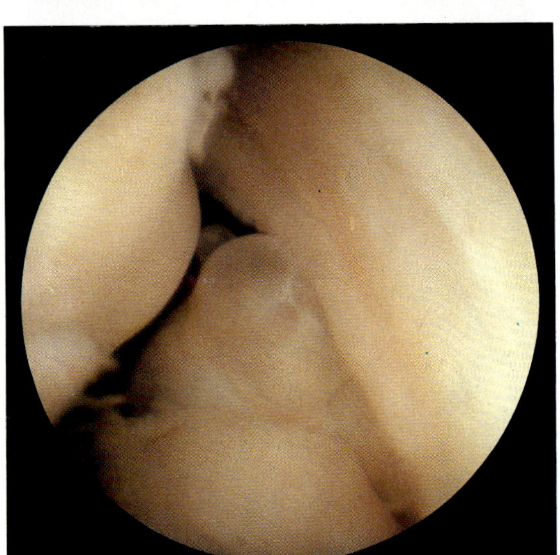

5.32

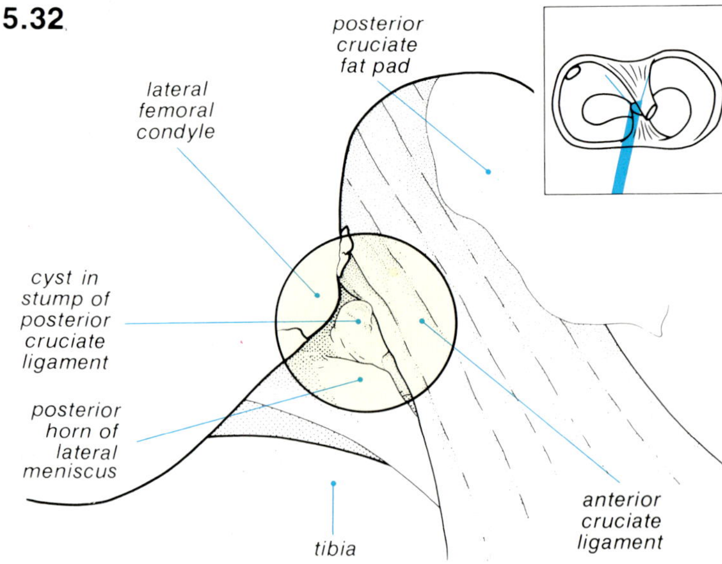

tear in the synovium through which the medial ligament can be seen at the level of the tibial plateau. This appearance is abnormal and is seen only in patients with ruptures of the medial collateral ligament.

The superior meniscosynovial junction is also affected when the medial ligament is torn. Fig.5.35 shows the superior meniscosynovial junction of a patient who had sustained an injury to the medial ligament and also had generalized ligamentous laxity. The synovium overlying the capsule has a tear through which the capsule can be seen. The meniscus, although abnormally mobile, was intact. Because the lesion is at the periphery of the knee, natural healing without surgical intervention is likely.

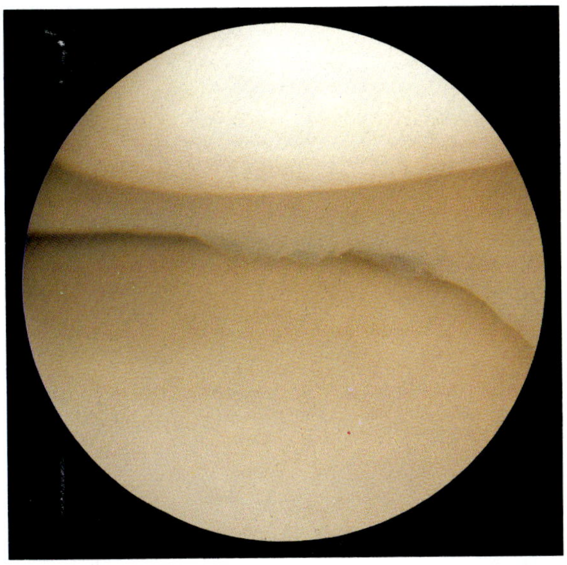

5.33

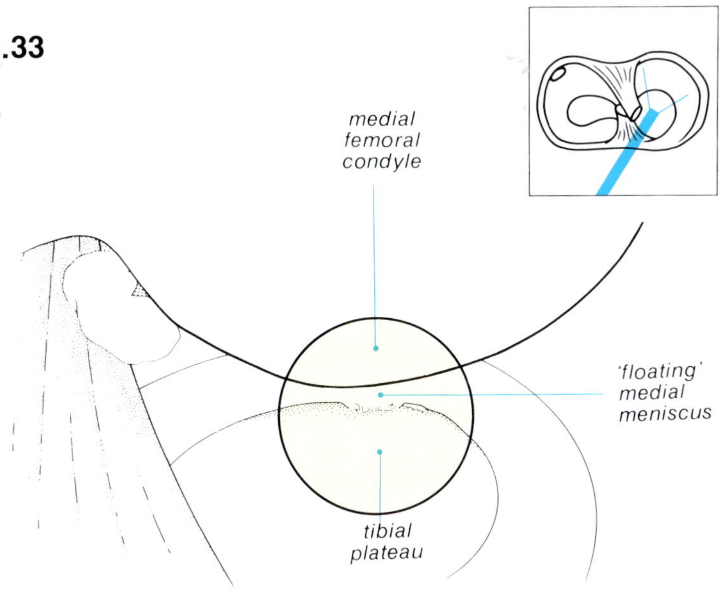

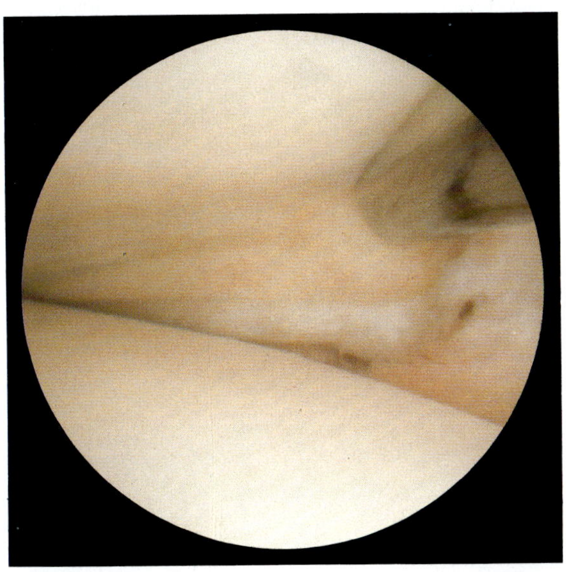

5.34

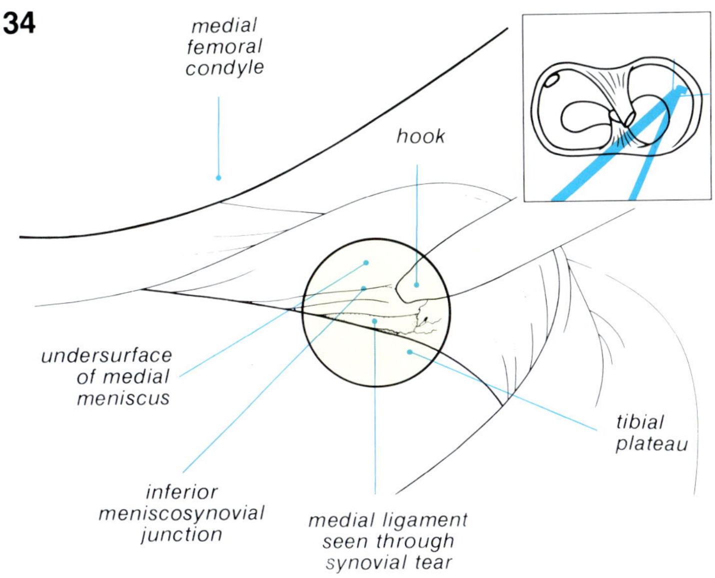

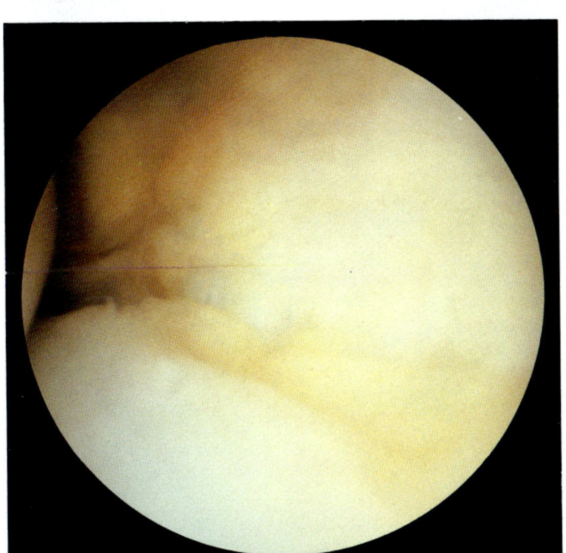

5.35

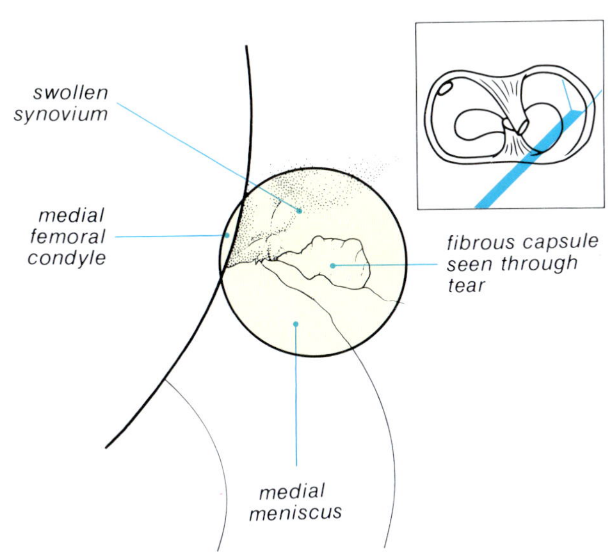

POPLITEUS TENDON

Despite taking a very curious course through the knee and having an intimate relationship with the lateral meniscus, the popliteus tendon very seldom gives rise to difficulties. However, there are occasions when symptoms do arise either from the tendon or its sheath. In Fig.5.36, the popliteus tendon is avulsed from the femur with a small block of bone which is being pulled forwards with a needle in the illustration. A narrow soft tissue band maintains some contact with the femur and has prevented the tendon from slipping completely down the popliteus tunnel.

Rupture of the popliteus tendon is rare, but the shape of the popliteus tunnel and its synovial lining make it a common site for synovitis. Fig.5.37 shows the insertion of the popliteus tendon and surrounding synovium in a knee that had been subjected to repeated small haemorrhages. The lining of the tunnel and the sheath covering the tendon are both intensely inflamed. The patient was troubled by discomfort around the lateral side of the joint, particularly when the tibia was rotated or the knee flexed.

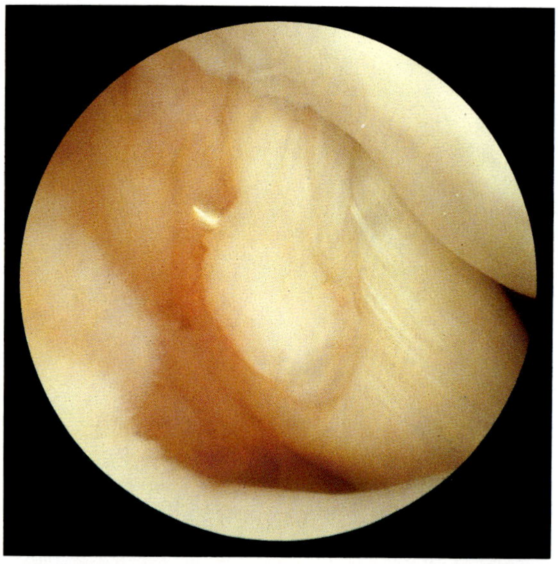

5.36

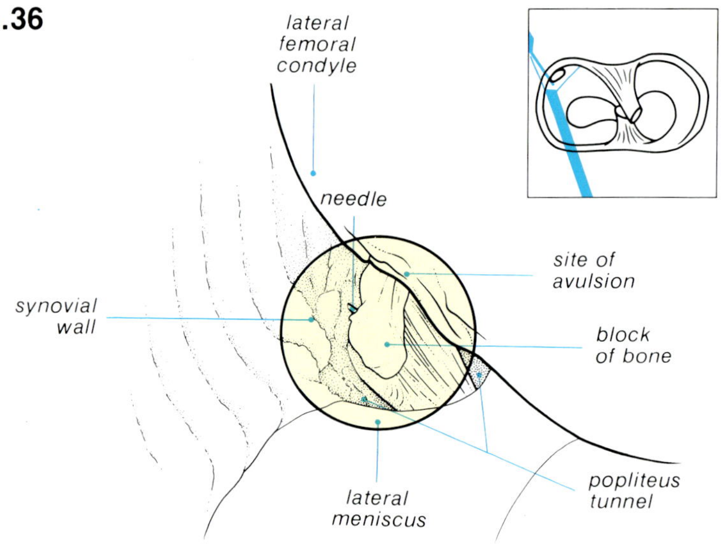

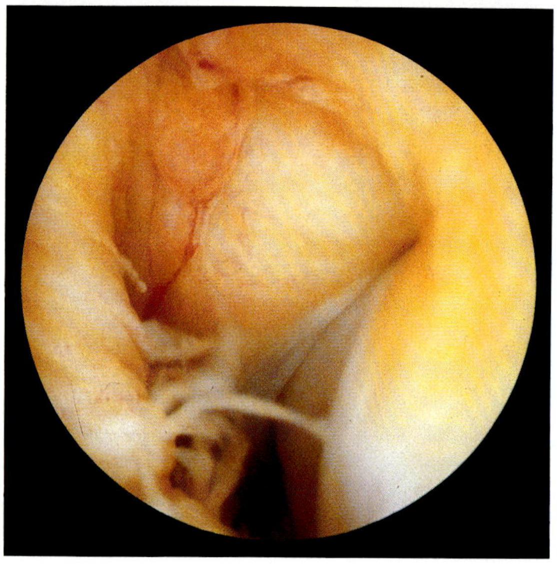

5.37

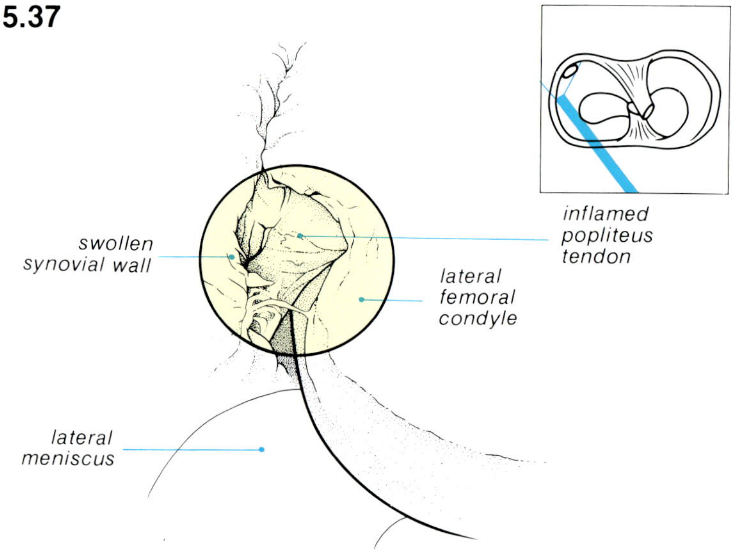

6
Pathology of the Menisci

I The Medial Meniscus

I. THE MEDIAL MENISCUS

Fig.6.1 is the knee of a patient who denied any history of operation and, indeed, no scar could be found around the knee. No symptoms were attributable to a meniscal lesion and the indication for arthroscopy was pain felt at the back of the knee on full flexion. At arthroscopy there was no sign of the medial meniscus in the normal position, the posteromedial compartment or anywhere else. Instead, a narrow knife-like rim was found in place of the medial meniscus (Fig.6.1). The patient had a positive pivot shift and jerk sign, but the anterior cruciate ligament appeared unusually slack although it was apparently intact within its synovial sheath. It may be that the patient had suffered a meniscal lesion early in life which was possibly accompanied by an anterior cruciate rupture or that there was true congenital absence of the medial meniscus and perhaps a dysplasia of the anterior cruciate ligament.

PATTERNS OF TEARS

Circumferential tears

Injuries of the medial meniscus are probably the most common internal derangement of the knee and the patterns of tear are numerous. In a patient who also had a ruptured anterior cruciate ligament from a fall when skiing, there is a peripheral detachment and tear in the medial meniscus at its vascular outer third, which is in close apposition to the vascular synovium (Fig.6.2). Peripheral detachments of this type are unusual but are most often seen in patients who also have ligament injuries. These lesions are very suitable for meniscal reattachment because at least one of the surfaces to be sutured has a vascular supply.

More commonly, the tear runs just inside the meniscosynovial junction. In Fig.6.3 there is considerable synovitis within the knee and pannus is extending onto the meniscus from the synovium. The unusually vascular synovium appears to be creeping across the meniscal surface towards the cleft. The distribution of the pannus, which is confined to the vascular outer third of the meniscus, may indicate the area in which repair or reattachment of the meniscus is a practical possibility. Alternatively, it may represent a process which could, if left undisturbed by arthroscopy or arthroscopic meniscectomy, result in natural healing of the meniscal lesion.

A more common appearance is a vertical split in the meniscal substance midway between its margin and the meniscosynovial junction (Fig.6.4). There is no sign of blood vessels anywhere so the two

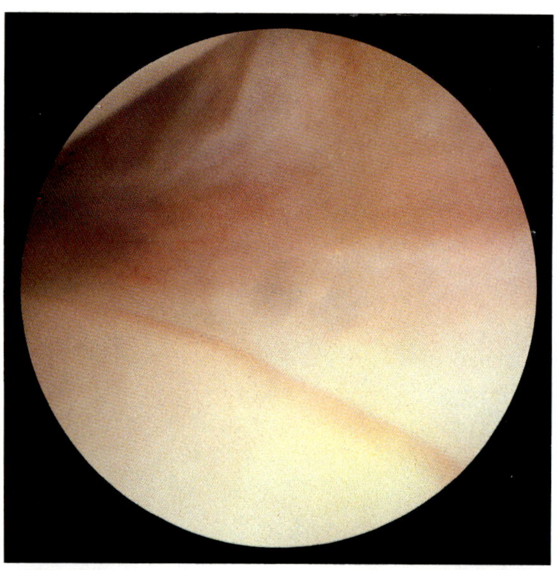

6.1

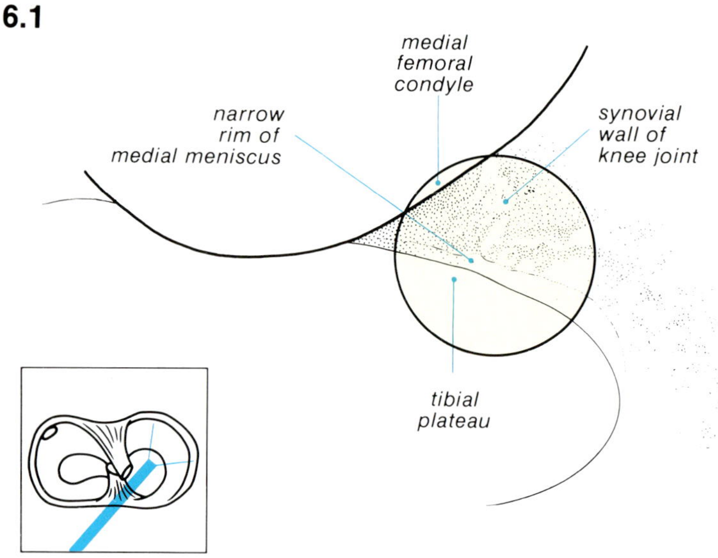

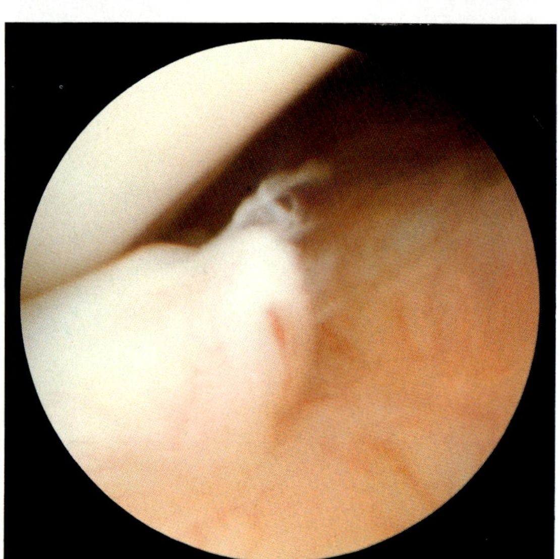

6.2

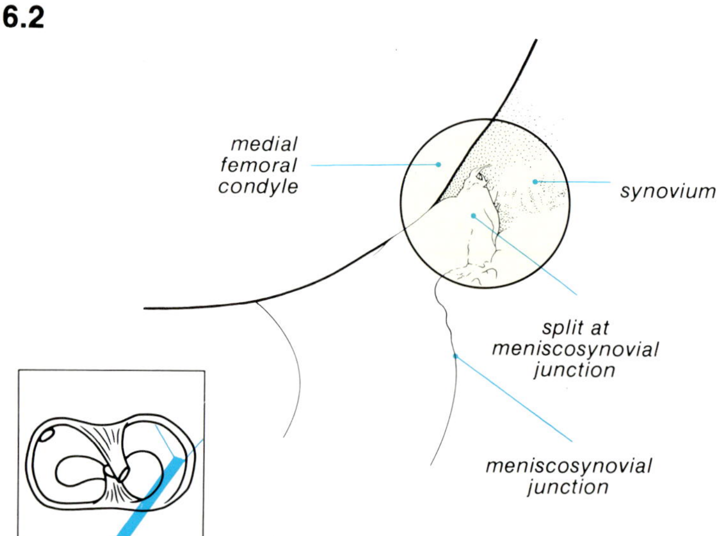

surfaces are avascular. The meniscal margins on both sides of the split are rounded, indicating an old lesion, and there are no signs of vascularity or healing at either edge of the meniscus. To demonstrate more clearly that the meniscal surfaces are avascular, the arthroscope can be passed directly into the cleft to inspect its sides (Fig.6.5). As no vascular markings can be seen, the potential for healing must be small indeed.

A constant feature of the rim of circumferential tears of the medial meniscus is the horizontal fissure, which lies at the centre of the meniscus and divides the rim into an upper and a lower leaf. In Fig.6.5 the fissure is so well marked that it appears almost as if there are two narrow meniscal rims stacked one above the other. The horizontal fissure may act as a natural plane of separation in the meniscus.

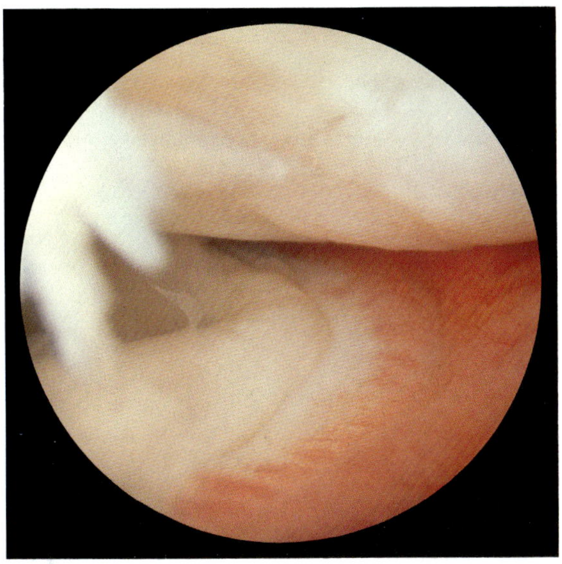

6.3

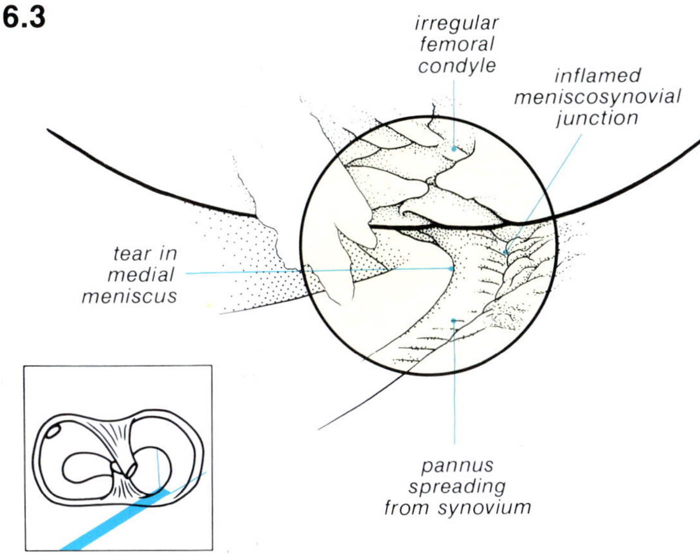

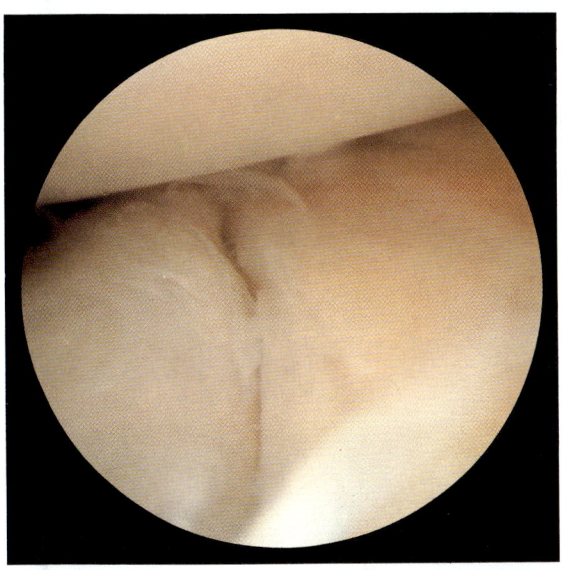

6.4

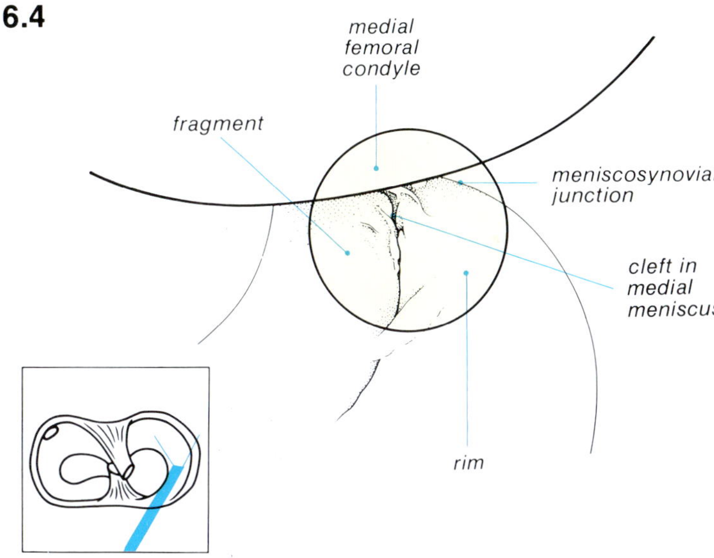

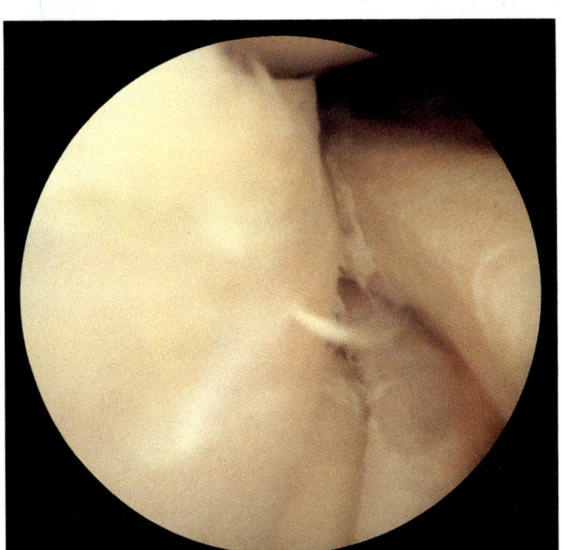

6.5

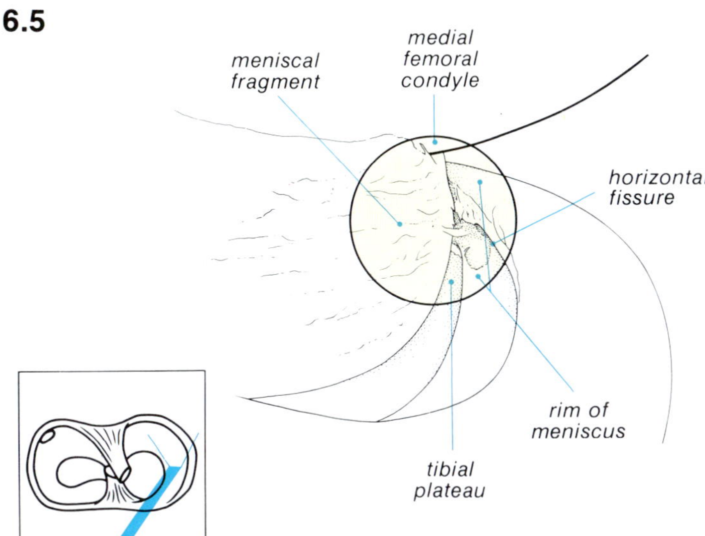

No horizontal fissure is seen in Fig.6.6 because the tear in the meniscus lies close to its free margin. The rim appears to be triangular with an intact vertical edge. Although this at first might be mistaken for an intact medial meniscus with an irregular rim, the vertical edge is invariably associated with a meniscal tear, most commonly of the bucket handle type. Occasionally the bucket handle fragment may rupture at its anterior limit so that the fragment falls into the posteromedial compartment and can escape notice. If the meniscal fragment is dislocated into the intercondylar notch or locked, a beam of meniscal tissue will be seen lying in front of the medial femoral condyle, obstructing the view of the posterior part of the medial compartment. In Fig.6.7, such a fragment of meniscus is locked into the intercondylar notch.

Circumferential tears of the medial meniscus almost always begin within a centimetre of the attachment of the posterior horn of the meniscus to the tibia and extend forwards for a variable distance. The extent of the tear and the anatomy of the meniscal fragment are of great importance during arthroscopic surgery and lesions of the medial meniscus can be divided into three categories. In the first, Type I or 'complete' tears, the tear extends along the entire length of the medial meniscus up to the anterior horn. The fragment from such a tear may lie so comfortably in the intercondylar notch that it gives rise to no symptoms and may be found quite unexpectedly. The fragment in Fig.6.7, which arose from a complete tear, caused only a slight block to extension and flexion and trivial disability.

The complete or Type I tear (Fig.6.7) is less common than an 'incomplete' or Type II tear in which the tear stops in the middle or anterior third of the meniscus. The term 'incomplete' is used not because the tear extends only part of the way through the meniscus but because it extends only part of the way along its length, stopping short of the anterior horn. In this type of tear (Figs.6.8 & 6.9) the meniscus is stretched tightly across the front of the knee and obstructs extension. The patient will usually complain of locking of the knee and an effusion.

In Fig.6.8 the fragment is riding unusually high and the posterior horn of the meniscus can be seen behind the medial femoral condyle. The torn surface of the meniscus has been twisted so that its hard central margin lies medial to the vertical surface facing the arthroscope, which was torn from the peripheral rim.

Fig.6.9 also shows a locked Type II fragment of meniscus. The fragment is a little broader than that in Fig.6.8 and is pushed so far forwards by the femoral condyle that it completely occupies the anterior part of the knee. These fragments can be so large and so close to the lens that they are difficult to assess arthroscopically. Attempts to pull the arthroscope away from the fragment may cause

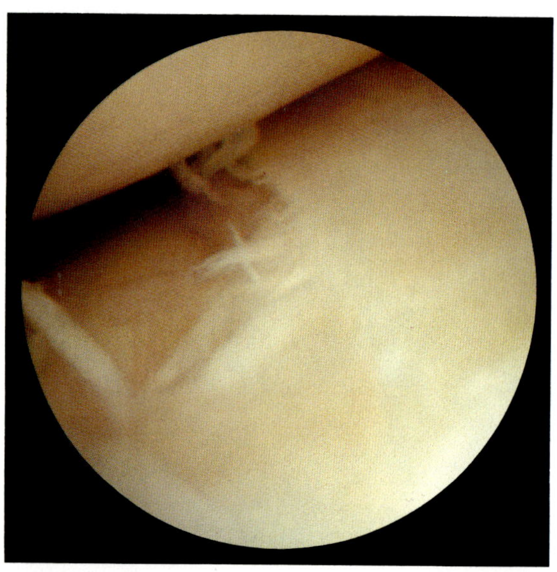

6.6

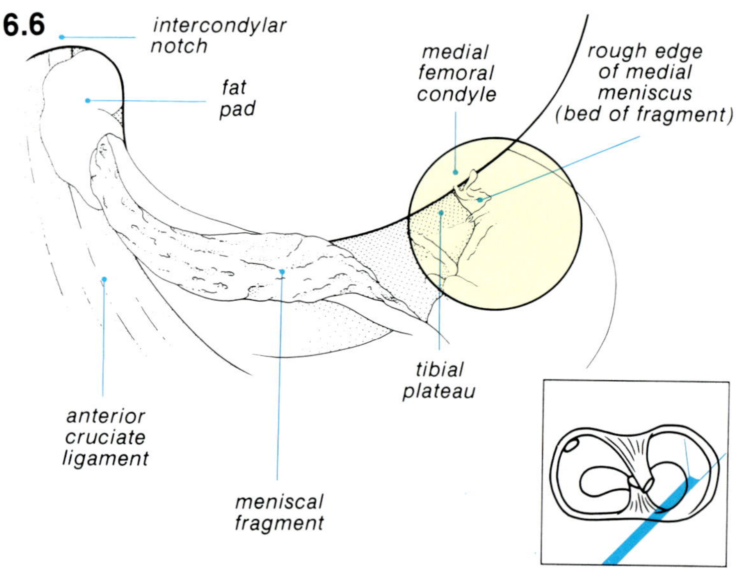

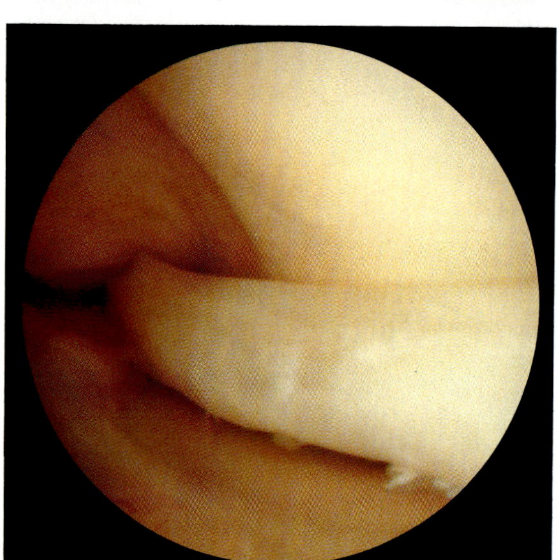

6.7

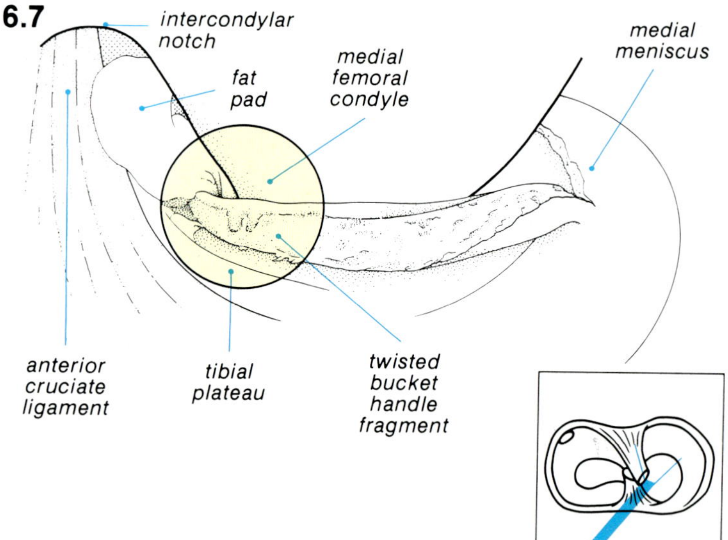

the tip of the sheath to lie in the infrapatellar fat pad which, in turn, may result in distension of the fat pad with saline and obliteration of the intercondylar notch by a soggy mass of distended tissue. This mishap can be avoided if care is taken to ensure that saline flows through the sheath only when its tip is lying within the synovial cavity.

When the meniscal margin lies in the intercondylar notch with the open surface of the tear lying laterally, a twist may be seen in the meniscus at its anterior limit (Fig.6.10). It is important to define this point precisely when performing an arthroscopic meniscectomy so that the fragment can be divided neatly at its anterior limit.

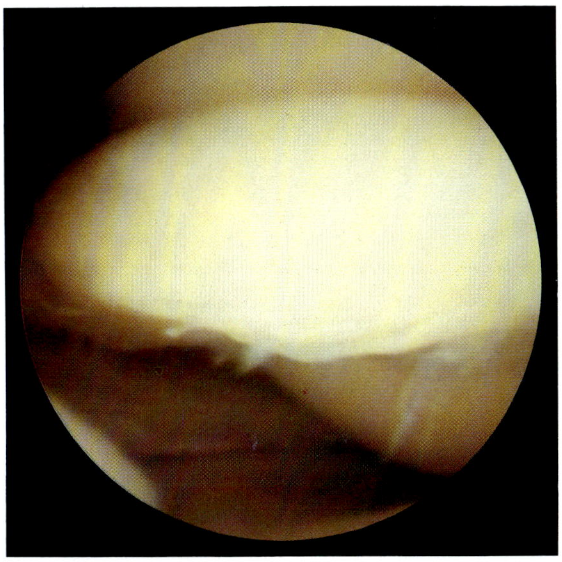

6.8

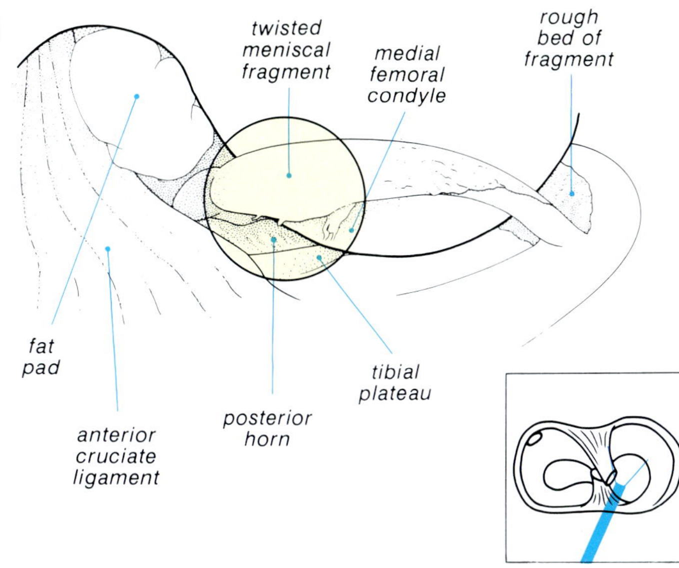

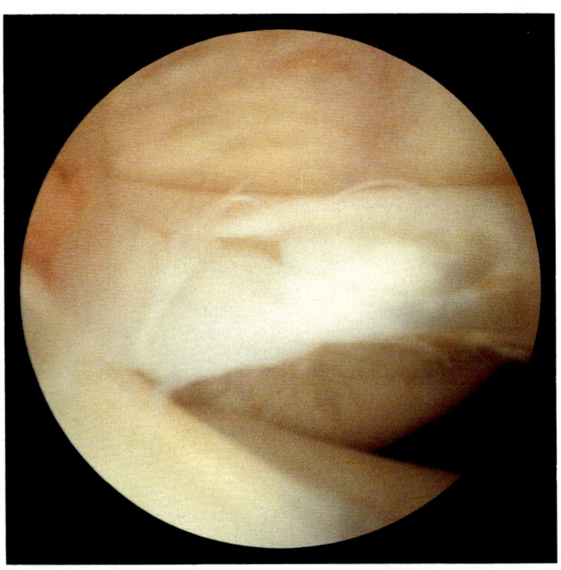

6.9

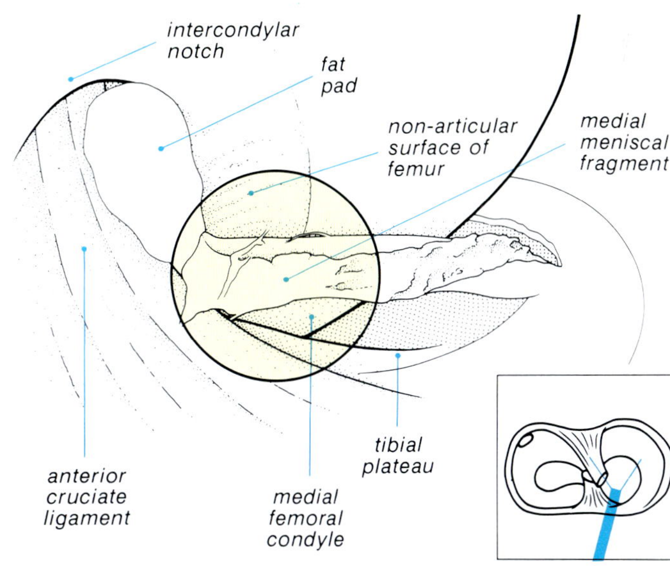

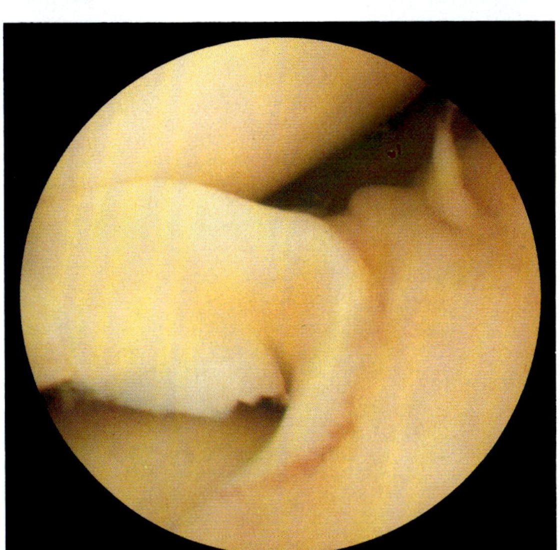

6.10

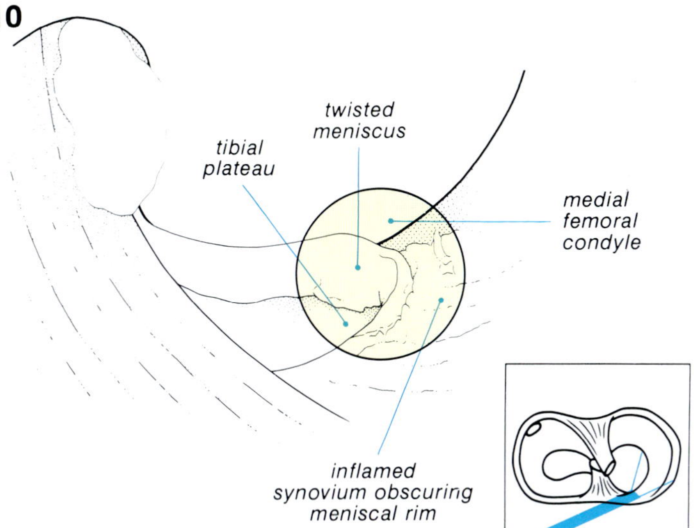

The line of cleavage of the meniscus does not always extend in front of the femoral condyle but may lie so far posteriorly that its anterior limit cannot be seen. Such a tear is termed a 'concealed' or Type III circumferential tear. In Fig.6.11 the fragment is jammed tightly in front of the femoral condyle, causing a marked block to extension. If the fragment is not dislocated in front of the condyle, the tear may escape notice because the fragment is not particularly mobile. A concealed tear may, however, be revealed by an unnatural prominence of the posterior third of the medial meniscus (Fig.6.12).

If the tear does not extend far enough forwards to create a fragment long enough to twist upon itself, the free margin will be stretched as it is pushed forwards by the condyle during locking episodes, producing the small radial tear seen in Fig.6.12.

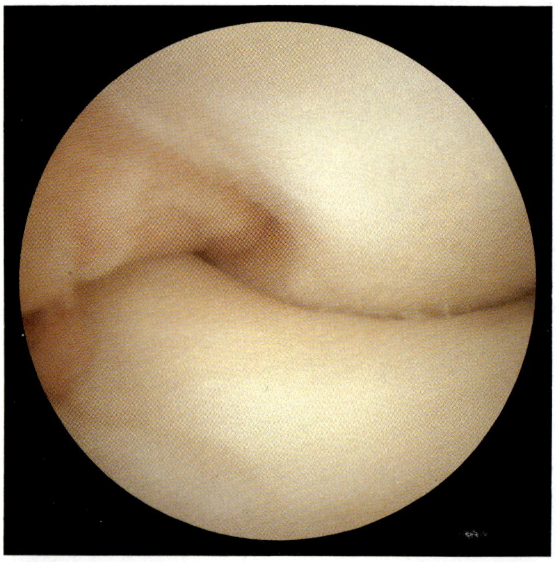

6.11

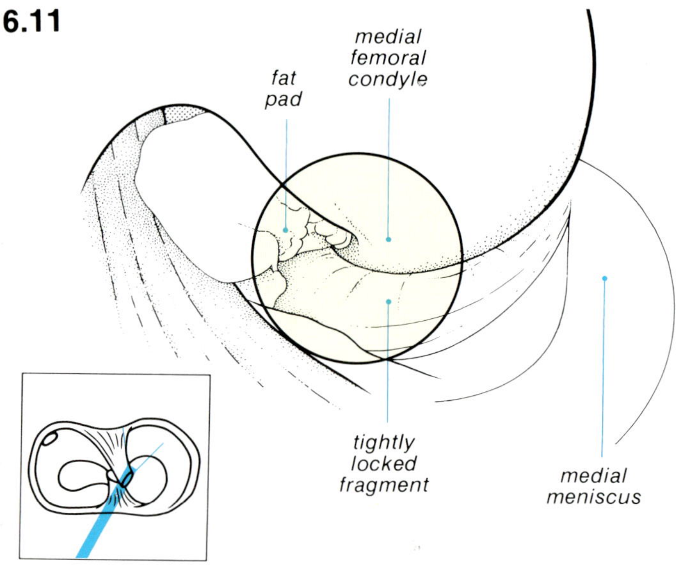

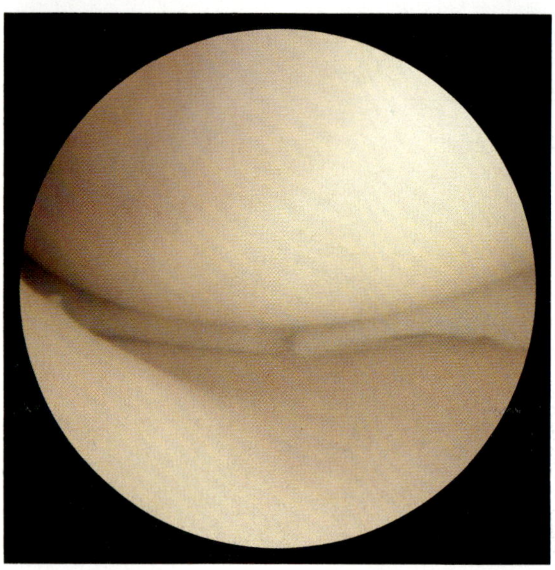

6.12

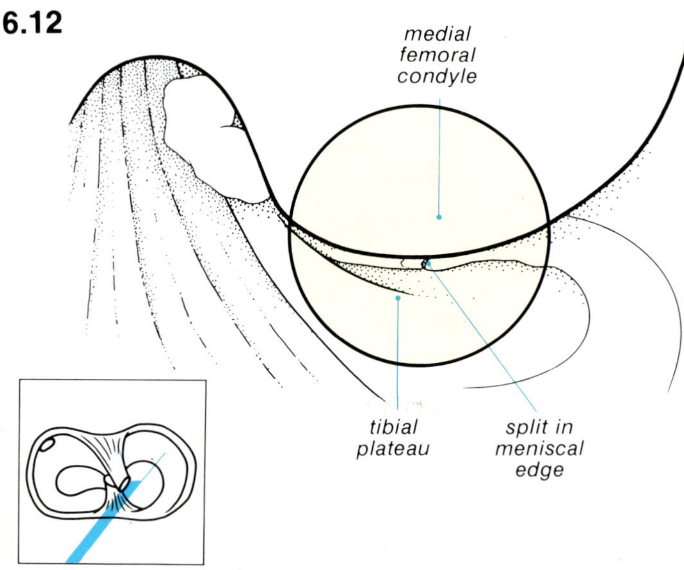

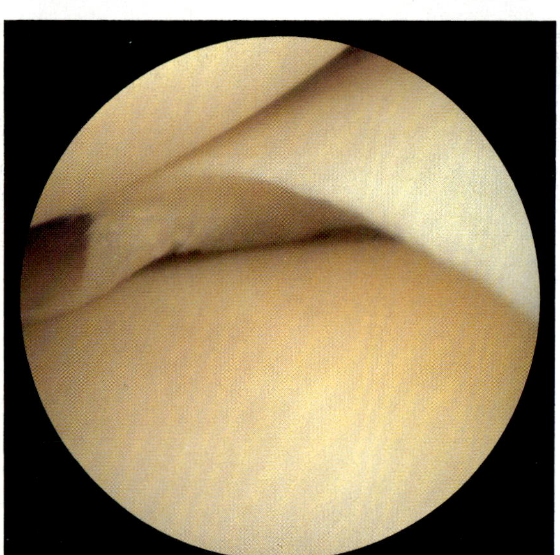

6.13

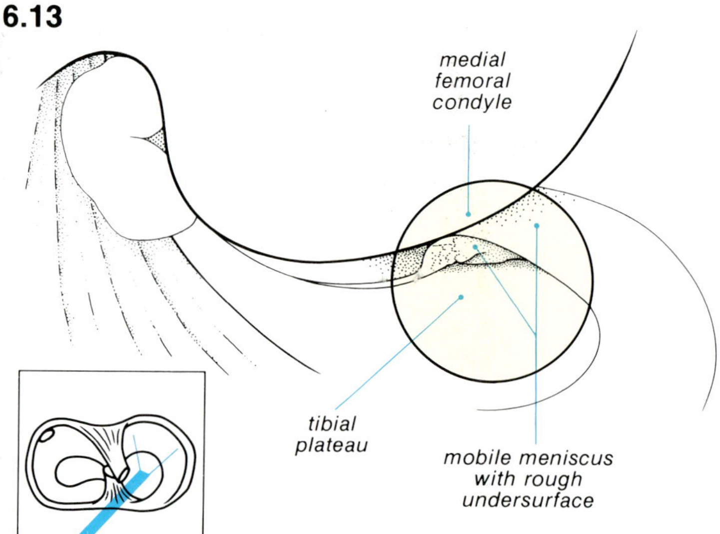

The natural history of the lesion in Fig.6.12 can proceed in one of two directions: either the tear may propagate forwards and produce a complete (Type I) or incomplete (Type II) tear; or the split may extend through the full width of the meniscal fragment and produce two short tags of meniscus.

Concealed (Type III) tears of the posterior third of the meniscus may also be revealed by unusual mobility of the posterior third even if no frank tear is present (Fig.6.13). The abnormal mobility of the meniscal fragment when probed with a percutaneous needle passed beneath the meniscal body into the fragment itself was so unequivocal that the presence of a tear was not in doubt and was confirmed by an irregularity of the undersurface of the meniscus.

Tears of the posterior third of the meniscus are especially common if the anterior cruciate ligament is ruptured because the meniscus is pulled forwards to lie beneath the weight-bearing arc of the medial femoral condyle (Fig.6.14). It is easy to see how continued or violent compression of the meniscus in this position could lead to a split in the posterior third, which could then extend forwards to form the more common incomplete (Type II) tear. This mechanism may well be the cause of most, if not all, circumferential tears of the medial meniscus. In Fig.6.14 the small loose body lying beneath the meniscus was removed arthroscopically.

The free margin of a meniscus with a concealed (Type III) tear may show slight irregularities. Fig.6.15 shows a tiny irregularity of the posterior horn, which might have been regarded as a trivial tear of no significance if it had not been for the patient's history of locking of the knee in flexion. The patient's history and clinical examination are of great importance because it is only possible to assess the significance of arthroscopic findings with full knowledge of the patient's symptoms together with the findings of clinical examination. To depend upon arthroscopic assessment alone in the management of a patient is no more sensible than to depend upon radiological examination alone.

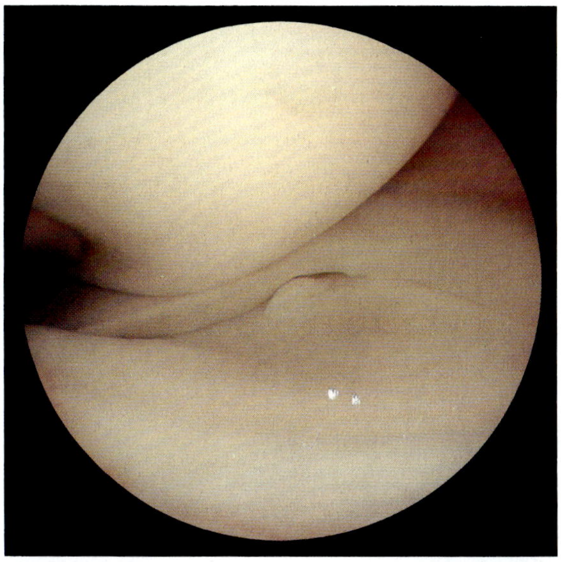

6.14

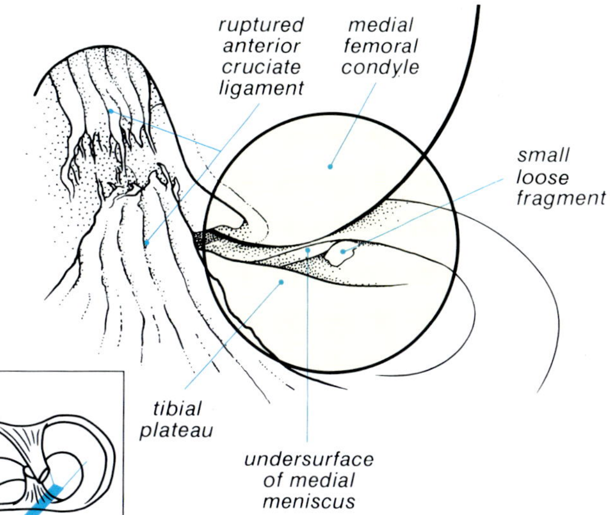

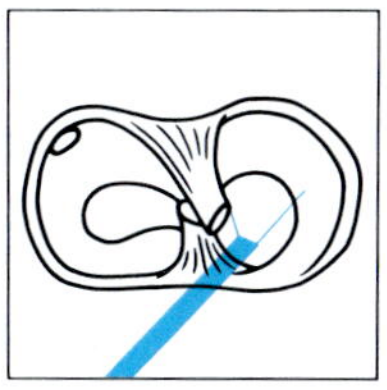

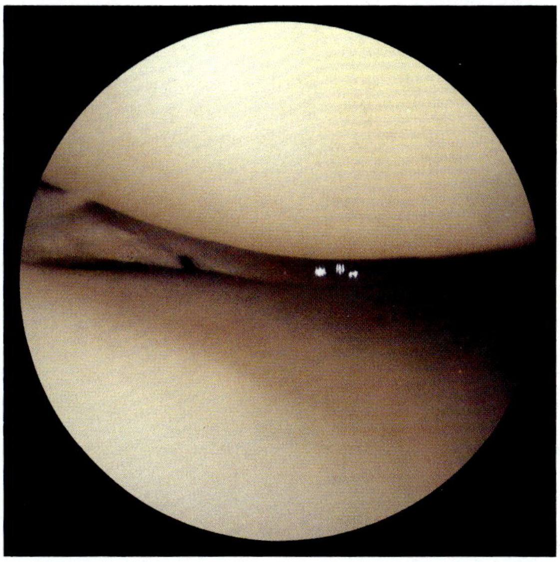

6.15

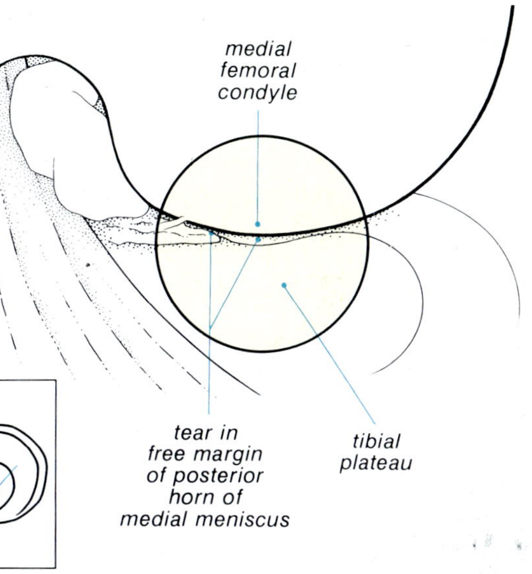

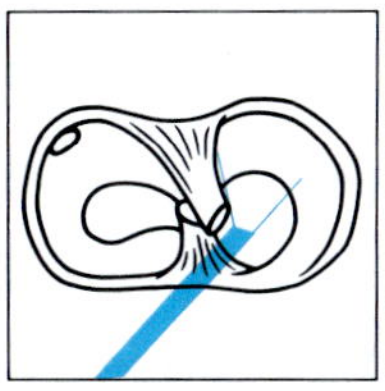

Tears in which the inferior surface of the meniscus has been disrupted but where the superior surface and meniscosynovial junction remain intact present particular problems for the arthroscopist, both in assessment and in management of the patient. The tear in Figs.6.16 and 6.17 cannot be seen from above and there is insufficient space beneath the meniscus to accommodate the arthroscope for examination from below. This patient experienced locking of the knee in full flexion. Only when a probing needle was passed beneath the meniscal body was a small tear seen on the undersurface. With the needle passed directly into the meniscal body so that it could be pushed forwards, the undersurface demonstrated abnormal mobility. Further investigation with a hook showed that the tear had extended approximately two-thirds of the way through

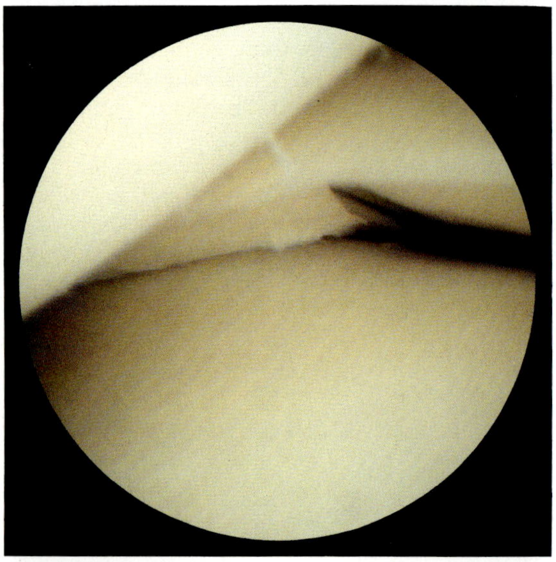

6.16

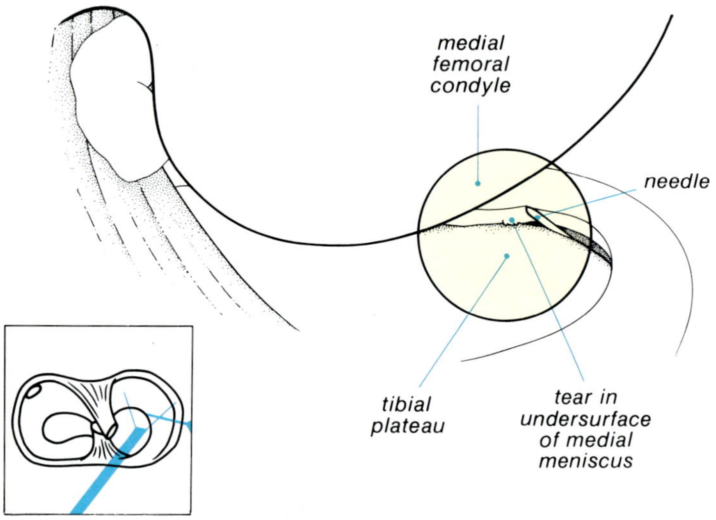

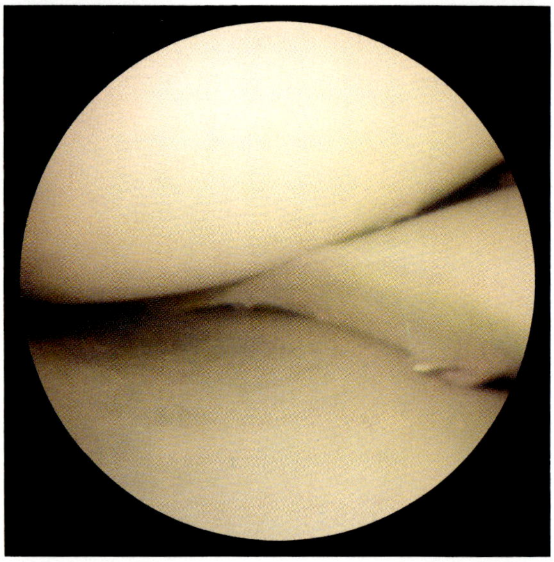

6.17

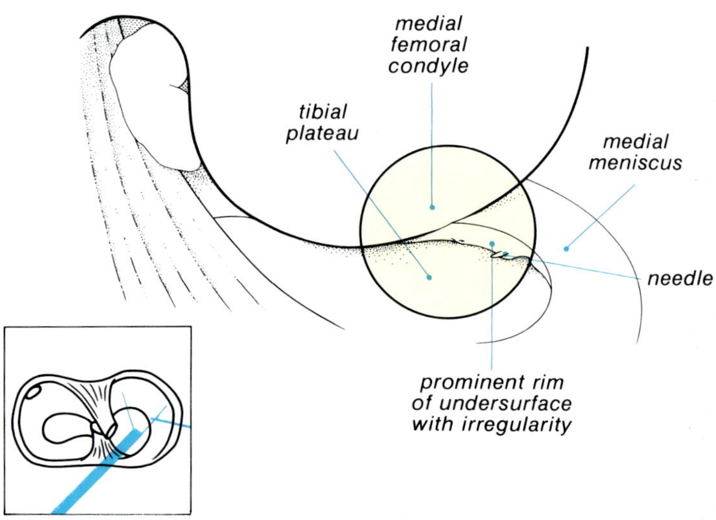

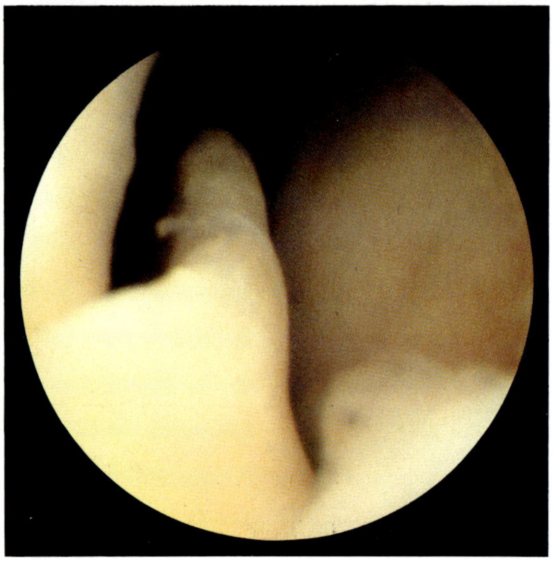

6.18

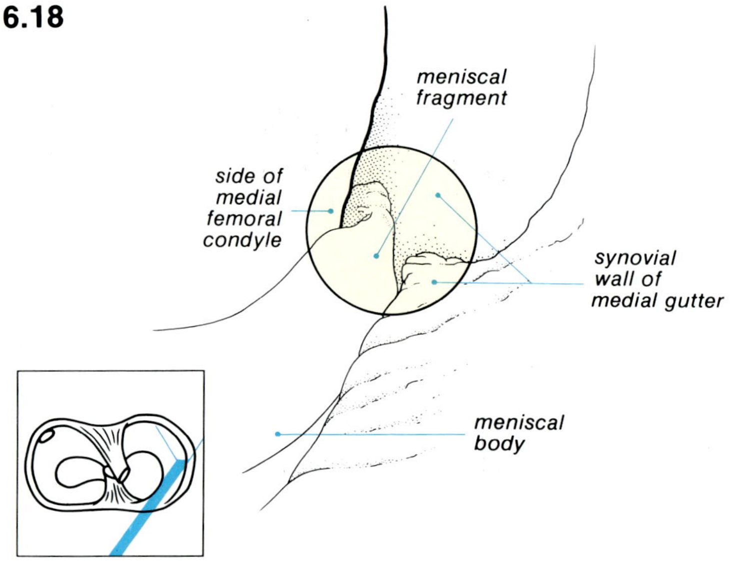

the meniscus from the inferior surface upwards. The loose portion of meniscus was removed arthroscopically.

These lesions probably represent the beginnings of a full thickness tear of the posterior third of the meniscus and should always be suspected if the patient complains of pain or instability of the knee on full flexion, even if there is no true mechanical locking. Such tears may be referred to as partial thickness tears of the posterior third to distinguish them from other patterns of lesion.

Although there is no conclusive evidence that partial thickness tears of the posterior third of the meniscus progress to full thickness Type III tears, the position of the lesion in the plane of weakness of the meniscus makes this possibility very likely.

Reattachment of the meniscal fragment either arthroscopically or at open operation is a difficult and uncertain procedure, while removal of the entire meniscus is unnecessarily radical. Removal of the mobile fragment alone presents technical difficulties but, despite this, is probably the treatment of choice at present.

Ruptured bucket handle fragments

Bucket handle fragments resulting from circumferential tears of the meniscus may rupture, producing long tags based anteriorly. Because the rupture usually occurs about 1cm from the posterior attachment, probably as the result of a radial tear (see Fig.6.12), the posterior stub of a ruptured fragment is usually less than 1cm in length while the anterior segment includes the remainder of the meniscus lying in the medial gutter. On clinical examination, the fragment could be felt as a mobile 'finger' in the medial gutter, moving in an arc based on its anterior attachment to the meniscus (Fig.6.19). As the anterior limit of the tear lies behind the anterior horn of the meniscus but in front of the medial femoral condyle, this represents an incomplete (Type II) tear. There is also a horizontal fissure in the peripheral rim (see also Fig.6.5).

Ruptured bucket handle fragments of this type may be multiple. In Fig.6.20 there are two bucket handle fragments, neither of which is lying along the full length of the medial gutter. The fragments must have arisen from the rupture of the components of a double bucket handle

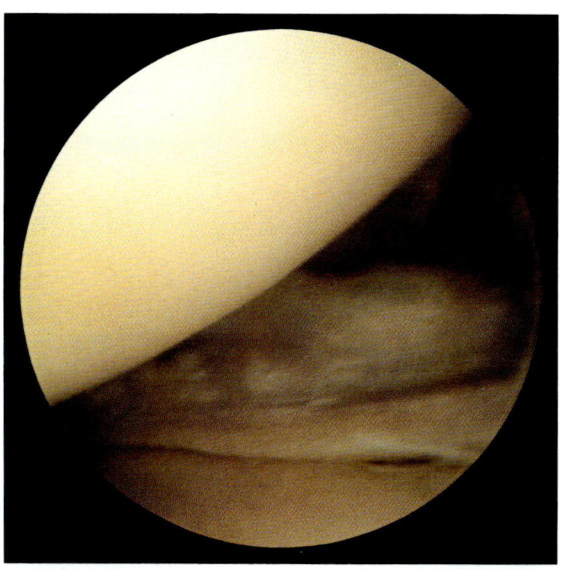

6.19

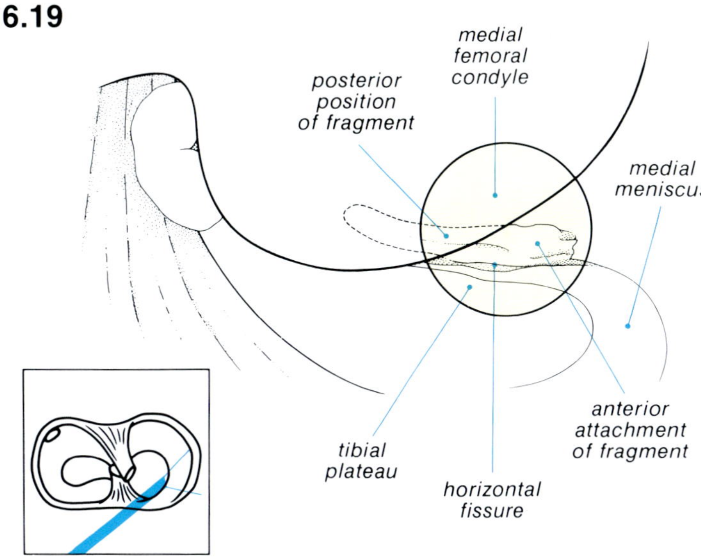

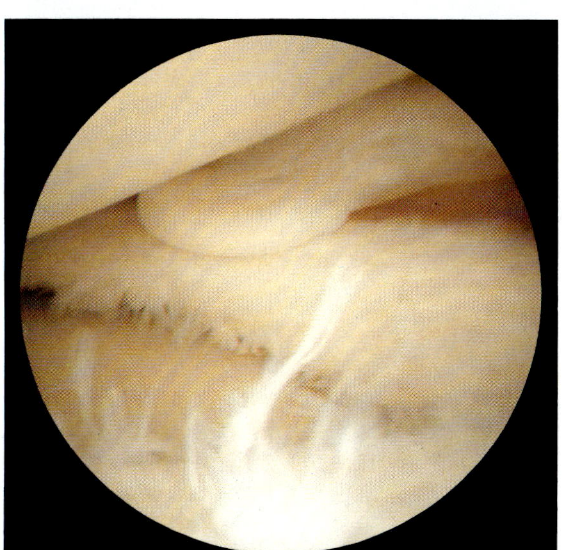

6.20

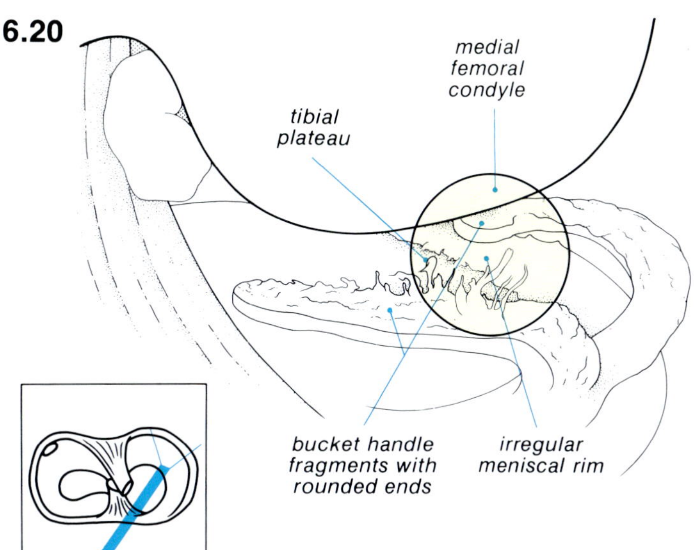

tear. It is interesting to note that the end of the meniscal fragment is smooth and rounded, which is a tribute to the efficiency of the natural healing process. This smooth finish was accomplished without the use of meniscal cutting instruments or powered shavers, the value of which must be seriously doubted in view of the excellent results achieved by nature alone.

Another variation of the detached bucket handle fragment is shown in Fig.6.21 where the fragment does not lie vertically in the medial gutter but behind the medial femoral condyle. At first sight the meniscus appears to have only the horizontal split in the rim, but closer inspection shows that the split does not continue along the full length of the meniscus and that the free edge is rising above the tibial plateau. A probing hook removed a large meniscal fragment from behind the femoral condyle. The anatomical pattern was similar to that of Fig.6.18 but the anterior limit of the tear lay more posteriorly, producing the somewhat confusing appearance of Fig.6.21.

Fig.6.22 shows another example of a ruptured bucket handle fragment from a Type II tear. The fragment has been pushed forwards rather than backwards or medially, and the fragment itself has become swollen and degenerate. Although most medial meniscal fragments retain their shape and consistency, this example shows the same appearance as a lateral meniscus which has undergone cystic degeneration. The tissue was friable and soft when grasped with arthroscopic instruments and lacked the normal firmness of a meniscal fragment. The articular surface of the femur adjacent to the fragment showed degenerative changes, perhaps the result of repeated contact with the degenerate fragment.

Flap tears

The circumferential tears demonstrated have all involved the full thickness of the meniscal substance and have arisen from a vertical split. Horizontal splits also occur in the posterior third of the medial meniscus and give rise to flaps of tissue that bear a superficial resemblance to detached bucket handle fragments. Close inspection, however, will demonstrate that these flaps lack the thickness of bucket handle fragments.

Fig.6.23 shows a meniscal flap with a clean detached end which is consistent with its having been caused by a radial tear (see Fig.6.12). Careful examination of the torn edge of the stump reveals a cross-section of the upper half only of the meniscus. If the fragment involves only part of the meniscal thickness, it may be considered a flap tear rather than a ruptured bucket handle fragment; but exact separation of these groups is not always possible and classification of the fragments may be difficult. The anterior limit of the circumferential tear,

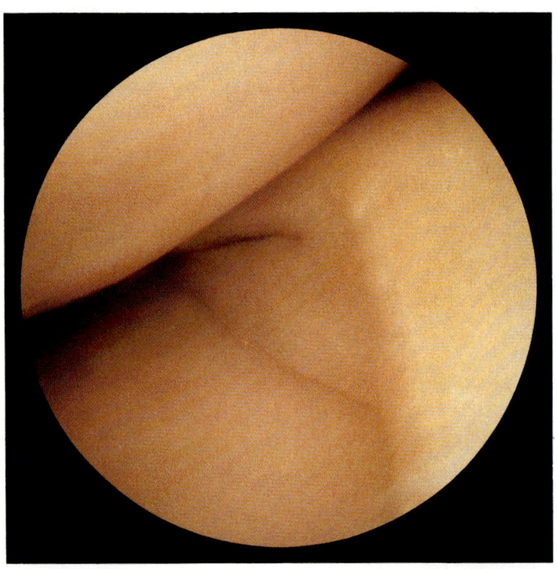

6.21

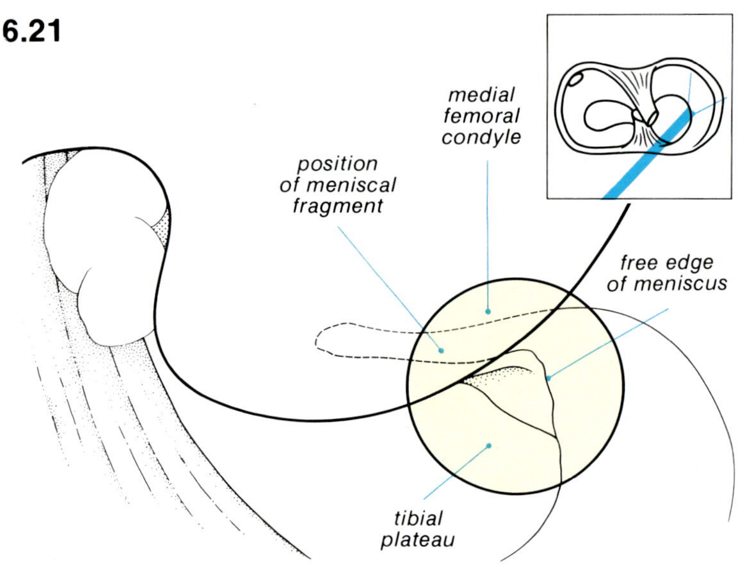

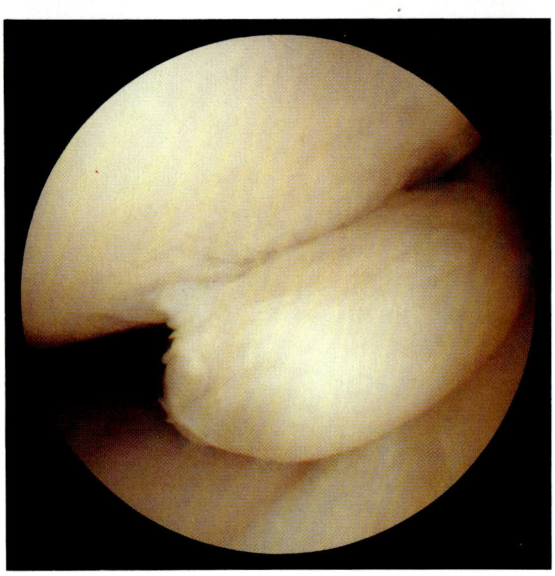

6.22

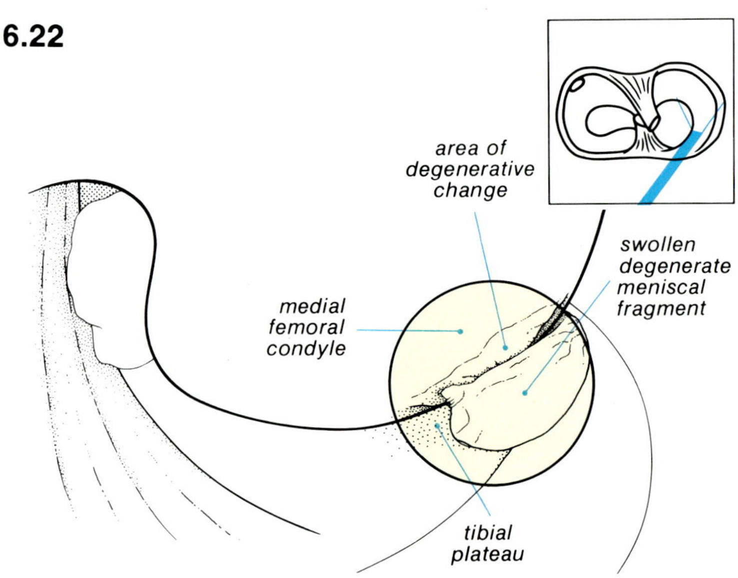

from which the fragment seen in Fig.6.23 arose, lies behind the femoral condyle so that it could be classified as a detached concealed (Type III) bucket handle fragment but it is perhaps best regarded as a thick flap.

The meniscal fragment shown in Fig.6.24 has been pushed forwards to lie in the medial gutter and is thinner than that in Fig.6.23. The ruptured end is more cleanly 'cut', but again it involves only the upper half of the meniscus. This fragment proved to be a flap tear.

In Fig.6.25 a similar small flap of medial meniscus is lying in the medial gutter. The flap is old, its edges rounded, and the patient was aware of the clicking and catching at the posteromedial corner of the knee. The symptoms were relieved by arthroscopic excision of the flap, leaving the rest of the meniscus intact.

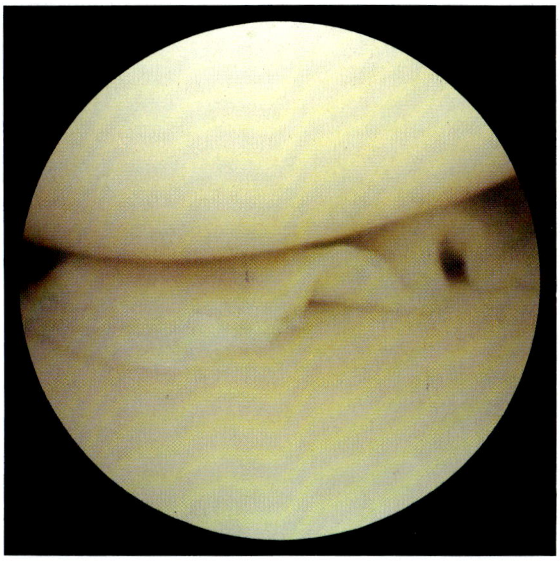

6.23

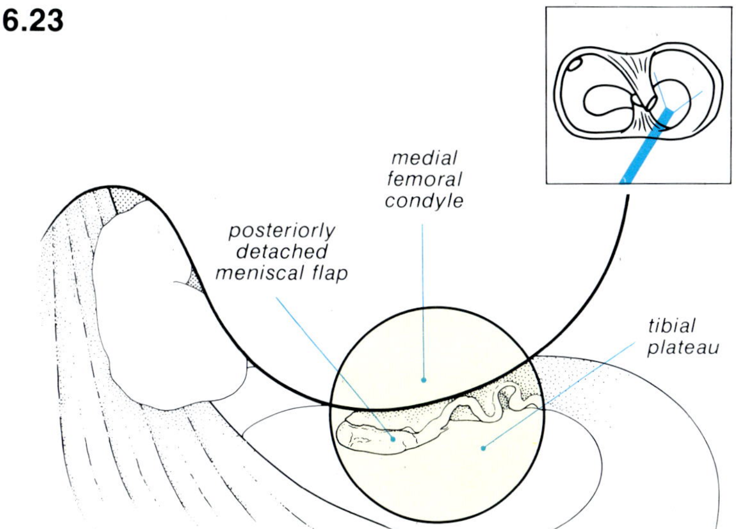

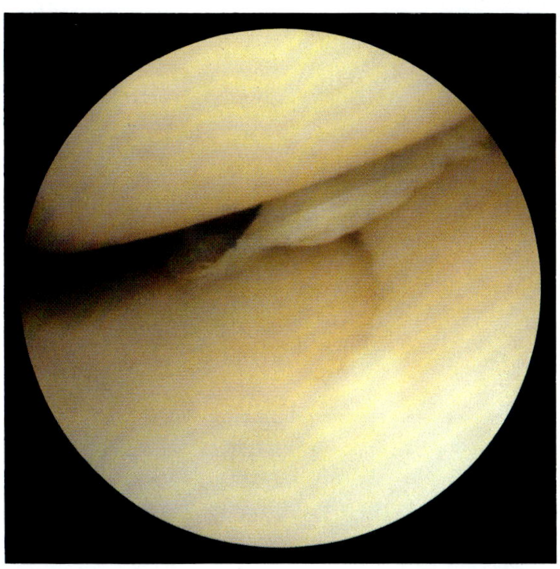

6.24

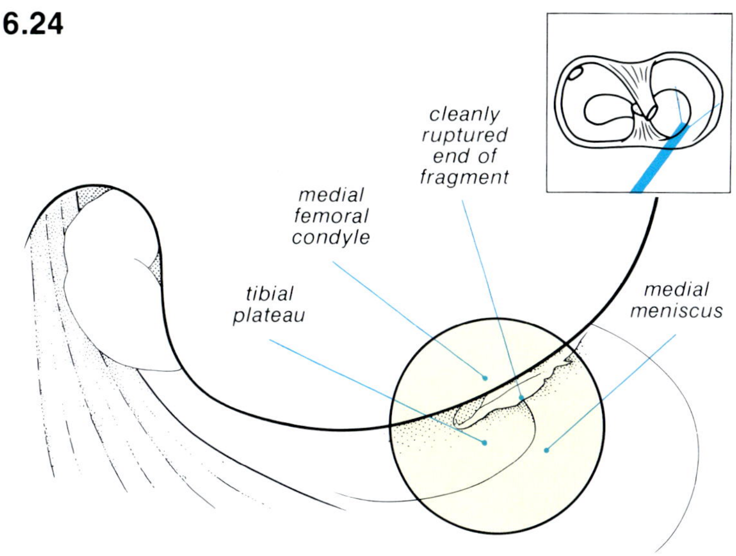

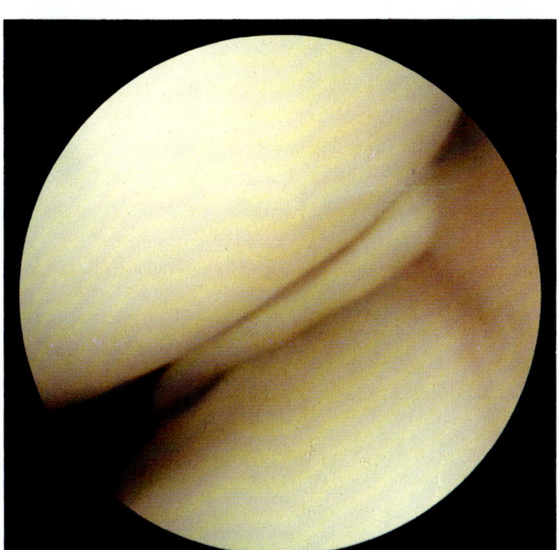

6.25

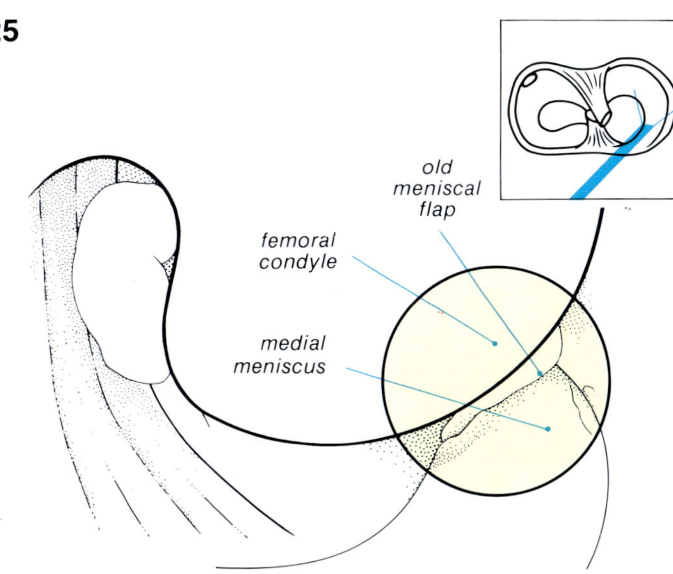

The meniscal fragment seen in Fig.6.26 also lies in the posteromedial corner of the knee, but the fragment is larger and is jammed not in the medial gutter but between the medial meniscus and the femoral condyle. The patient's symptoms were also of clicking and catching at the posteromedial corner of the knee but were more severe, and the fragment itself could be felt moving in the posteromedial corner of the knee. The fragment is unusually thick for a flap tear and may well have resulted from the rupture of a full thickness concealed (Type III) bucket handle fragment.

When the flap was pulled forward with rongeurs, the meniscal remnant came away smoothly, leaving the meniscal body intact (Fig.6.27). Apart from roughness indicating that the superficial layers of the meniscus have been peeled away, the meniscus could pass for normal. This appearance is unusual when full thickness bucket handle fragments are removed, the usual result being a clean vertical edge to the meniscus. Assessment of the anatomy of flaps and detached bucket handle fragments of the posterior third of the knee can be difficult and precise anatomical definition of the lesion may be impossible until the fragment has been removed and the meniscal rim can be examined.

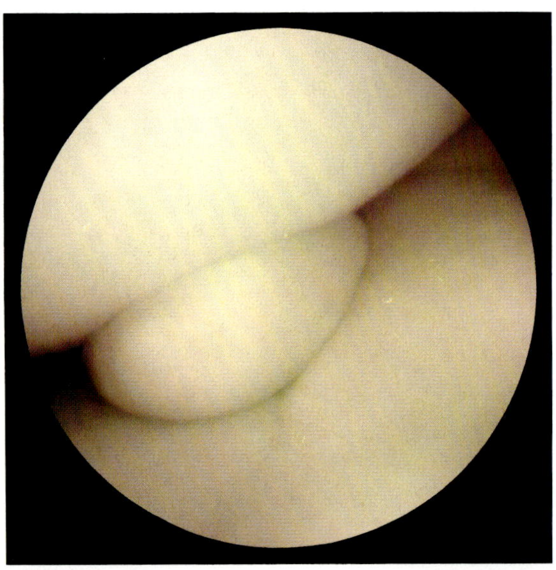

6.26

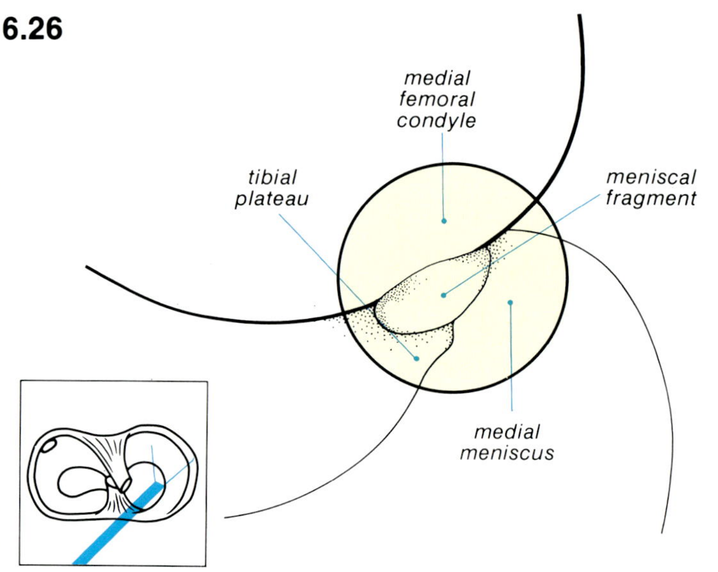

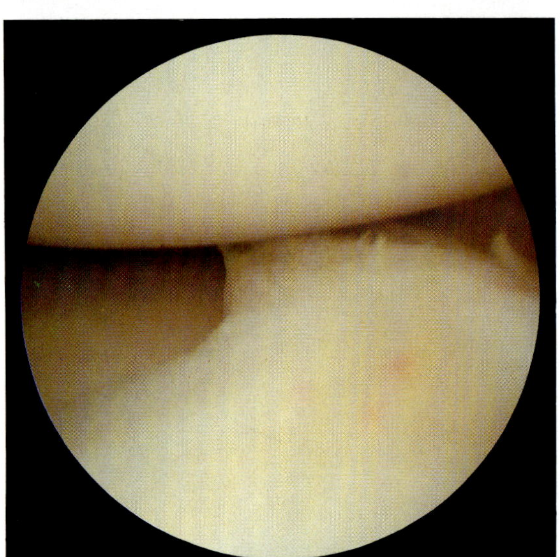

6.27

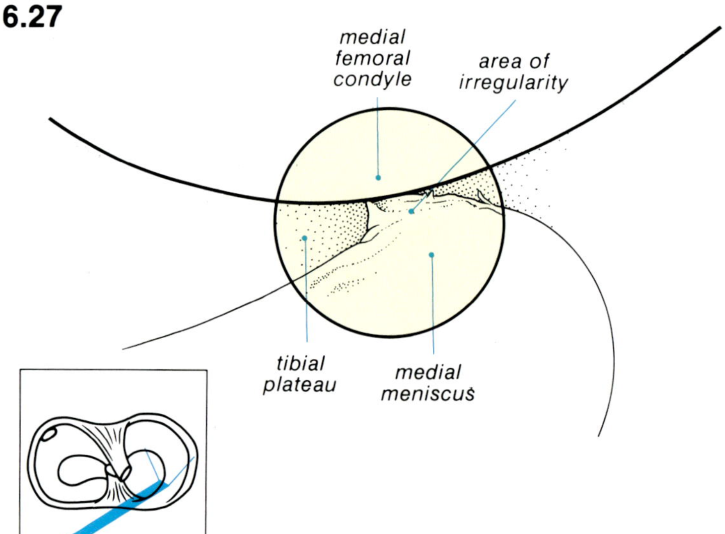

Meniscal flaps can sometimes become tucked under the main meniscal body. Fig.6.28 shows a rounded or rolled edge of meniscus which on superficial inspection might be regarded as normal, but this appearance is always pathological and invariably associated with a tucked-under flap. The flap is usually stiff and may be difficult to extract. In Fig.6.29 a needle has been pushed through the meniscus in an attempt to push the flap out from beneath the meniscus, but the resilience of the fragment pulled it back as soon as the needle was removed.

Most inverted or tucked-under flaps can be extracted without difficulty (Fig.6.30) but flaps are not always as

6.28

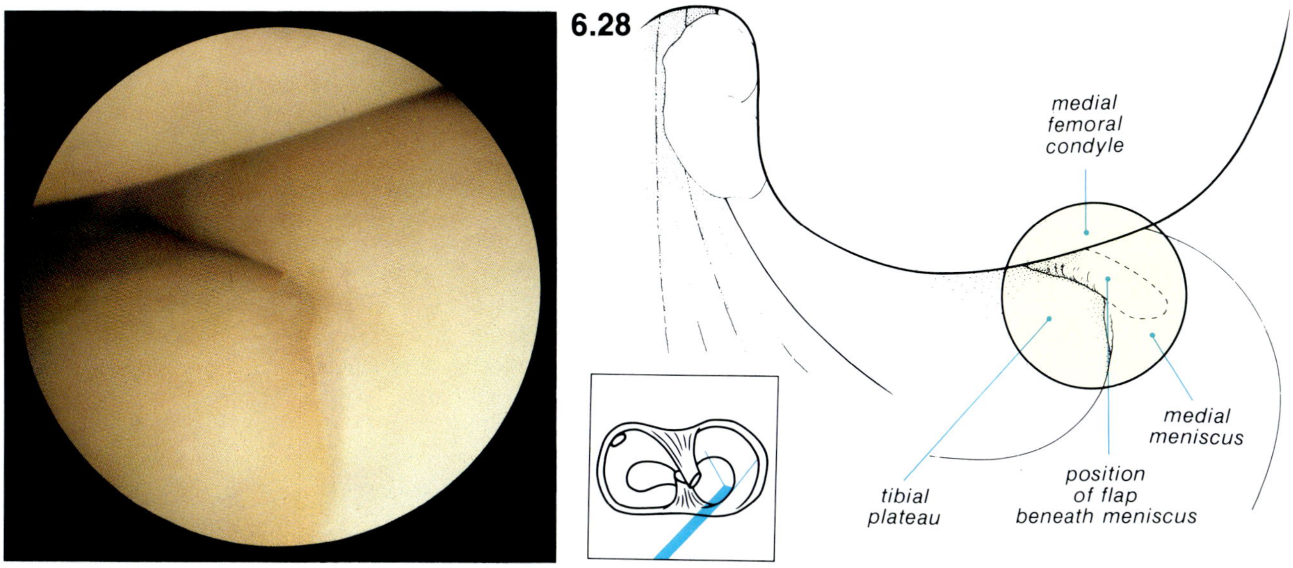

6.29

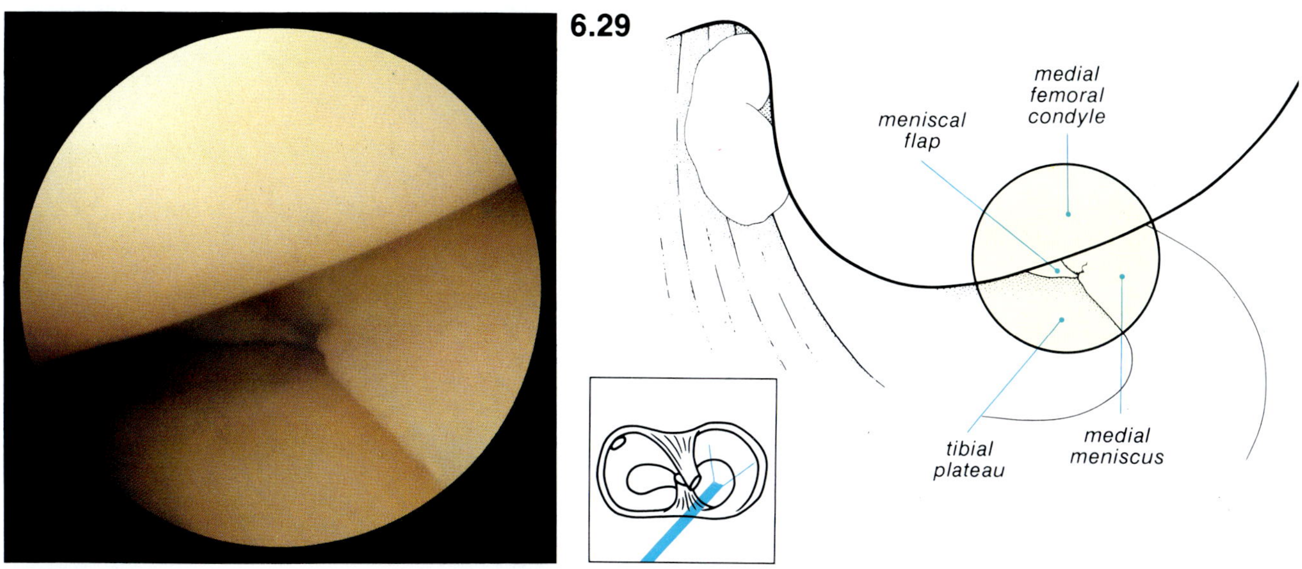

6.30

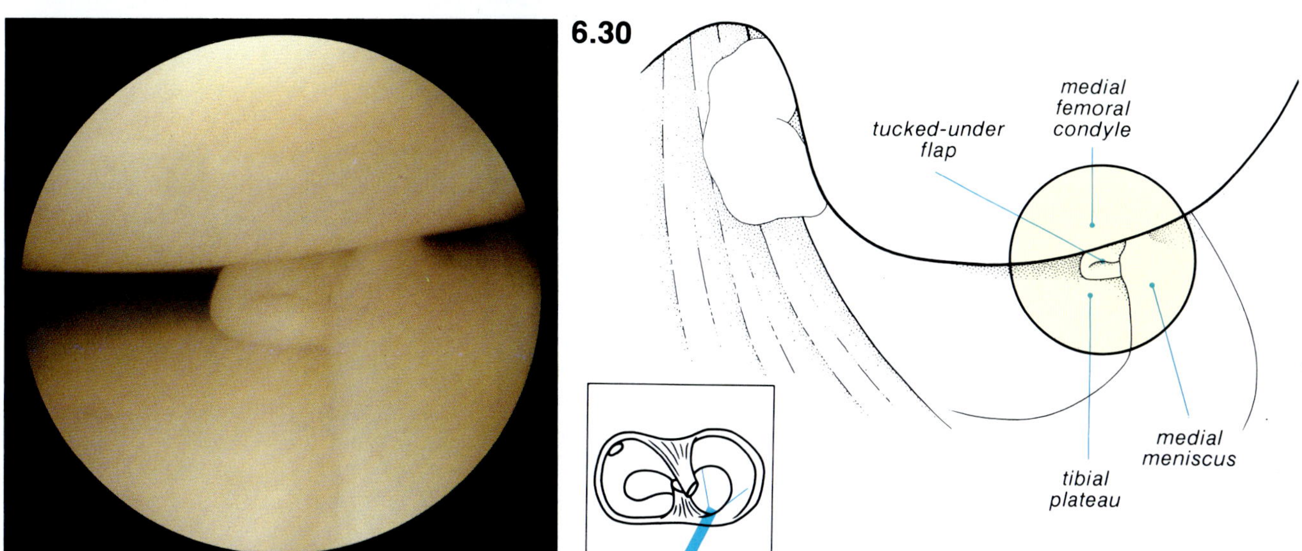

thin as that in this illustration. Fig.6.31 shows a thick meniscal flap tucked beneath the posterior third of the meniscus. The point at which these meniscal flaps become inverted is quite constant and lies where the medial meniscus sweeps away from the capsule of the knee to run behind the medial femoral condyle.

In Fig.6.32 the arthroscope has been slipped beneath the medial meniscus, revealing a flap between the tibial plateau and the meniscus. There is intense synovitis with large pendulous masses of inflamed synovium. This appearance is exaggerated by the proximity of the fronds to the lens of the arthroscope; a true impression of their

6.31

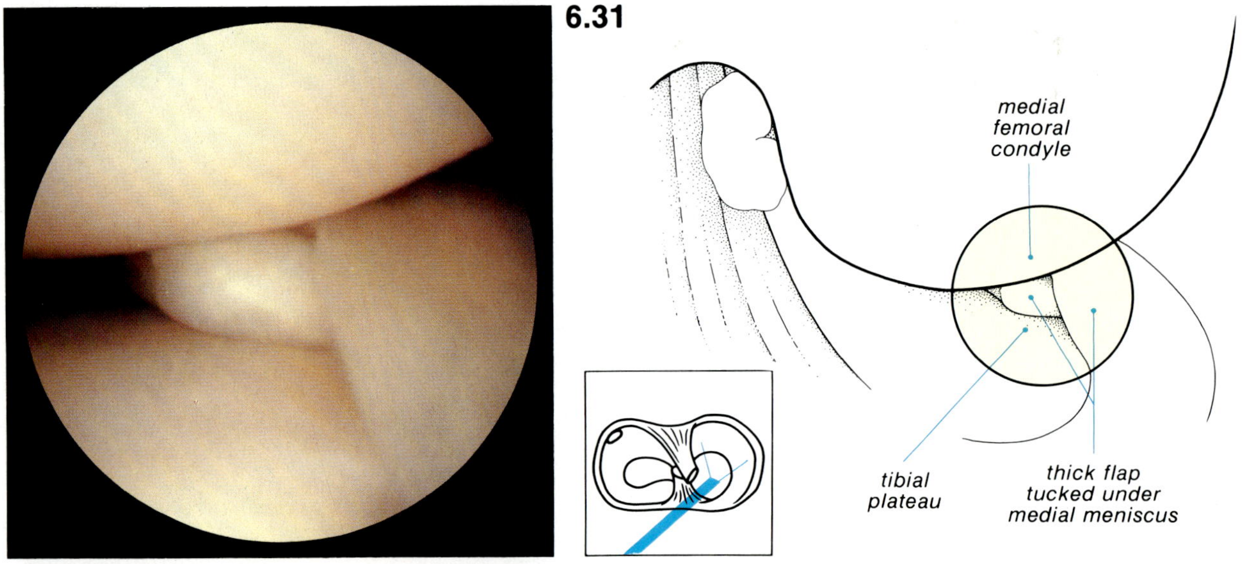

6.32

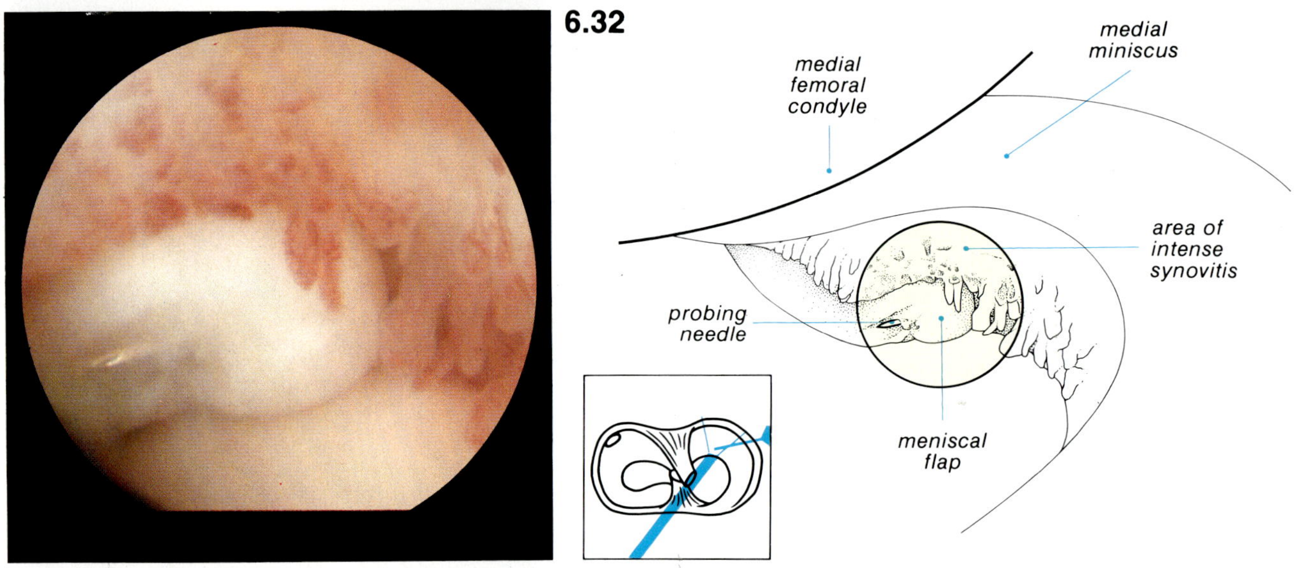

6.33

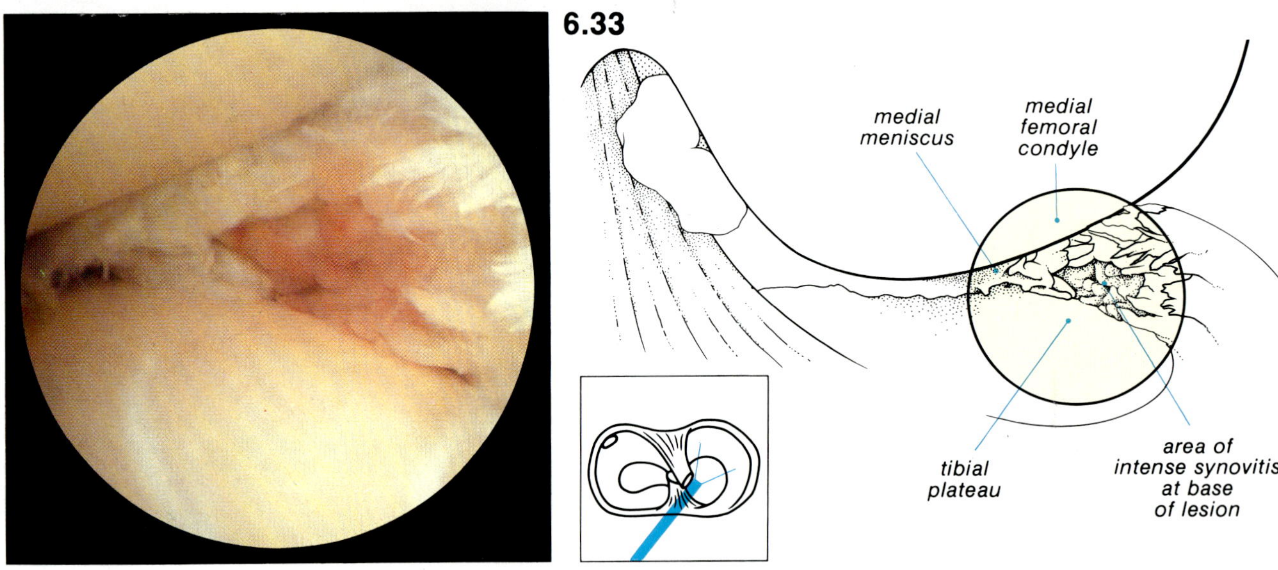

size can be obtained by comparison with the probing needle.

If the posteromedial joint line is particularly tender before meniscectomy and synovitis is present, the synovitis is likely to persist after operation and the patient may be disappointed that the pain does not disappear immediately. In Fig.6.33 an inverted fragment has been removed from the inferior meniscosynovial junction, but the synovitis in the cleft is so intense that it resembles granulation tissue and such synovitis is slow to resolve.

Not all meniscal flaps come to lie in the medial gutter or beneath the medial meniscus; many of them remain free in the joint space. Fig.6.34 shows a long flap from the undersurface of the posterior third of the meniscus which was the result of a split along the cleavage in the centre of the horizontal plane of meniscus. The flap was unusually long and had a slightly rounded or bulbous end, a feature more usually seen at the ends of ruptured bucket handle fragments (see Fig.6.20).

To illustrate further the importance of the rounded meniscal rim as an indication of a meniscal tear, Figs.6.35 and 6.36 show a particularly large meniscal fragment that has become inverted at the usual site, the junction of the middle and posterior thirds of the medial meniscus. The meniscal margin is rounded with a small fissure at the anterior limit of the abnormal edge (Fig.6.35). A needle is passed beneath the meniscal body,

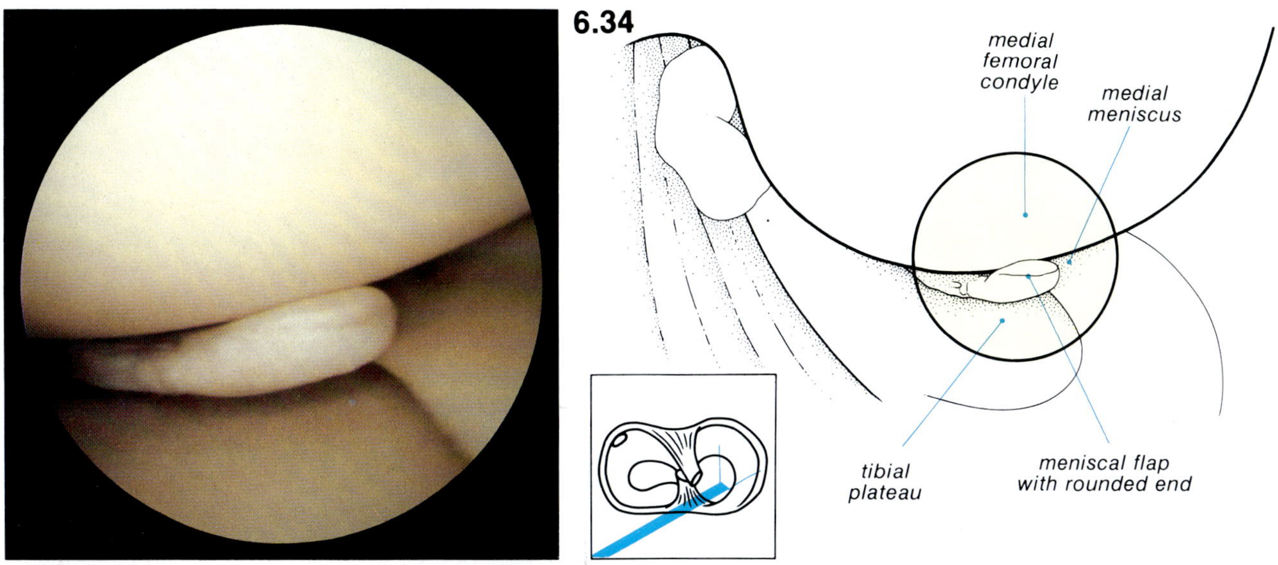

6.34

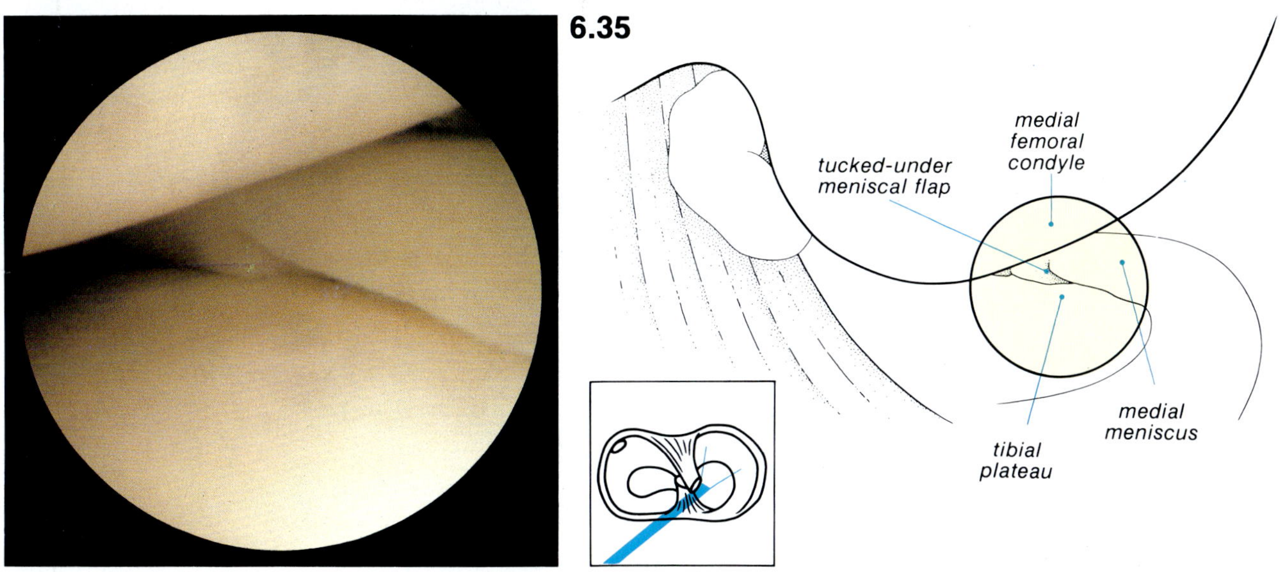

6.35

moving the fragment which is now seen to be a long stub, representing a ruptured bucket handle fragment well over 1cm in length (Fig.6.36). The fragment was stiff, as is usual, and its base had to be excised to achieve a smooth meniscal rim.

Concern is often expressed about the 'retained posterior horn fragment' of the medial meniscus. In the past it was often believed that such fragments were responsible for persistent symptoms following meniscectomy. Since the more widespread use of arthroscopy, however, many other causes of problems following meniscectomy have been recognized, particularly degenerative osteoarthritis.

The meniscal stub that remains at the posterior horn following meniscectomy has the same capacity for remodelling as the anterior horn. The stub of meniscus in a patient with a ruptured bucket handle fragment (Fig.6.37) represents the natural end result of a 'retained fragment'. When these fragments are seen immediately after rupture, they measure approximately 1cm in length and are seldom shorter. When the fragments are seen later (Fig.6.37) they appear as a rounded nubbins of material, from which it may be concluded that the original longer fragment has contracted to form a much smaller mass. It is difficult to see how such a small swelling could be the cause of symptoms in the knee.

Fig.6.38 shows the appearance before removal of the main meniscal fragment. The posterior stub is similar to that in Fig.6.37 but has neither the size nor the position to interfere with function of the knee. The main meniscal fragment, however, is lying beneath the femoral condyle and is well placed to cause mechanical symptoms.

Fig.6.39 shows the posterior limit of a ruptured bucket handle fragment with a stub of about 1cm in length. Although such a fragment is preferably removed at operation, it is reassuring to know that in time the

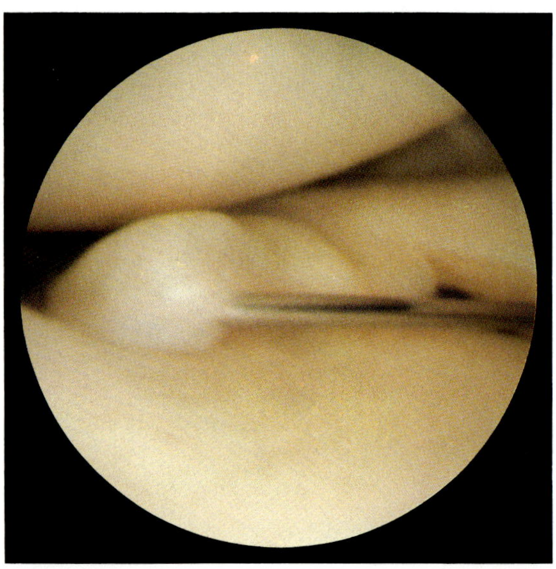

6.36

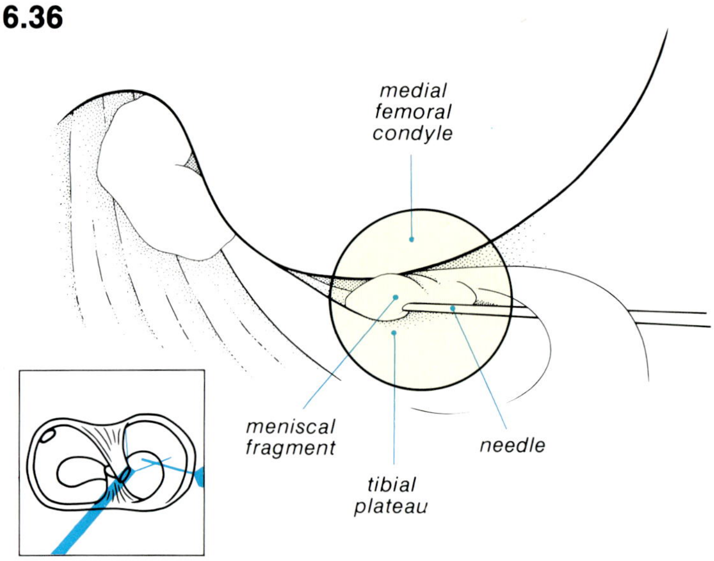

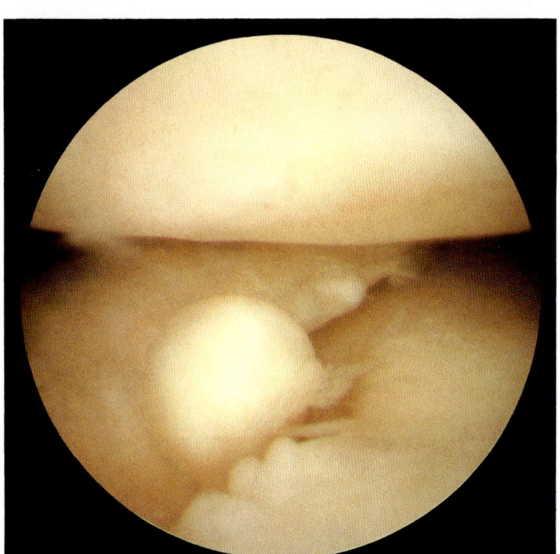

6.37

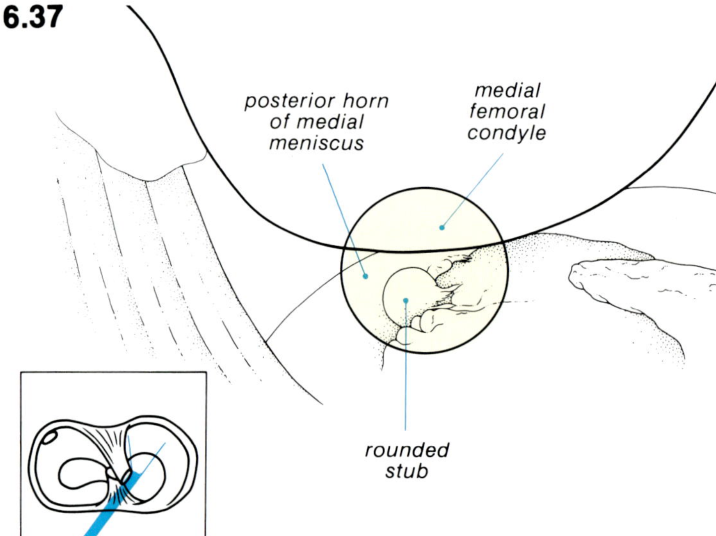

fragment is likely to contract into the rounded stub seen in Figs.6.37 and 6.38. Access to the posterior horn of the meniscus may be difficult and it is unwise to prolong an operation unnecessarily and perhaps risk articular cartilage damage only to remove a small posterior-third fragment that is unlikely to cause problems if left alone.

Although it is usual for a bucket handle fragment to rupture near its posterior horn, rupture at the anterior limit does occasionally occur. Fig.6.40 shows a circumferential tear of the medial meniscus in which the fragment has ruptured at its extreme anterior limit, leaving a step in the contour of the meniscus.

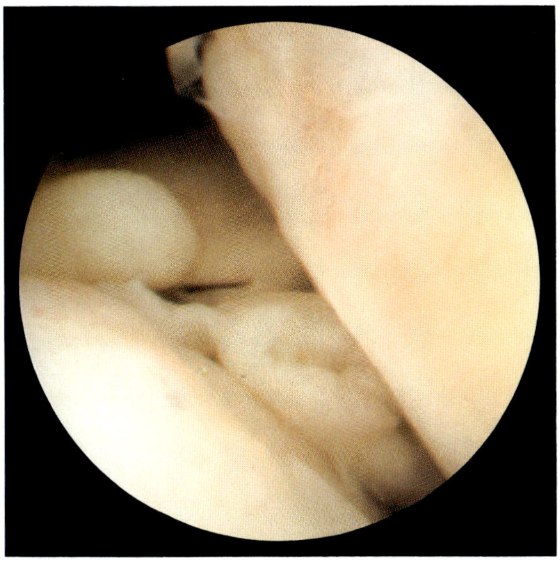

6.38

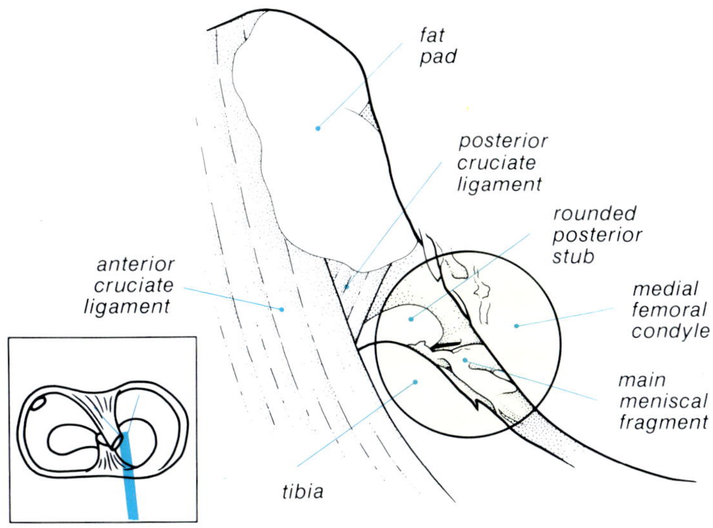

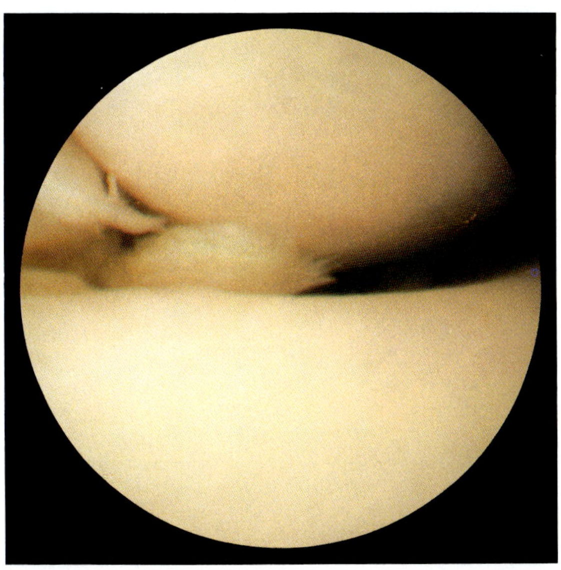

6.39

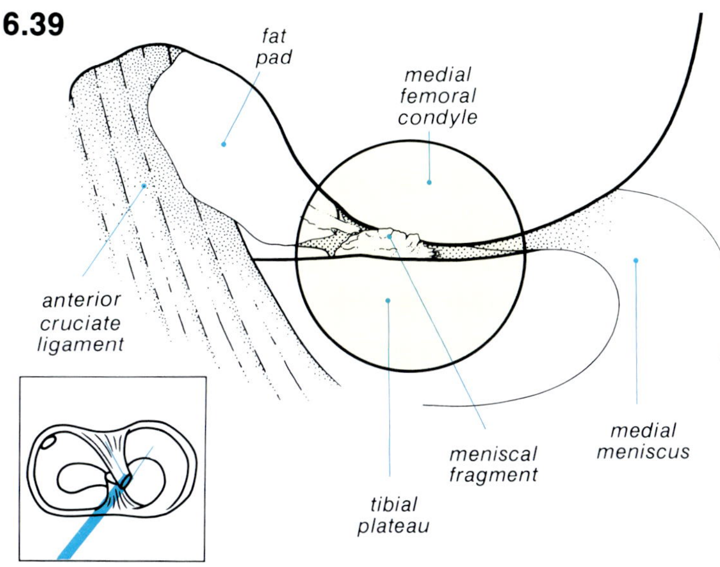

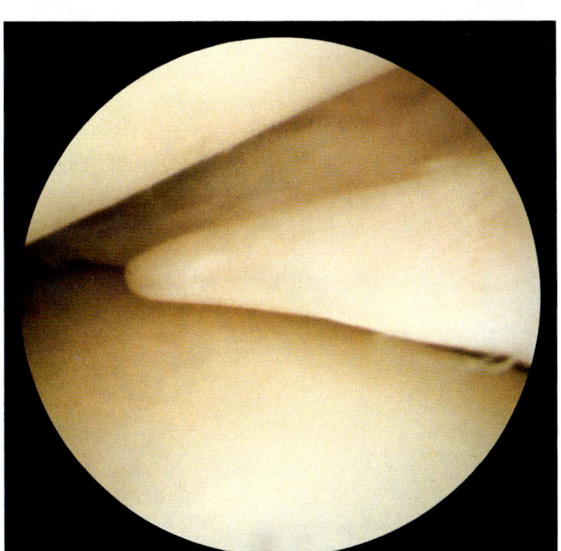

6.40

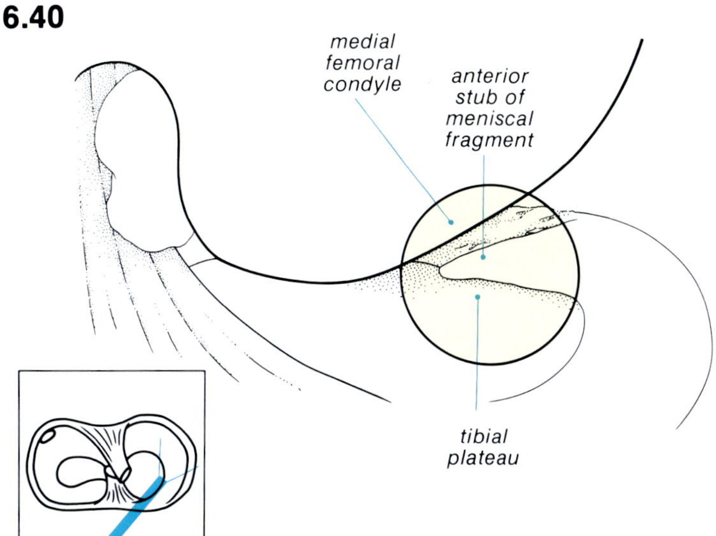

Fig.6.41 shows the main body of a meniscus torn in a manner similar to that in Fig.6.40. The meniscal fragment sweeps backwards over the posterior horn and is lodged in the posteromedial compartment. Unless special care is taken to examine the posterior horn of the meniscus, large fragments of this type can escape detection. Fig.6.42 shows another example of a meniscal fragment lying in the posteromedial compartment. A hook was used to probe the posterior horn and a large fragment was retrieved from the posteromedial compartment (Fig.6.43) which proved to be an incomplete (Type II) fragment that had ruptured at its anterior end and was over 2cm in length.

While meniscal fragments usually rupture at the posterior end or occasionally at the anterior limit, ruptures in the centre of the fragment are most unusual in the medial compartment. The result of such ruptures, when they do occur, is a pair of stubs of roughly equal length (Fig.6.44). The anterior fragment had an irregular margin and could be felt in the medial gutter. The other half of the lesion was lying beneath the medial femoral condyle and interfered with normal function of the knee.

Inspection of the posterior horn of the medial meniscus and the posteromedial compartment is an essential part of the arthroscopic assessment of any meniscal tear. Not only may meniscal fragments be concealed in the posterior compartment, but some tears of the posterior horn cannot be identified from the front of the knee nor exposed with either the manipulating hook or the needle.

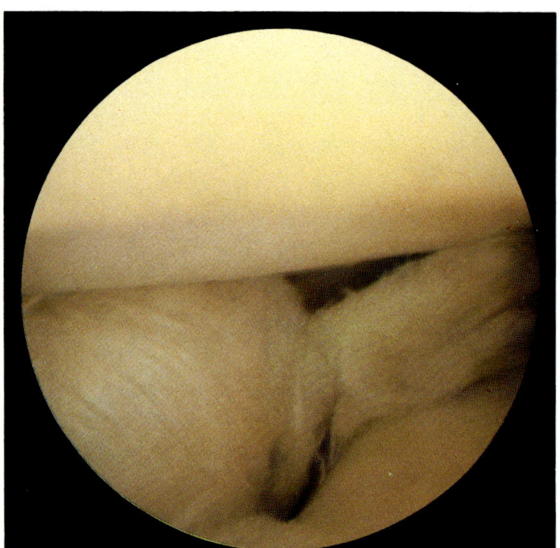

6.41

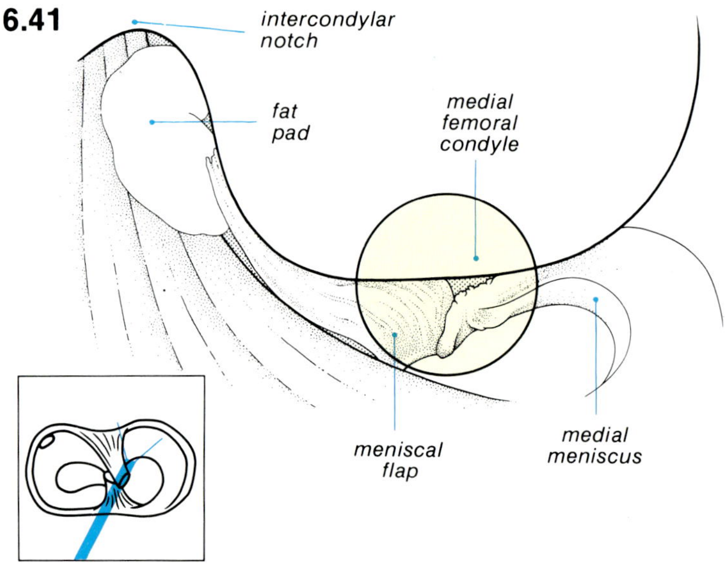

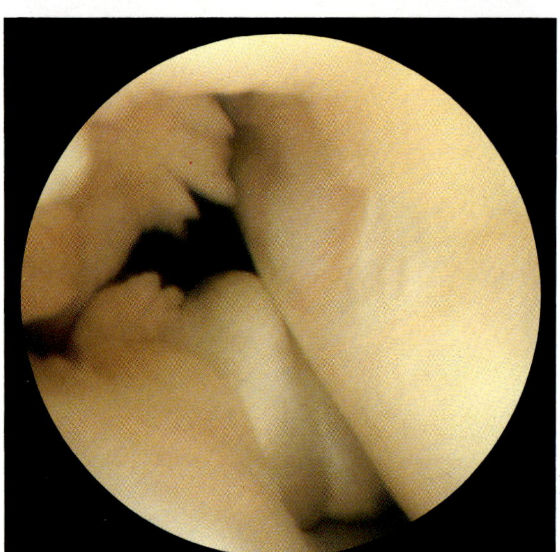

6.42

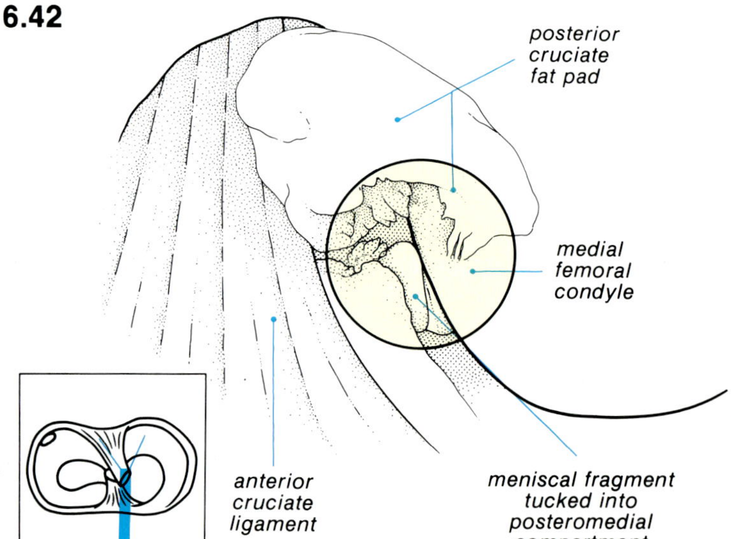

Fig.6.45 shows the posterior horn of the medial meniscus in a knee with a ruptured anterior cruciate ligament. No tear of the meniscus could be demonstrated despite careful probing with a needle and hook, but there is subsynovial staining over the posterior horn of the meniscus and small punctate haemorrhages are seen. These appearances are strongly suggestive of subsynovial bleeding at the attachment of the posterior horn to the tibia which in turn suggests that the meniscotibial attachment has been subjected to considerable strain even though no tear has occurred. Lesions such as that in Fig.6.45, which lack a definite tear, will probably heal spontaneously and excision of such a meniscus would be difficult to justify.

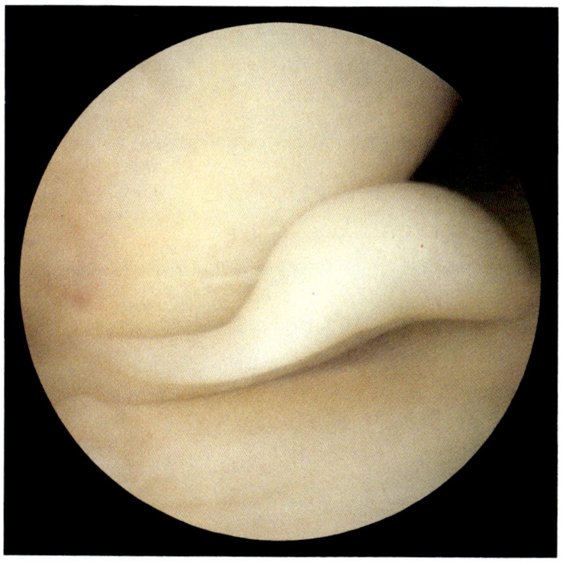

6.43

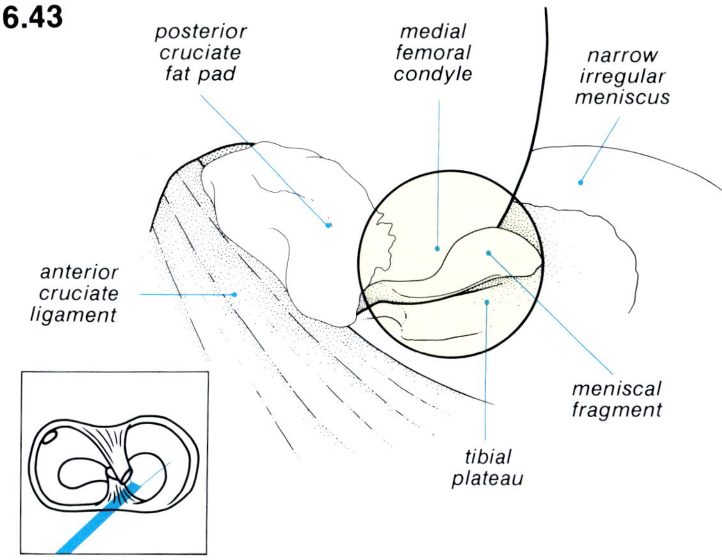

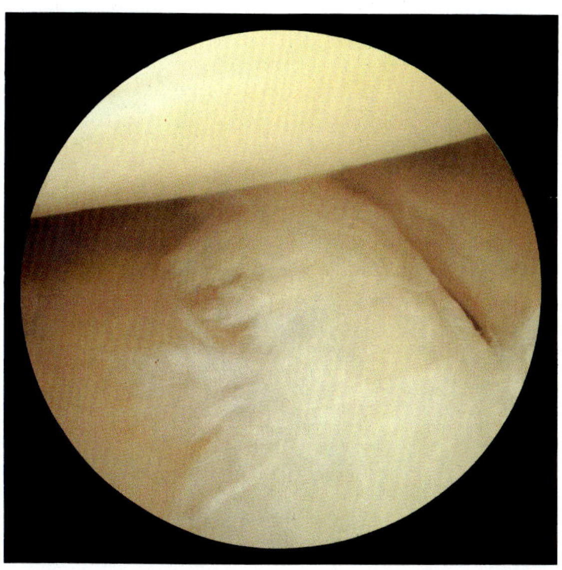

6.44

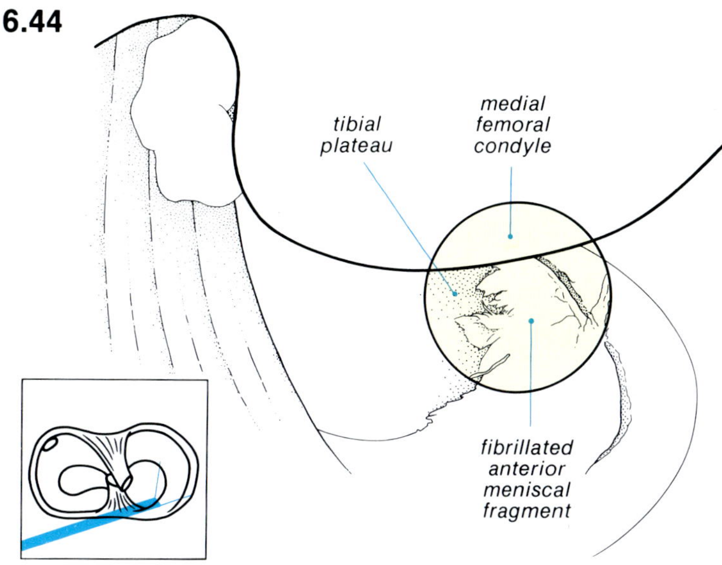

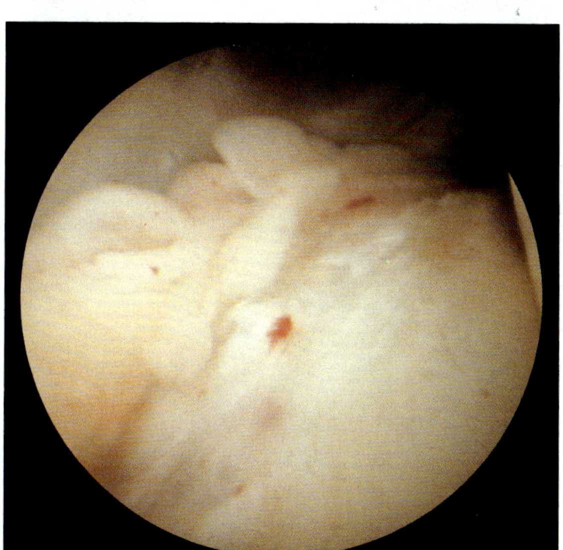

6.45

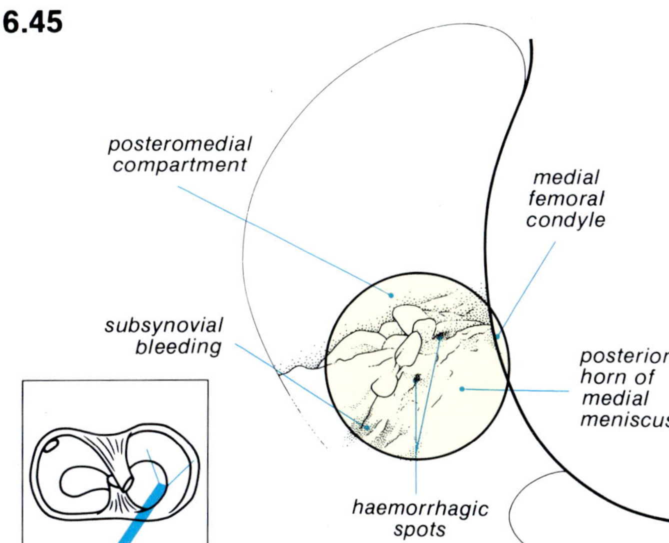

In Fig.6.46, which also shows the posterior horn of the medial meniscus in a knee with a ruptured anterior cruciate ligament, the same punctate haemorrhages and subsynovial bleeding are seen but there is also a definite tear of the medial meniscus running parallel to the meniscal rim just behind the femoral condyle. The tear was not seen on initial inspection from the front of the knee but was suspected because the posterior horn of the meniscus was a little more mobile that usual. The meniscal fragment was excised arthroscopically.

In Fig.6.47, a tear in a similar situation is clearly demonstrated with a probing needle and, unlike that in Fig.6.46, lies close to the posterior meniscosynovial junction. Because this area has a good blood supply, the

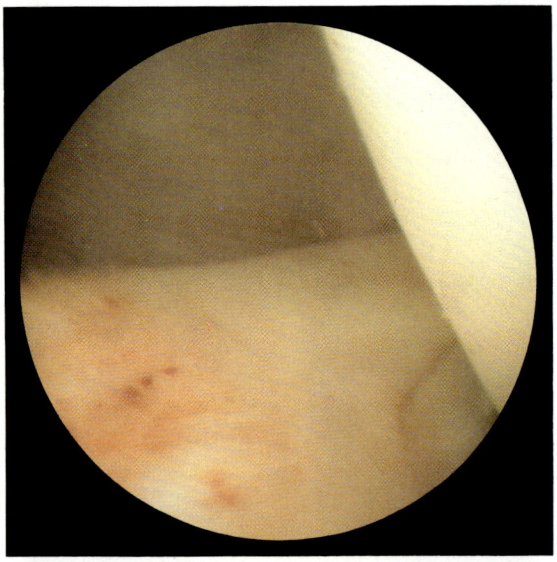

6.46

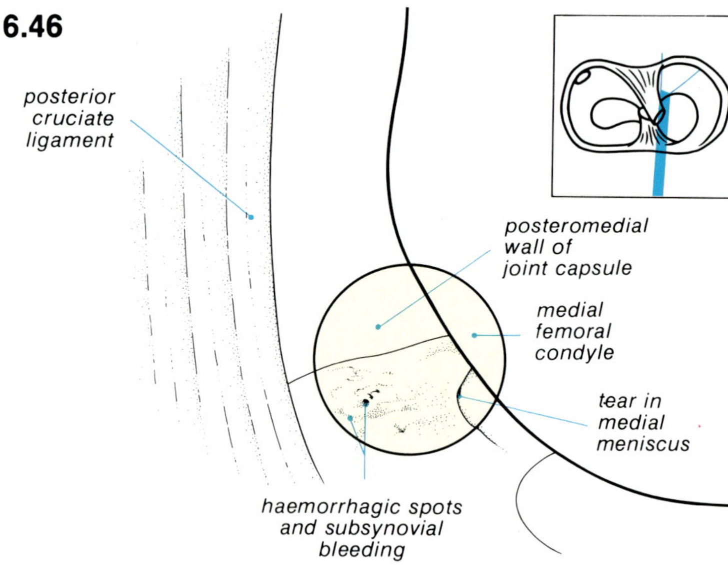

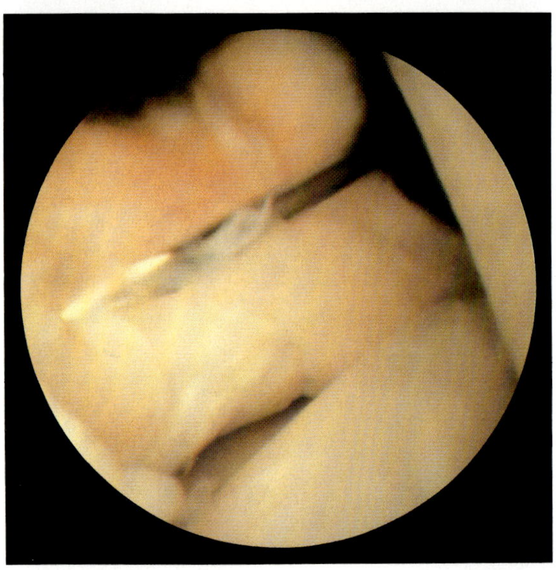

6.47

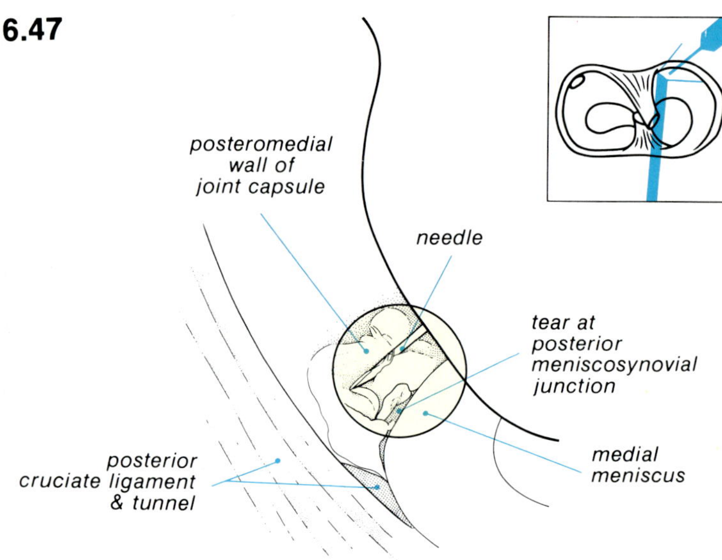

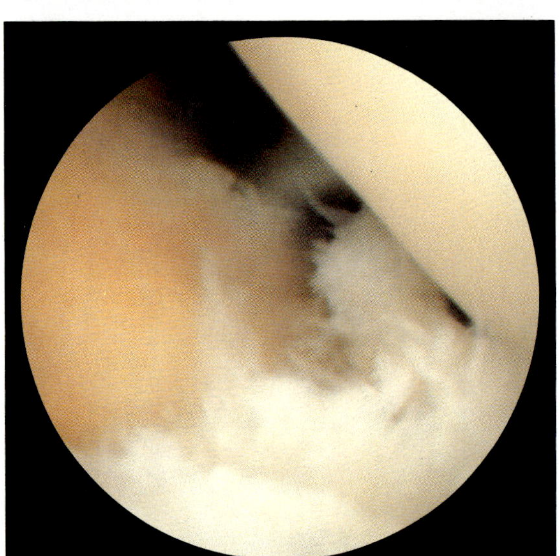

6.48

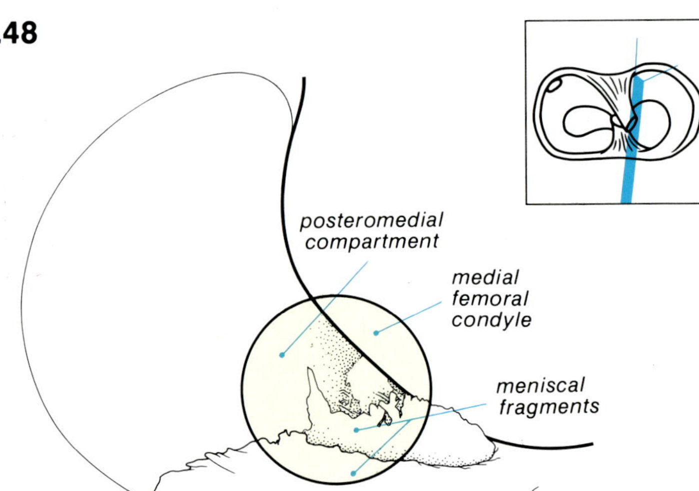

lesion is perhaps suitable for meniscal reattachment. There is no sign of vascularity in the meniscal tissue on either side of the tear, but excision of the avascular meniscal portion of the posterior surface of the tear might bring enough blood into the line of repair to ensure healing. These are speculative comments only, but pose questions on the management of meniscal tears that will one day receive answers.

In Fig.6.48, a large meniscal fragment is seen in the posteromedial compartment. The patient had two parallel circumferential tears of the meniscus creating two bucket handle fragments; after removal of one, the second fragment was eventually located in the posteromedial compartment and removed from the posteromedial approach.

POSTMENISCECTOMY APPEARANCES

If a total meniscectomy has been performed, only a fibrous rim of meniscus remains. In Fig.6.49 the rim has been grasped with forceps inserted from the posteromedial approach to expose the posterior surface of the tibia. The meniscectomy was carried out through a standard anterior arthrotomy, but the same operation is possible under arthroscopic control using cutting instruments inserted through the same approach as the forceps in Fig.6.49.

The rim that remains after meniscectomy depends on the shape and size of the excised meniscal fragment. In Fig.6.50 an open subtotal meniscectomy had been performed. There is no sign of a newly formed meniscus but in its place is a very narrow fibrous crescent with a

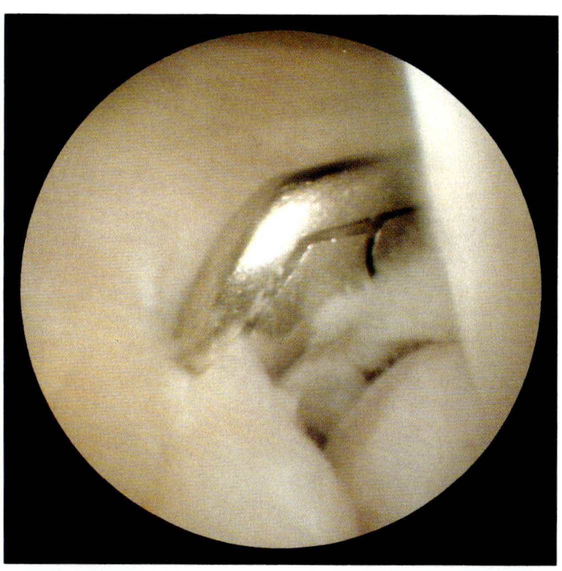

6.49

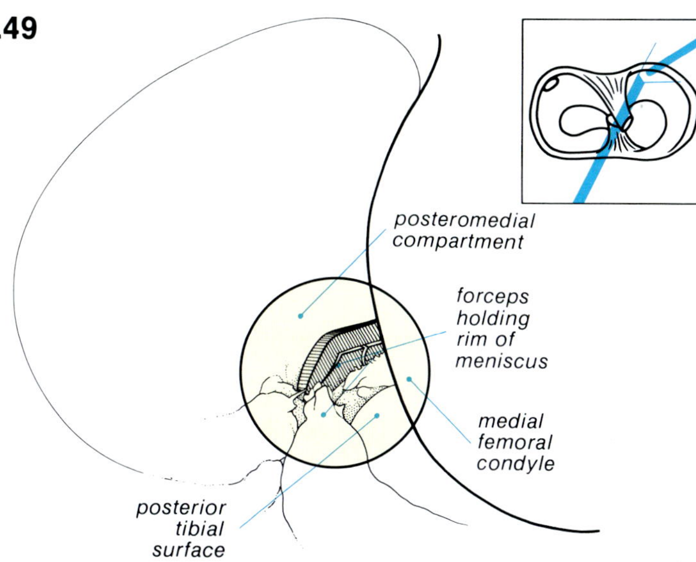

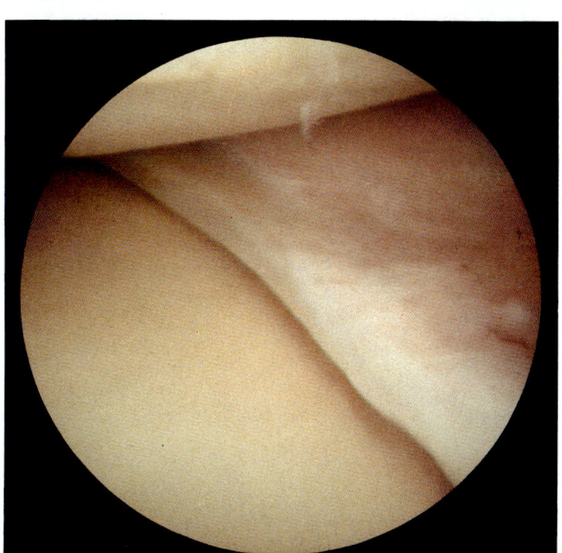

6.50

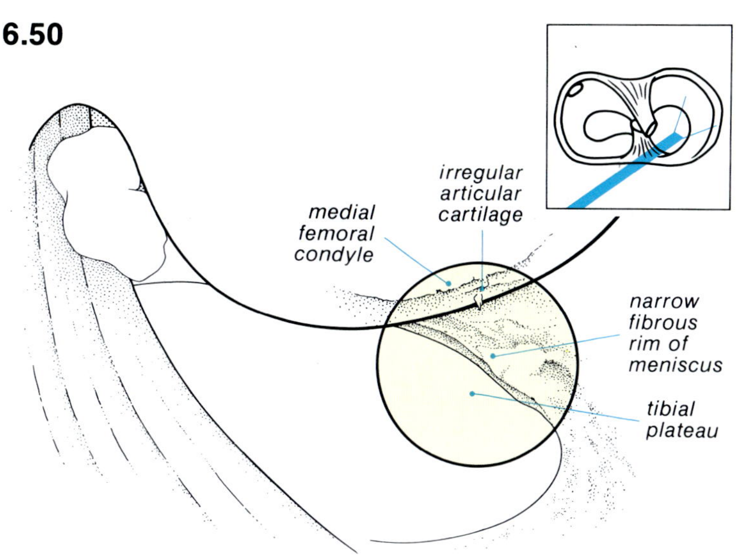

knife-like edge, a structure that can have little mechanical function. After excision of an incomplete (Type II) bucket handle fragment, the difference between the original meniscal tissue and the fibrous rim that has formed in the defect resulting from removal of the fragment can be clearly seen (Fig.6.51). The attempt at 'regeneration' of a new meniscus appears to be just as effective after partial meniscectomy (Fig.6.51) as after subtotal meniscectomy (Fig.6.50).

Fig.6.52 shows the rim of the medial meniscus following the removal of a narrow bucket handle fragment that arose from a slightly oblique tear. The meniscal rim is smooth and even and closely resembles the original; the only abnormality is a slight irregularity of the torn surface which would be difficult to improve surgically. Fig.6.53 shows a smooth and level meniscal rim after arthroscopic removal of a narrow bucket handle fragment. Even in the anterior horn, where the tissue lies so close to the lens that any irregularity is greatly magnified, the surface is remarkably smooth. For practical purposes, the meniscus following the removal of a narrow fragment is normal.

If the fragment arises from a vertical split, the meniscus will probably not have a sharp crescentic margin and the horizontal plane of cleavage that separates the upper and lower halves of the meniscus will be clearly visible (Fig.6.54). The meniscal tissue has been remodelled above and below this plane of cleavage, giving the appearance of two small menisci, one above the other. The horizontal fissure of the meniscal rim does not

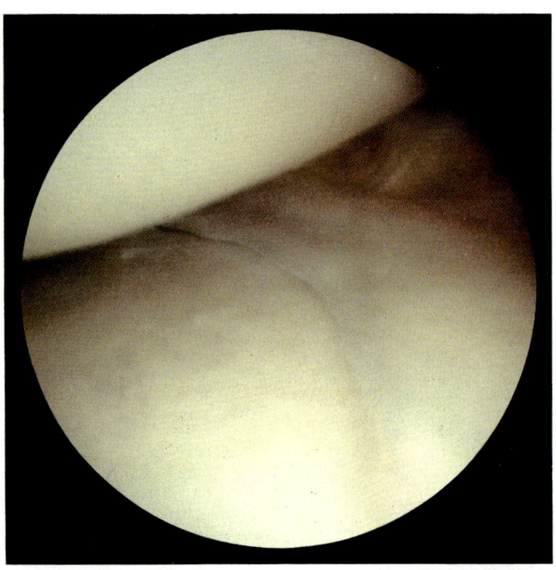

6.51

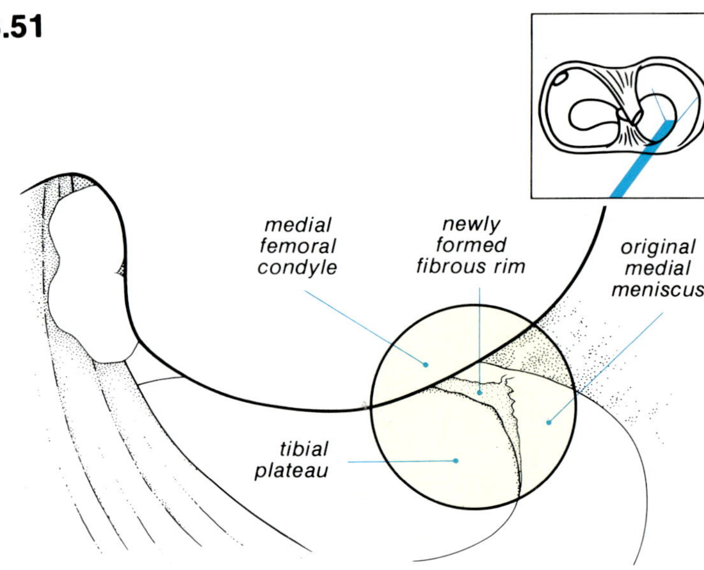

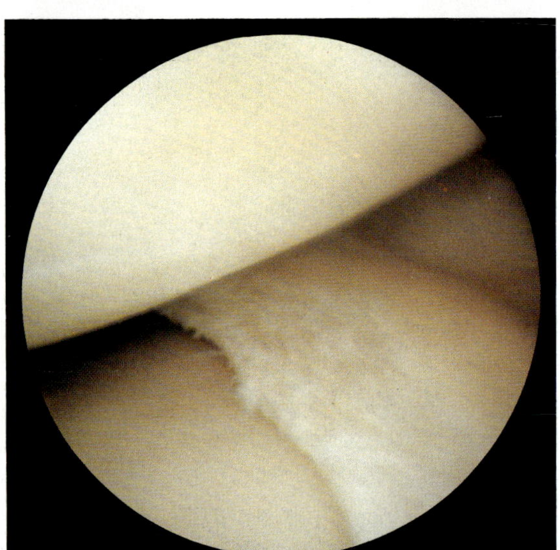

6.52

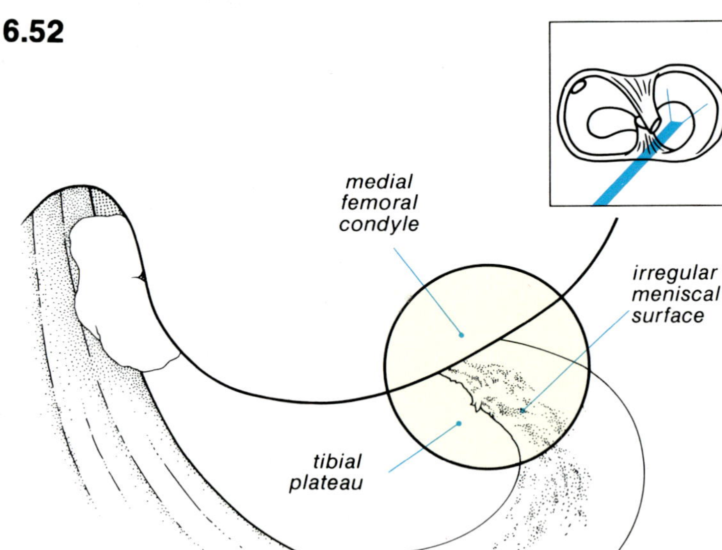

weaken the circumferential stability of the meniscus and does not extend through the full width of the meniscus.

Fig.6.55 shows the knee of a patient who had previously undergone an open medial meniscectomy and complained of persistent catching and clicking. The rim appeared satisfactory except for a small tag less than 5mm long. The flap was removed. The patient's symptoms were relieved and did not recur; but why such a small fragment should be the cause of symptoms is not clear.

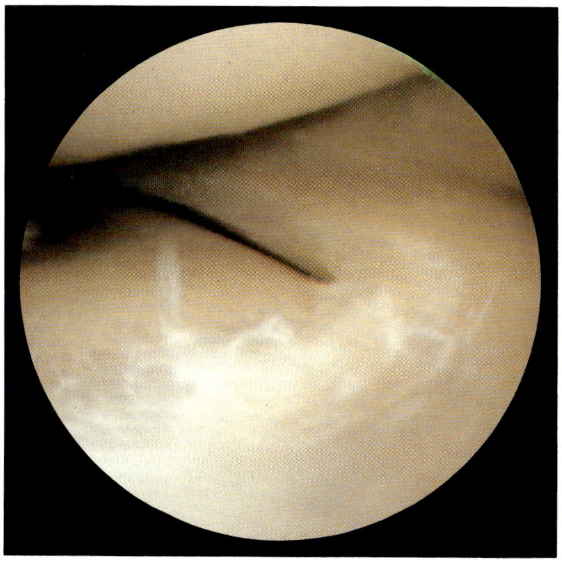

6.53

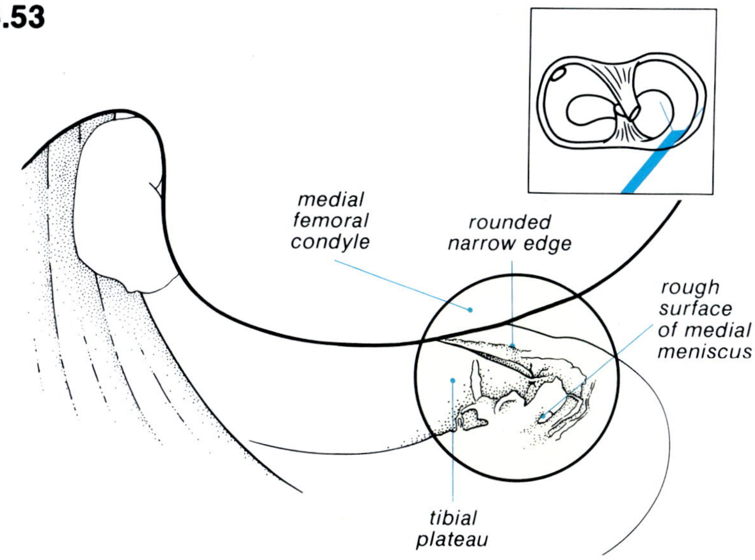

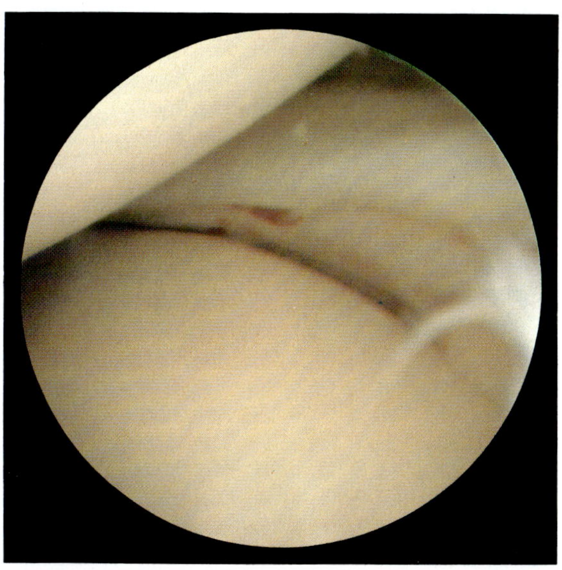

6.54

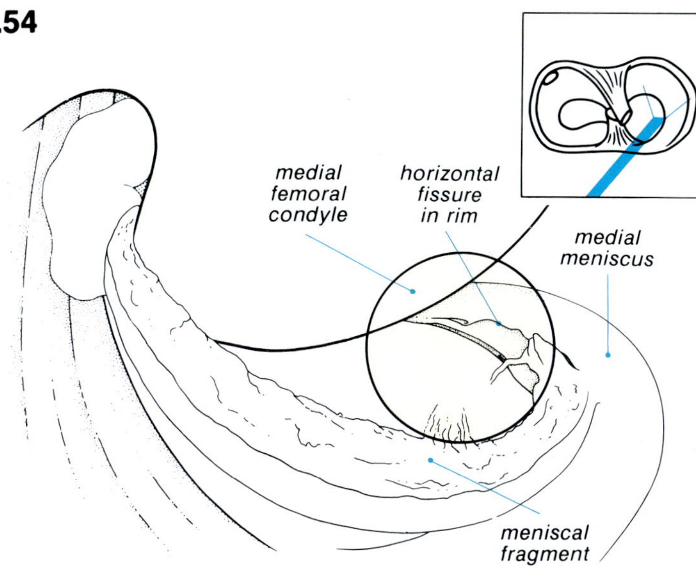

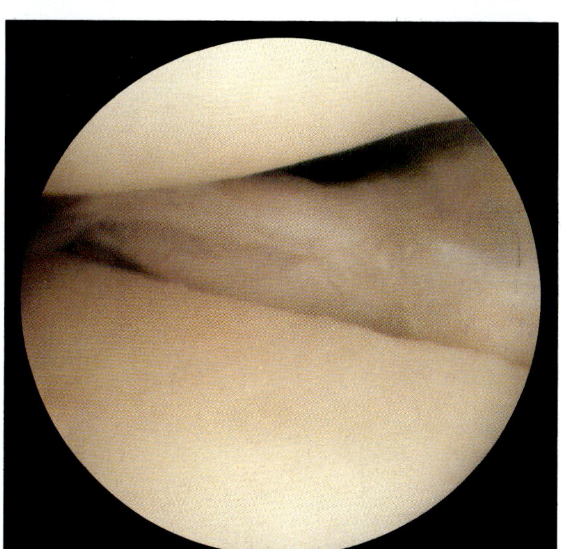

6.55

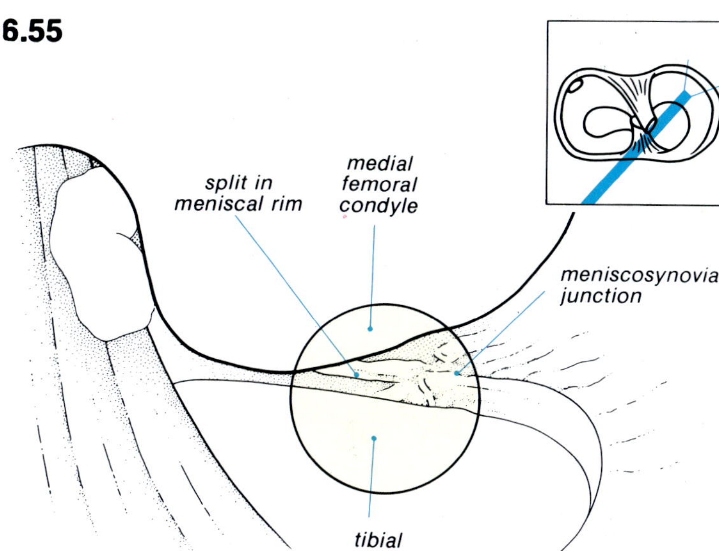

Fig.6.56 shows the rim of a circumferential tear of the medial meniscus. The knee also had a ruptured anterior cruciate ligament, two bucket handle fragments and an unusual pearl-like nodule midway along the meniscal rim. It may be that this swelling represents the former site of attachment of the more peripheral of the bucket handle fragments which had torn away, leaving a small stub which subsequently contracted down. Apart from this nodule, the medial meniscus has rounded off well. In the presence of two larger bucket handle fragments and a torn anterior cruciate ligament, it is impossible to know if any of the patient's symptoms were due to the small swelling.

The role of tears of the medial meniscus in patients with osteoarthritis is unclear, but as has already been suggested, the meniscus probably has a protective function in the osteoarthritic knee. Accordingly, the medial meniscus should be preserved if possible in patients with degenerative changes. On the other hand, there is no reason to suppose that the presence of osteoarthritis renders all meniscal tears asymptomatic.

Fig.6.57 shows the medial compartment of a patient who has osteoarthritis and exposed subchondral bone. There is also a flap tear involving the upper surface of the meniscus but the main body of the meniscus is intact. The flap, which is superficial, was well placed to cause mechanical problems and possibly to aggravate the already considerable damage to the articular surface. The flap was assessed carefully using a hook and probe to determine how much of the meniscus should be removed to relieve the mechanical symptoms without endangering the meniscal rim. After cautious trimming of the flap, the patient's symptoms of catching and unsteadiness on the medial side of the knee were improved but the ache and swelling of osteoarthritis remained unchanged.

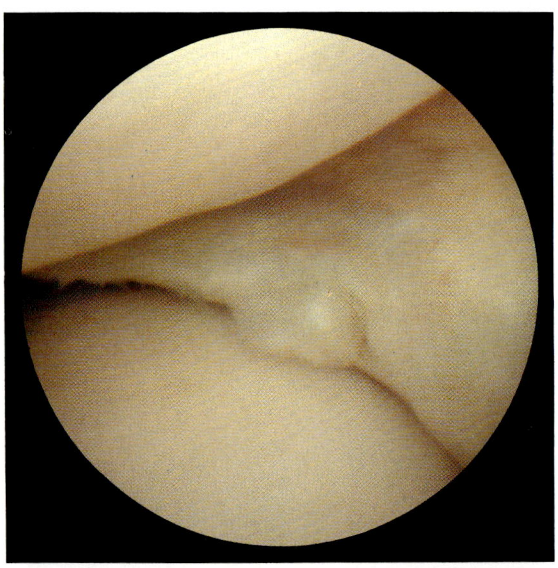

6.56

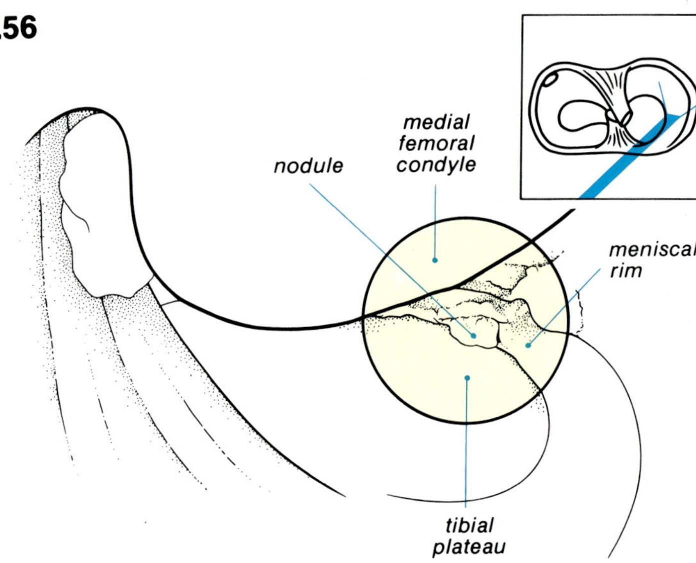

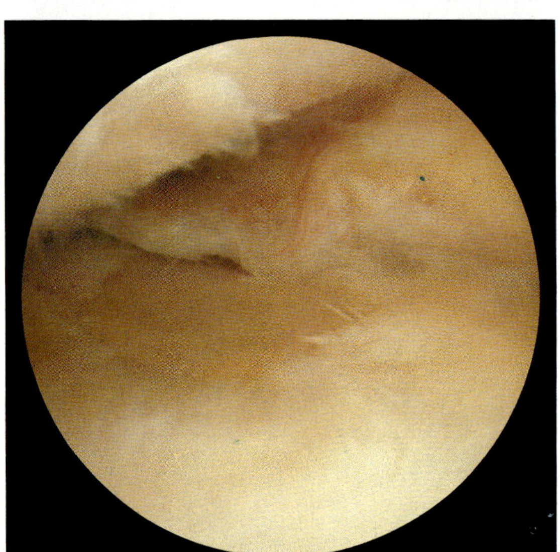

6.57

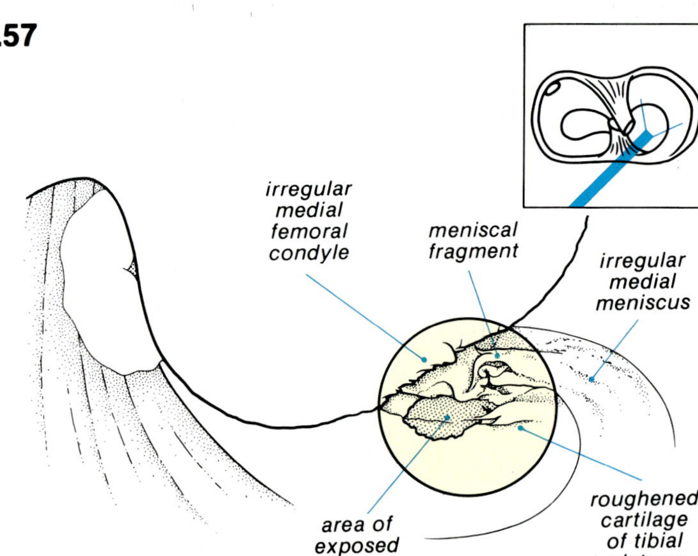

6
Pathology of the Menisci

II The Lateral Meniscus

II. THE LATERAL MENISCUS

Tears of the lateral meniscus are radically different from those of the medial meniscus. The lateral meniscus is shorter than its medial counterpart and its tibial attachments are closer together. The lateral compartment also has the popliteus tunnel which influences the patterns of tears that occur in the lateral side of the knee.

PATTERNS OF TEARS

The lateral meniscus often bears small tags on its edge which can be misinterpreted as indicating the presence of a larger tear and can lead to an unnecessary lateral meniscectomy. Fig.6.58 shows a minor irregularity in the posterior horn of an otherwise normal lateral meniscus. In view of the poor long-term results of lateral

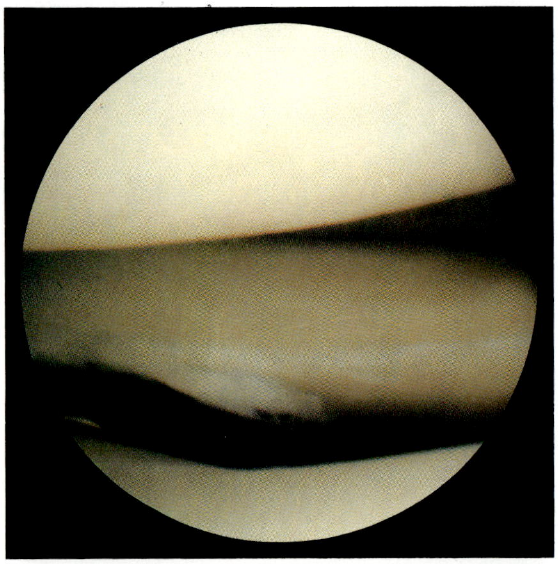

6.58

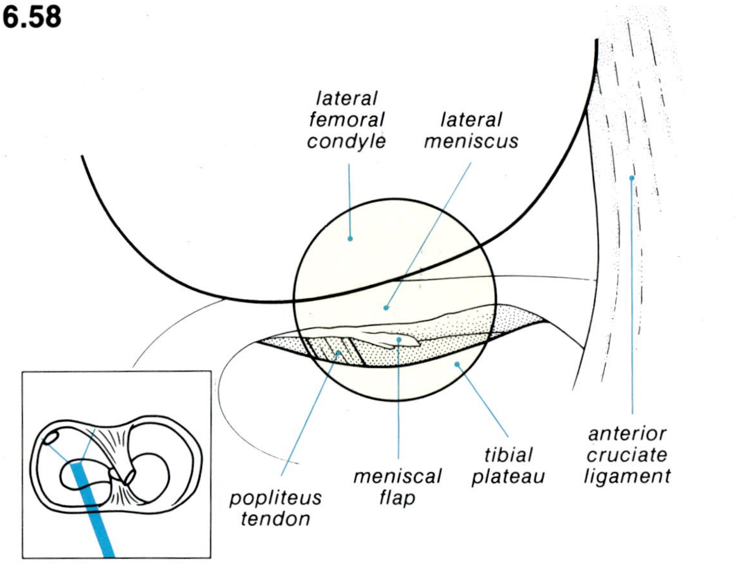

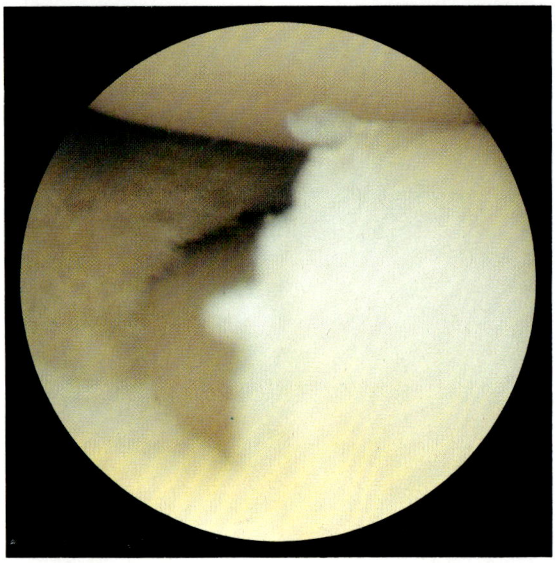

6.59

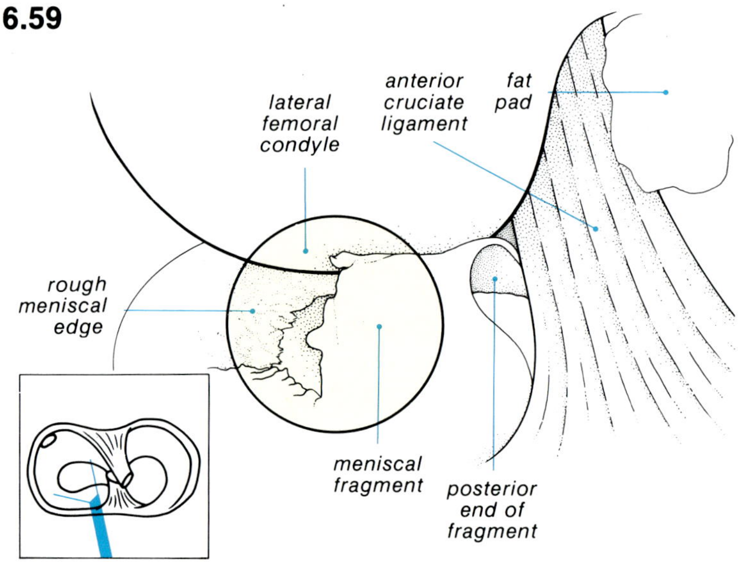

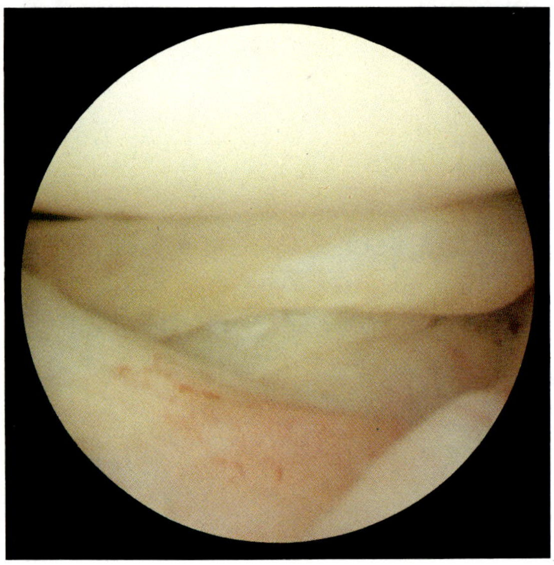

6.60

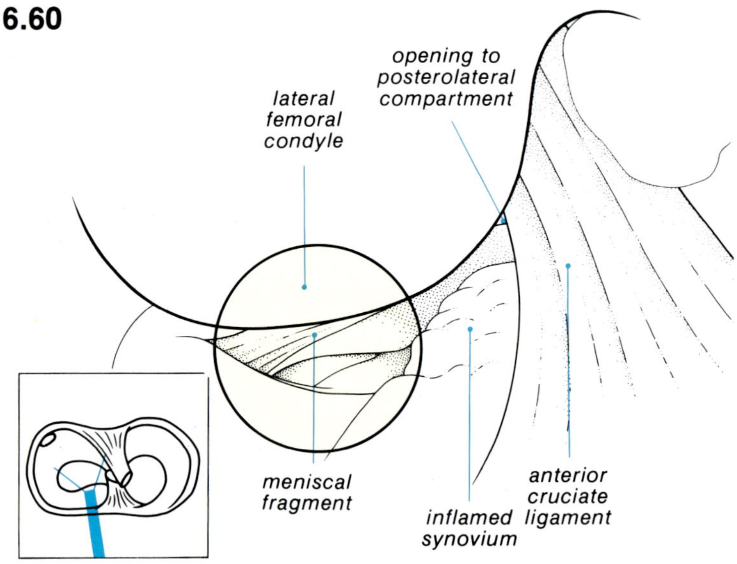

meniscectomy, the temptation to excise the entire meniscus because of this small irregularity must be resisted. If necessary, the tag could be gently trimmed, but division of the meniscus across its entire width will have unfortunate consequences for the long-term prognosis of the knee.

Bucket handle tears

Bucket handle tears of the lateral compartment follow a different pattern from those of the medial. Although, as in the medial compartment, the tears almost always begin posteriorly, they seem to extend forwards either as far as the popliteus tunnel or to the anterior horn and do not stop at any point in between. The tears may involve the whole of the meniscal substance or only half of it. If the fragment involves only half the meniscus, the split may be vertical, as commonly seen in the medial compartment, or oblique, which leaves an intact meniscal rim closely resembling the original except that it is narrower and has an uneven upper surface. Fig.6.59 shows a bucket handle fragment in the lateral meniscus involving the full length of the meniscus but only half its thickness. The line of cleavage is such that the remaining meniscal rim is identical to the original meniscus except that it is narrower and slightly thinner.

Fig.6.60 shows a bucket handle fragment that involves only the posterior half of the lateral meniscus with the tear stopping at the popliteus tunnel. The meniscus has been split vertically by a circumferential tear similar to those seen in the medial compartment and only the anterior half of the meniscus has dislocated forwards. The fragment is twisted upon itself, presenting the torn surface anteriorly, and is tightly locked in front of the condyle, bent almost double at its anterior limit which lies at the level of the popliteus tendon. This must be a point of considerable stress to the meniscus.

In Fig.6.61, another lateral meniscal tear involving only the posterior half of the meniscus, the split is horizontal and not vertical. The fragment involves the upper half of the meniscus only, is thinner than that in Fig.6.60, and is irregular and torn.

A fragment that involves the full thickness of the lateral meniscus presents special problems at arthroscopy. The bulk of the fragment is so great that the fragment is tightly locked and lies close to the lens, obscuring vision. Fig.6.62 shows a fragment involving the posterior half of the meniscus only but its entire width. The fragment is thicker than that in Fig.6.60 and is clearly holding the tibiofemoral joint surfaces apart. In the front of the joint there are a few strands of intensely inflamed synovium which can further obscure vision and hamper arthroscopy and arthroscopic meniscectomy.

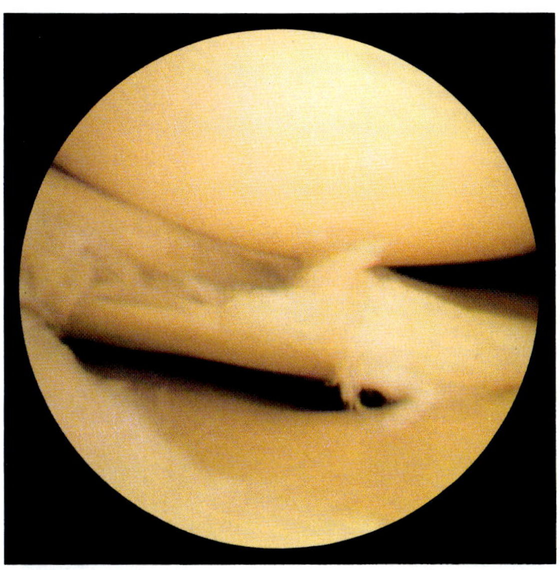

6.61

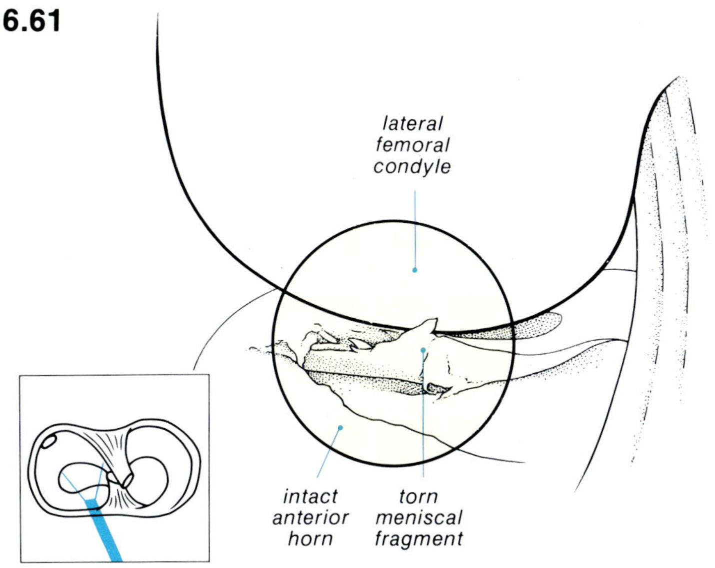

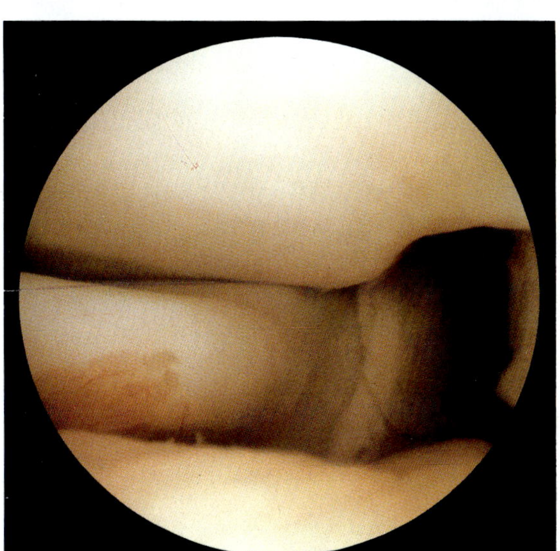

6.62

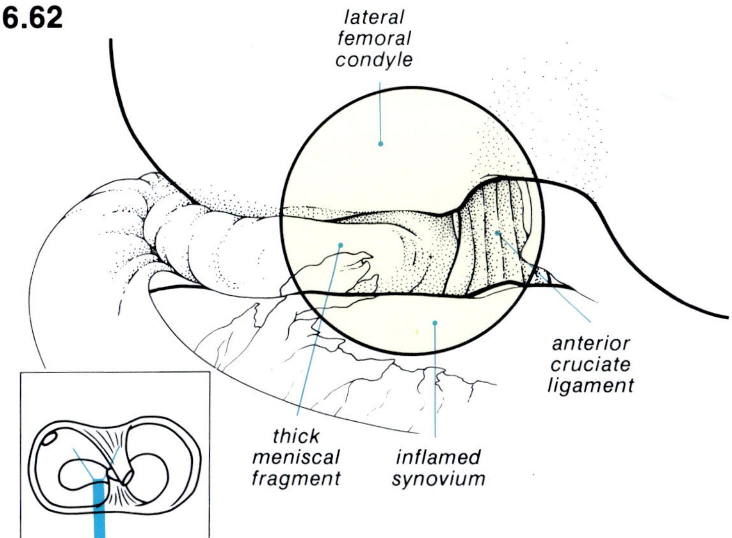

Fig.6.63 shows a tear of the posterior half of the lateral meniscus with the meniscal fragments lying in the reduced position. The tear runs from the posterior attachment of the meniscus to the tibia and as far forwards as the popliteus tunnel, at the junction of the posterior and middle thirds of the meniscus (see also Fig.6.60). This tear is comparable to the concealed (Type III) tear of the medial meniscus but, while the presence of such a tear may be suspected in the medial compartment because of the unusual prominence of the meniscal edge, no such prominence is seen in the lateral compartment.

In Fig.6.63 the meniscal margin is lying in its normal position. The presence of the tear was suspected because of a history of recurrent locking of the knee in full flexion. The suspicion was increased by the slight articular cartilage irregularity on the posterior part of the

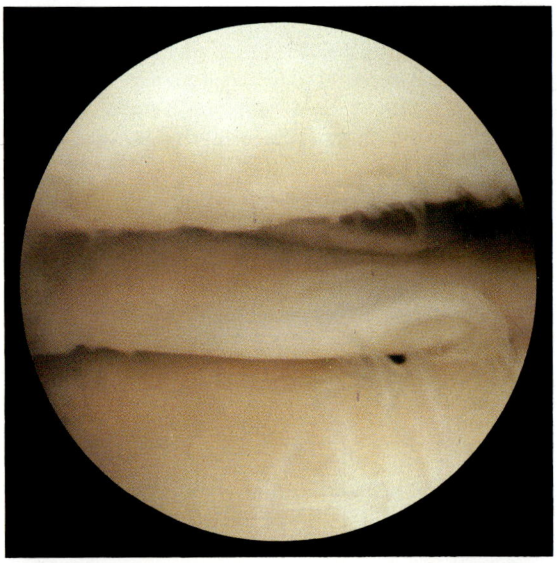

6.63

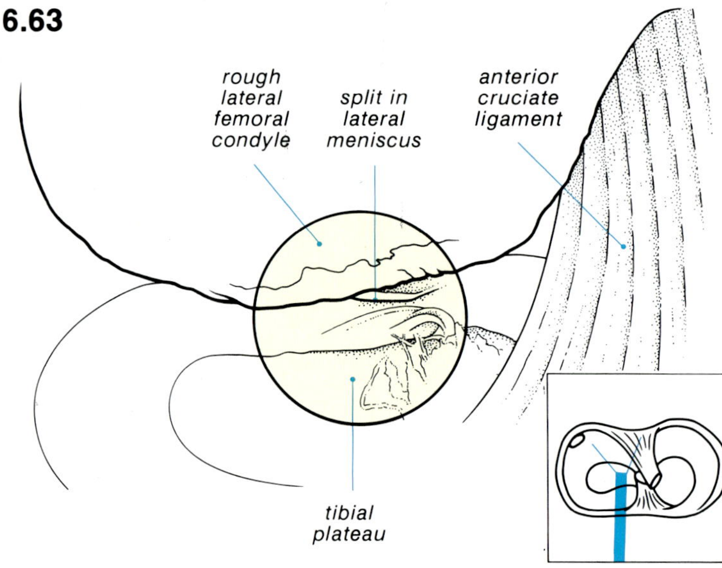

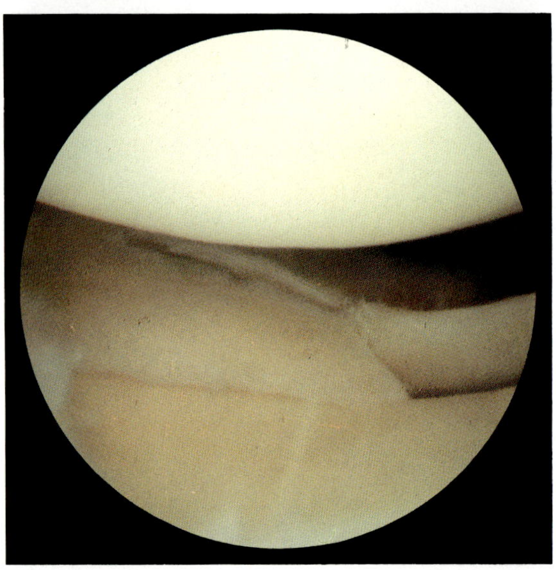

6.64

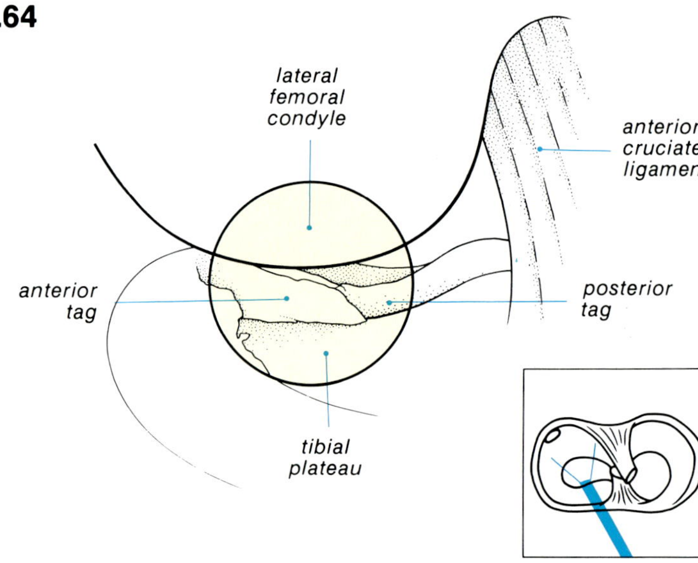

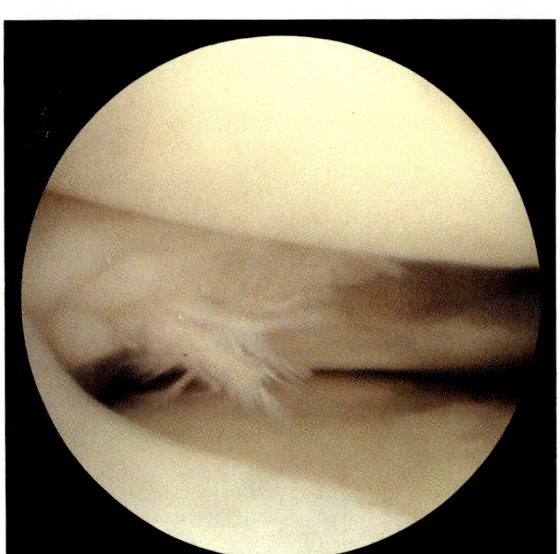

6.65

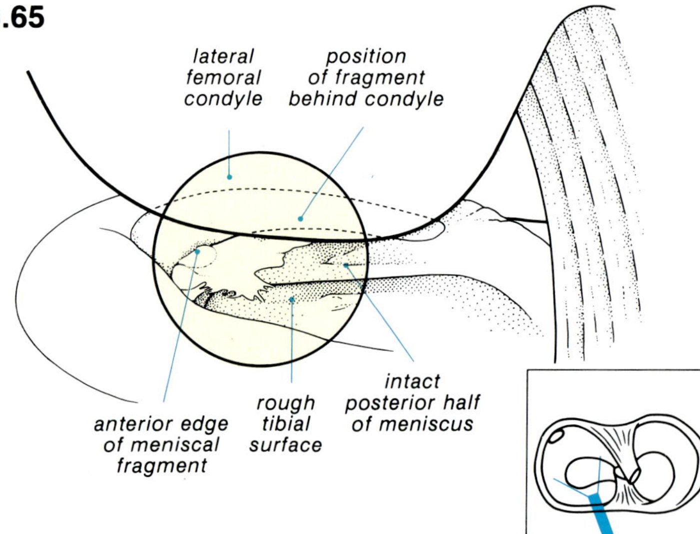

lateral femoral condyle. The presence of the tear was confirmed by direct inspection and careful examination with a probing hook and needle.

Whereas bucket handle fragments in the medial compartment will almost always rupture at their posterior limit and leave a long anterior stub, the site of rupture in the lateral compartment is much less predictable and no consistent pattern of meniscal tear has been recognized.

Fig.6.64 shows a bucket handle fragment involving half the length and half the width of the lateral meniscus which has ruptured at its centre to produce two tags of approximately equal length. The tags have clean edges and the posterior tag is twisted upon itself, showing its undersurface. No articular cartilage damage is seen.

Not only do the bucket handle fragments in the lateral compartment rupture less predictably than those in the medial compartment, but their effects upon the articular surface can be much more serious. Figs.6.65 and 6.66 show a fragment involving half the length and half the width of the meniscus. The fragment has ruptured at its posterior end and is lying in the lateral gutter (Fig.6.65). The anterior limit of the tear can be seen and the posterior half of the meniscus is intact. When removed from the gutter, the fragment proved to be over 1.5cm long.

Fig.6.66 shows a defect in the lateral femoral condyle, with exposed bone at its base, above the posterior attachment of the meniscal fragment. The position of the defect corresponds to the area that came into contact with the meniscal fragment in the reduced position, suggesting that the meniscal fragment was, at least in part, responsible for the damage to the articular cartilage. Such a knee has a poor prognosis however it is managed.

Figs.6.67 and 6.68 show a tear of the posterior half of the lateral meniscus. The fragment has arisen from a vertical tear similar to that in Figs.6.65 and 6.66 and has ruptured at its anterior limit to produce a short anterior stub and a long posterior stub, the opposite of the tear shown in Figs.6.65 and 6.66. In Fig.6.67 the short anterior stub is lying beneath the femoral condyle and a little articular cartilage irregularity is seen immediately above the meniscal fragment, but the changes are not gross. A short anterior stub such as this could well cause mechanical symptoms such as catching and instability.

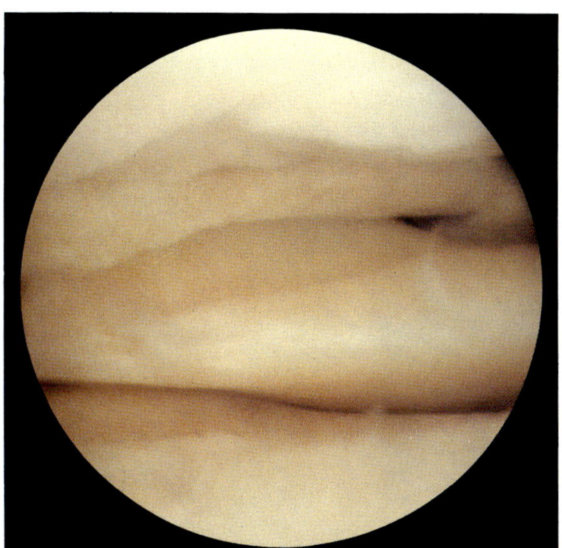

6.66

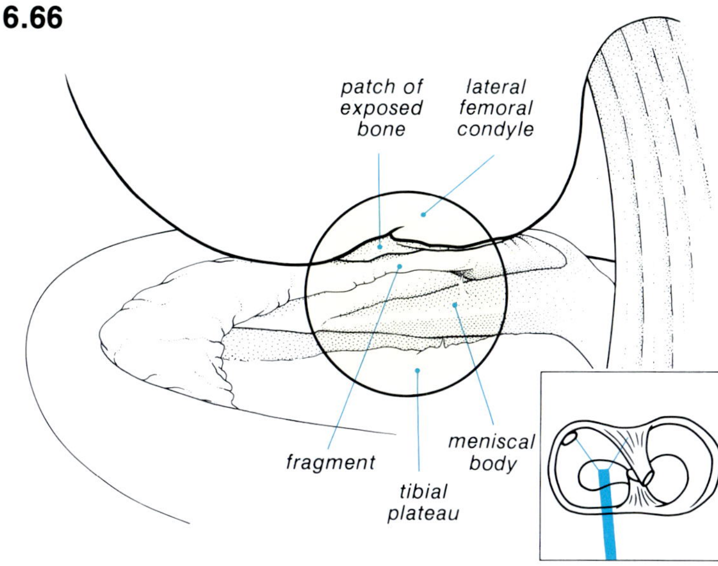

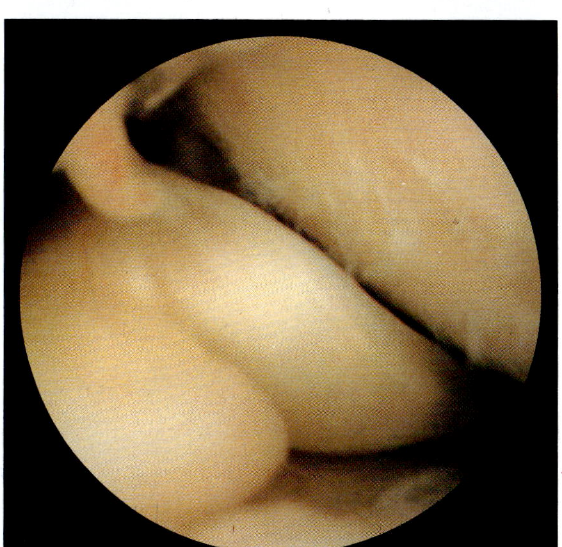

6.67

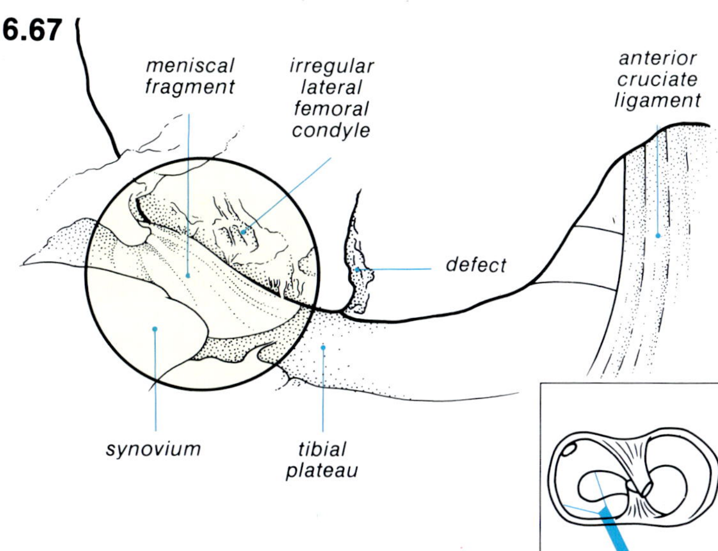

Fig.6.68 shows the base of the posterior remnant being probed with a needle. The fragment has fallen backwards into the posterolateral compartment, just as the comparable medial meniscal fragment falls into the posteromedial compartment. Immediately above the meniscus is a defect in the articular cartilage which extends down to subchondral bone. The chondral defect is linear and lies in the anteroposterior direction, similar to the chondral separation seen in Fig.3.13 (see Chapter 3). It may be that the abnormal height of the posterior horn of the lateral meniscus has caused constant abrasion of the lateral femoral condyle during flexion and extension, but the meniscal fragment may also have come forward into the anterior part of the knee and damaged the femoral condyle by direct contact.

A further example of the curious behaviour of ruptured bucket handle fragments in the lateral compartment is seen in Fig.6.69 which shows a bucket handle fragment involving the full length of the lateral meniscus. The tear is almost horizontal, similar to that seen in Fig.6.59, and has ruptured at its posterior end. The fragment is lying in the anterior part of the knee, curling round the lateral femoral condyle with its tip tucked under the posterior horn. Definition of the anatomy of this tear was particularly difficult because the anterior limit of the tear lay close to the arthroscope. Until the attachment was identified, the fragment presented the appearance of an elongated loose body.

Tags

Figs.6.70 and 6.71 show a pattern of tear that has only been seen in the lateral compartment. A radial tear has developed near the junction of the middle and posterior thirds of the meniscus and extends forwards to the anterior horn. This pattern is remarkably consistent and is probably the result of a specific injury. A fragment of this type often causes symptoms which are out of proportion to the size of the lesion and the fragment itself can also appear unduly magnified because of its proximity to the arthroscope lens. On removal the fragment often appears to be disappointingly small, although the results of excision are very satisfactory.

Fig.6.70 shows the bed from which the fragment arose. The posterior limit is marked by a clean radial tear and the anterior surface shows a vertical cliff-like edge. The fragment can often be made to fit neatly into its bed but usually is floating free, often in the intercondylar notch.

Fig.6.71 shows the anterior attachment of such a lesion but in a different knee from that in Fig.6.70. The stem of the fragment is attached to the anterior insertion of the

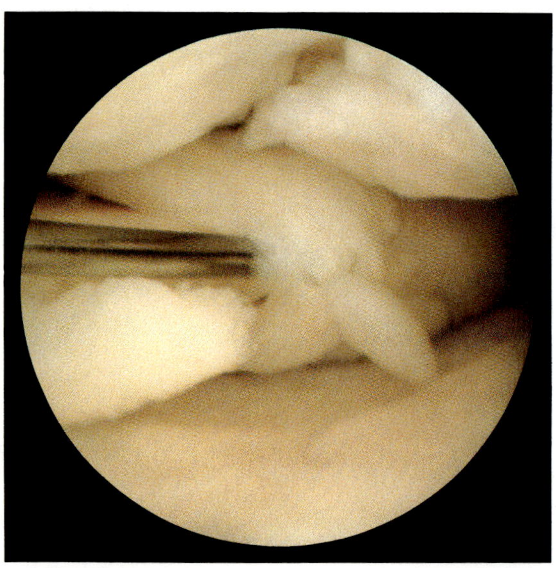

6.68

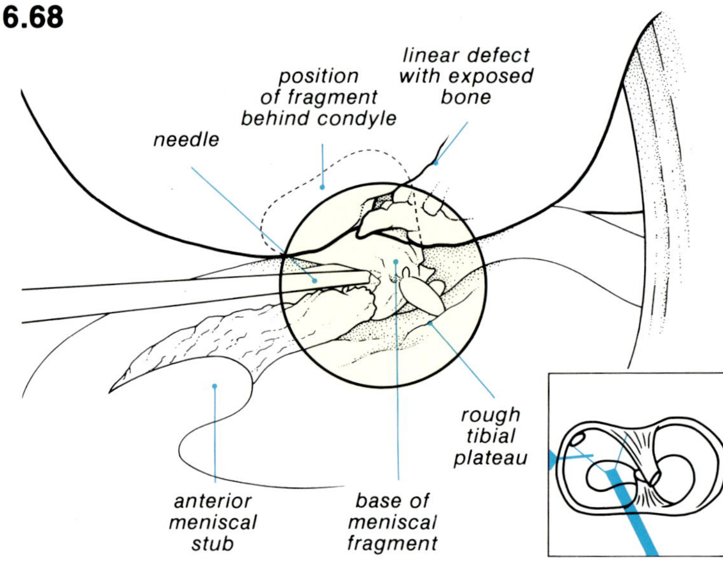

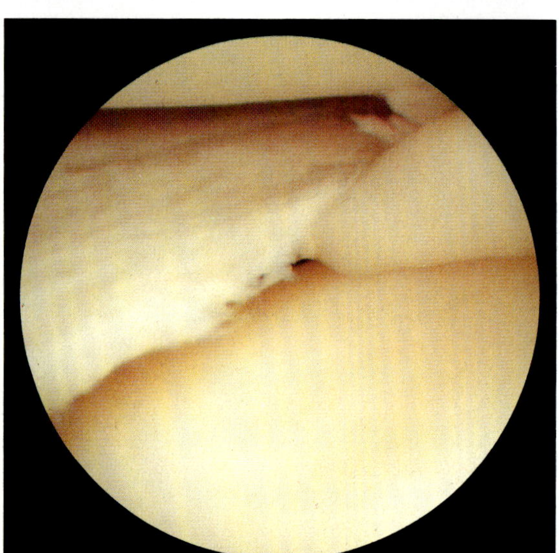

6.69

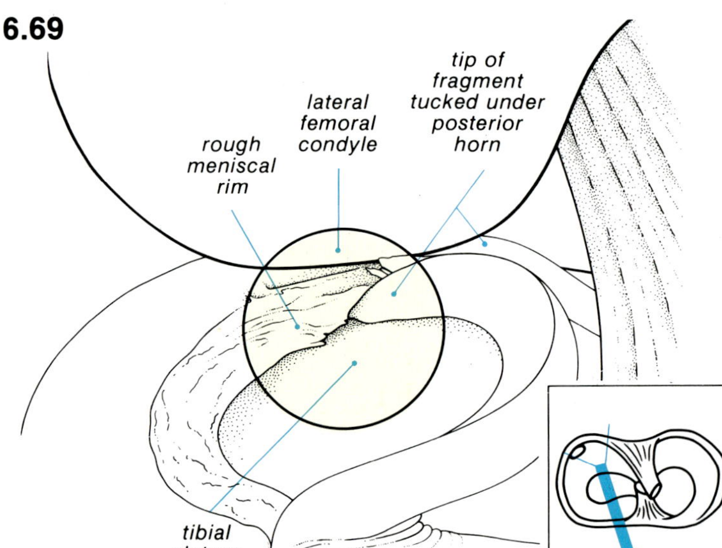

meniscus on the tibia and the tip of the arthroscope has been drawn back to lie on the upper surface of the lateral meniscus, just inside the synovial cavity.

A similar tear may be seen in the posterior half of the meniscus, but anterior tags (Figs.6.70 & 6.71) are much more common. Fig.6.72 shows a meniscal flap lying beneath the meniscus. The flap could not be found at first, but it was known that a fragment must be present because there was a defect in the meniscal margin and an irregularity in the surface of the meniscus itself. The meniscal fragment was located with a probing needle beneath the posterior third of the meniscus, in the same space occupied by the foreign body in Fig.4.35 and the loose body in Fig.4.36 (see Chapter 4). The fragment was easily removed arthroscopically and the patient's progress was satisfactory.

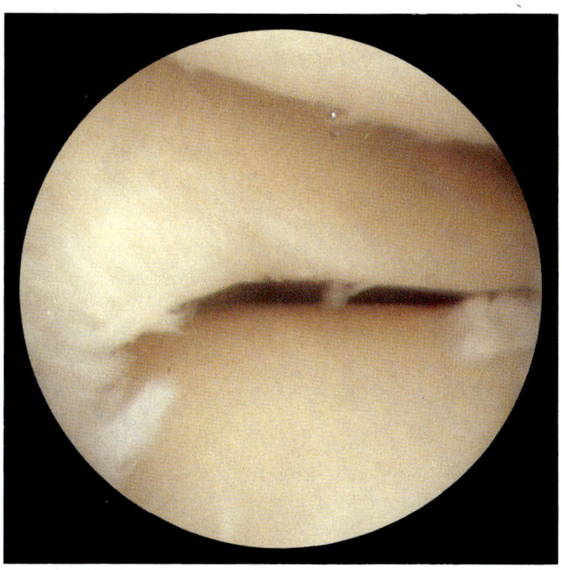

6.70

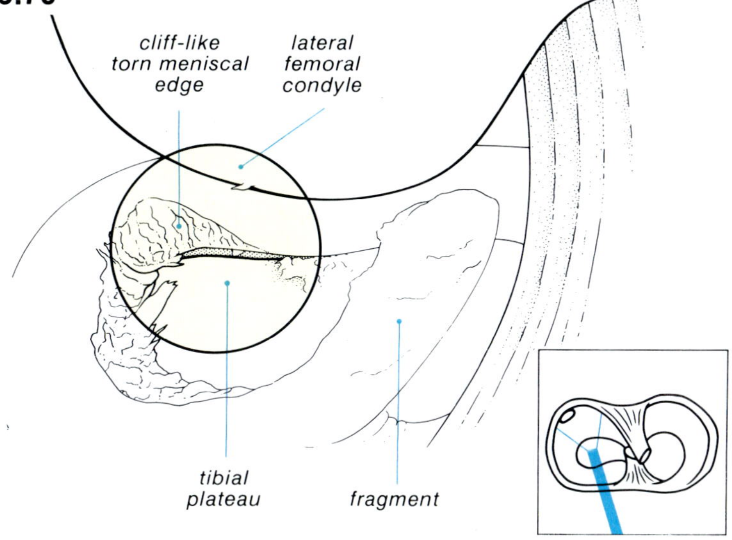

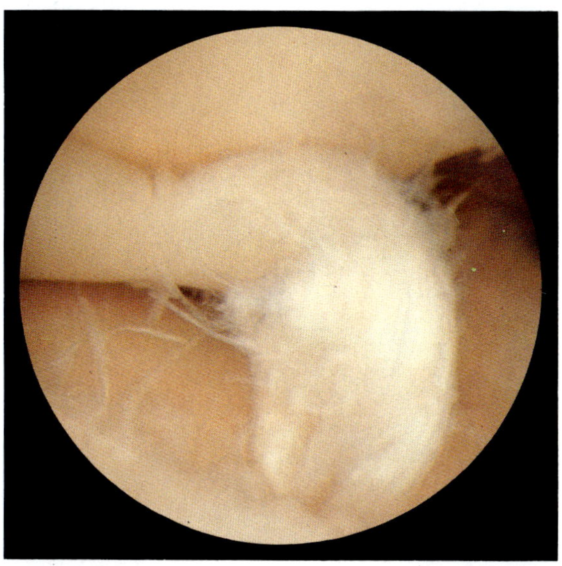

6.71

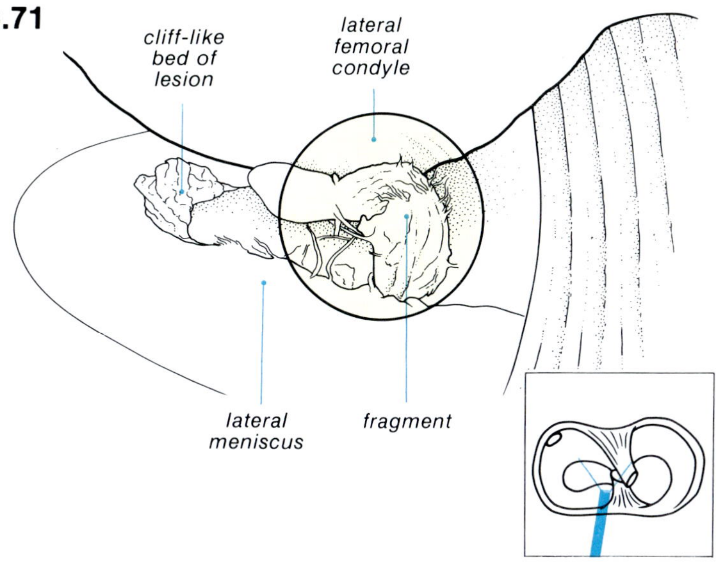

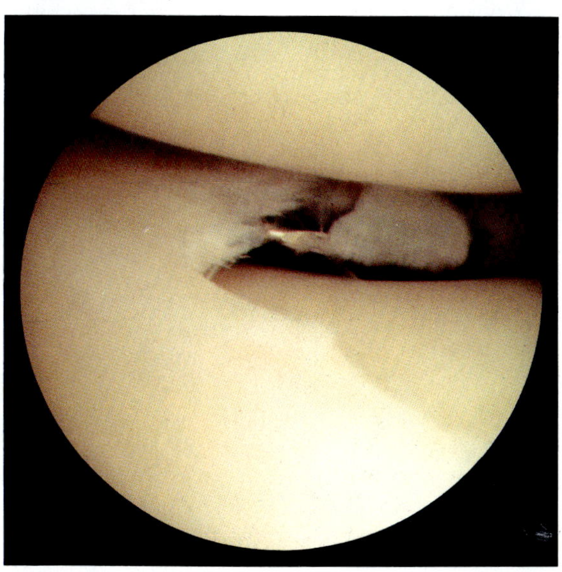

6.72

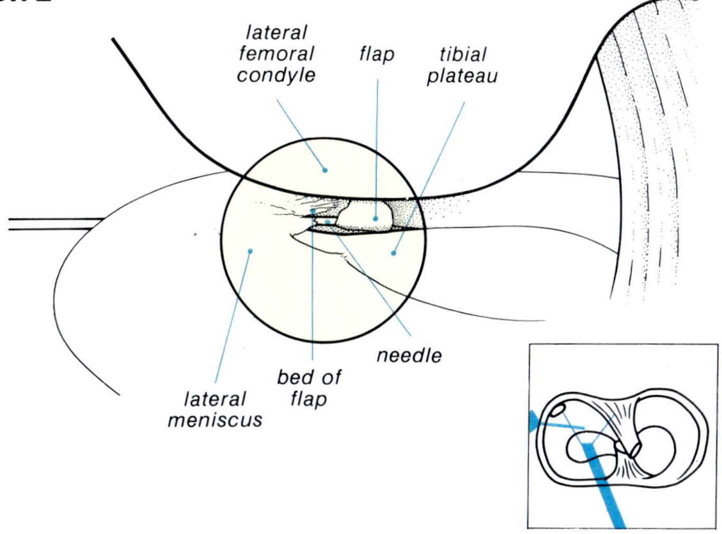

Three years later, the opportunity arose to re-examine the joint when the patient was suffering from anterior knee pain. At arthroscopy the site of the tag was found (Fig.6.73). The base of the flap had rounded off well; the meniscus was intact and the articular surfaces of both the femur and the tibia were normal in all areas with no sign of degenerative change. It is not clear how these tears arise but, like the tear in Figs.6.70 and 6.71, a specific injury is probably the cause.

Fig.6.74 may perhaps be an early stage of the same lesion. The posterior margin of the meniscus is seen with the needle lying beneath the meniscus in a plane of cleavage just in front of the vascular portion of the popliteus tendon, the upper limit of which is clearly seen. There is a radial tear in the free margin of the meniscus, but the meniscal fragment is not completely mobile. It was considered that the portion of meniscus in front of the circumferential tear and medial to the radial tear was abnormally mobile and only this portion was removed, preserving the rest of the meniscus intact.

Complex oblique tears

Complex oblique tears, sometimes known as parrot-beak tears, are peculiar to the lateral meniscus. These tears run obliquely from the upper to the lower surfaces of the meniscus but vary in pattern according to the exact relationship of the line of cleavage to the popliteus tunnel. Usually, the posterior limit of the tear on the superior surface lies behind the anterior limit of the tear on the undersurface, creating a triangular flap of meniscus that extends forwards on the undersurface of the meniscus.

The mechanism of these tears is unclear, but the patient can usually remember the moment of injury distinctly and will often describe a sharp twisting movement of the knee in the extended or almost extended position.

As has already been suggested (see page 1.28), these tears may be centred on the popliteus tunnel because the meniscus is forced firmly against the tibia by the popliteus tendon which lies on its lateral side. If the knee is twisted in extension while the meniscus is held against the tibia, an oblique tear centred on the popliteus tendon would be the likely result. The meniscus that crosses the popliteus tunnel is avascular, but the peripheral third of the lateral meniscus in front of and behind the tunnel has a good blood supply which may also influence the behaviour of these tears.

The exact shape of the tear depends on its precise relationship to the popliteus tendon. Fig.6.75 shows an oblique tear in the anterior horn of the lateral meniscus which does not enter the popliteus tunnel. An oblique flake of tissue has been raised from the upper surface of the meniscus and runs down towards the inferior surface. In this case the tear did not extend through the full meniscal thickness either radially to the

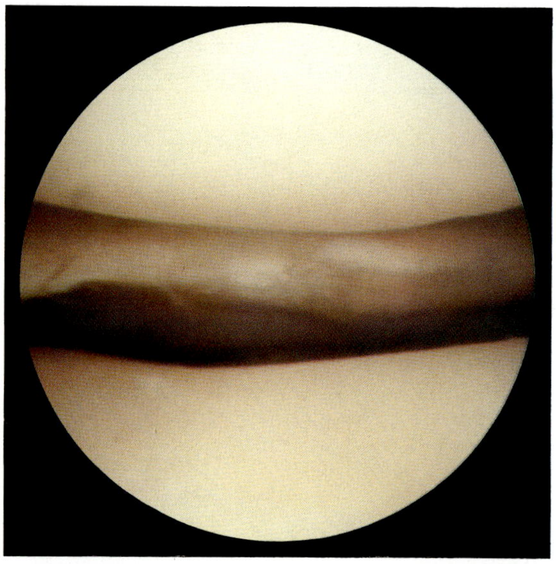

6.73

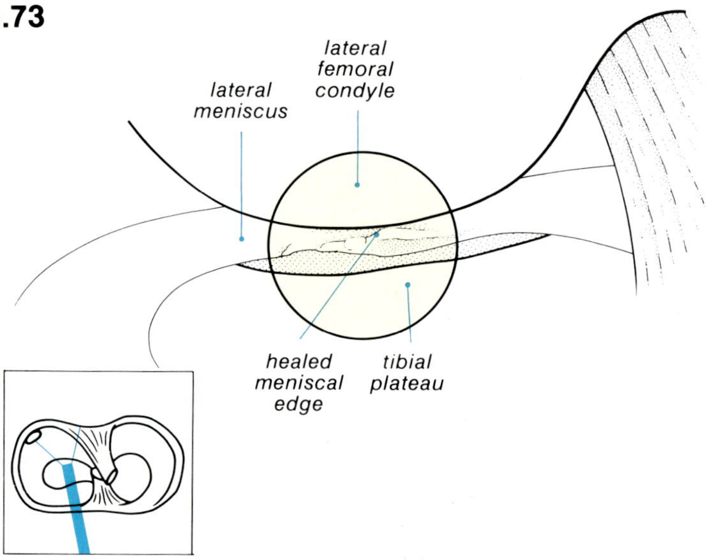

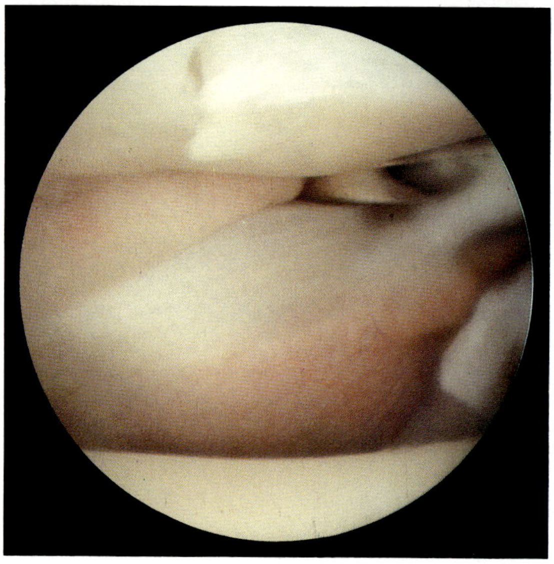

6.74

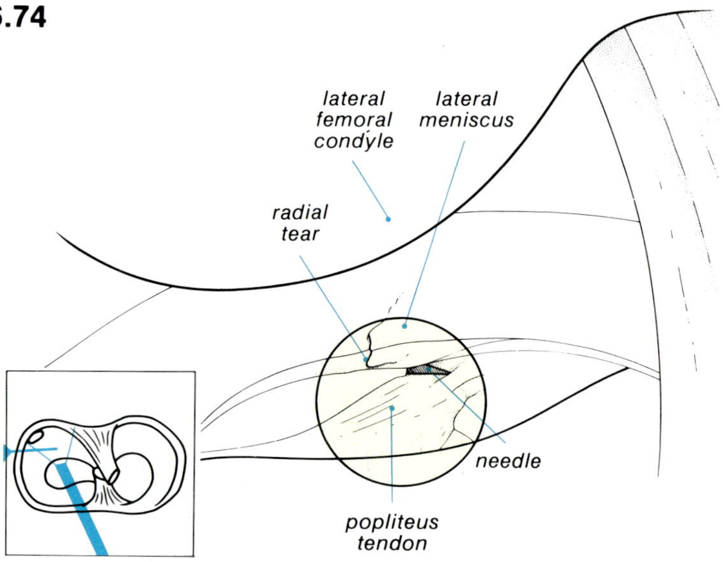

meniscosynovial junction or inferiorly to the lower surface of the meniscus and it was possible to remove the flap and leave a meniscal surface that appeared to be almost normal. This type of tear is unusual, perhaps because the patient also had a tear of the medial meniscus and a ruptured anterior cruciate ligament.

Figs.6.76 and 6.77 show a tear in the undersurface of the anterior part of the meniscus only. The tear extends through to the upper surface of the meniscus, and the fissure can just be seen (Fig.6.76). The bulk of the meniscal tissue, however, is firmly tethered to the undersurface of the meniscus and can be seen when pushed forwards with a probing needle (Fig.6.77). Because this flap lay entirely in front of the popliteus tunnel, the inferior flap was tethered anteriorly, limiting its mobility.

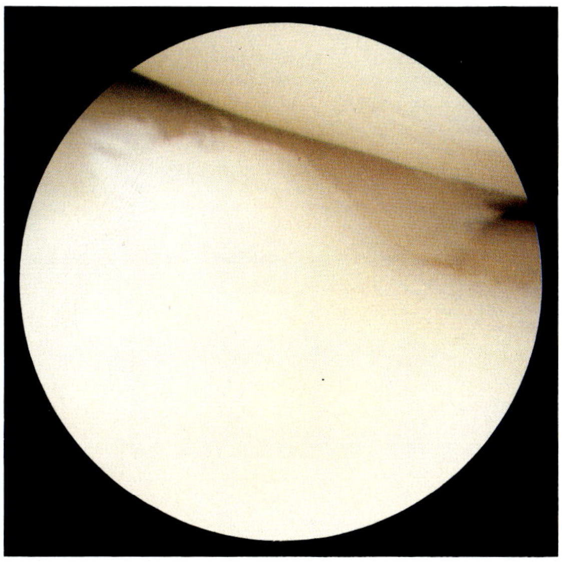

6.75

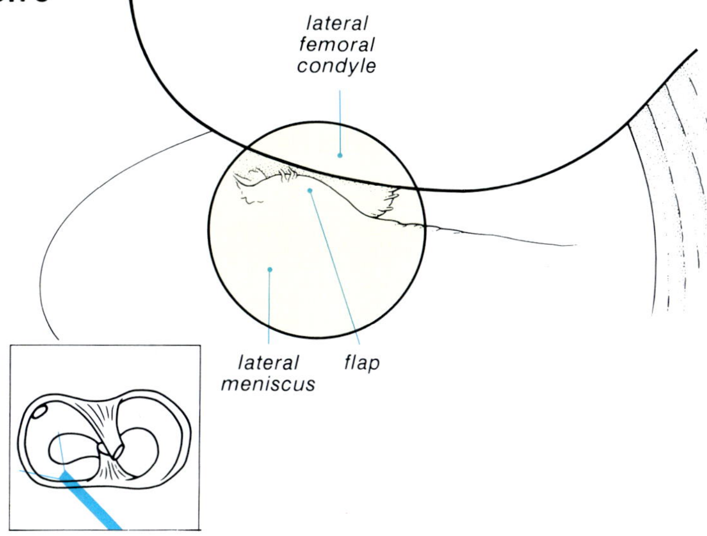

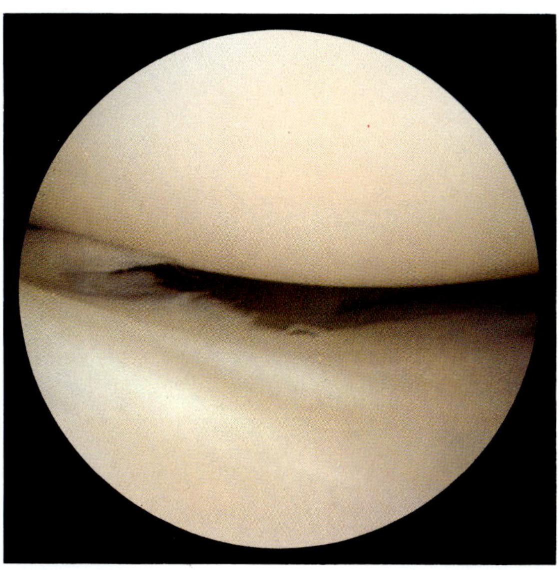

6.76

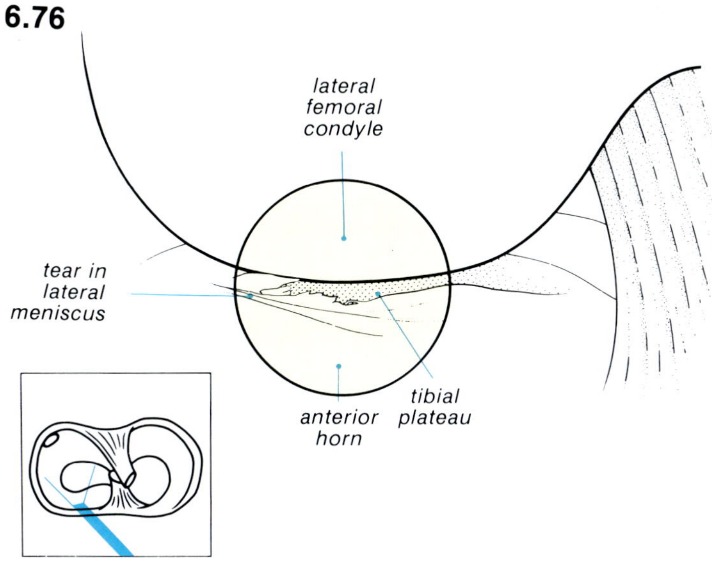

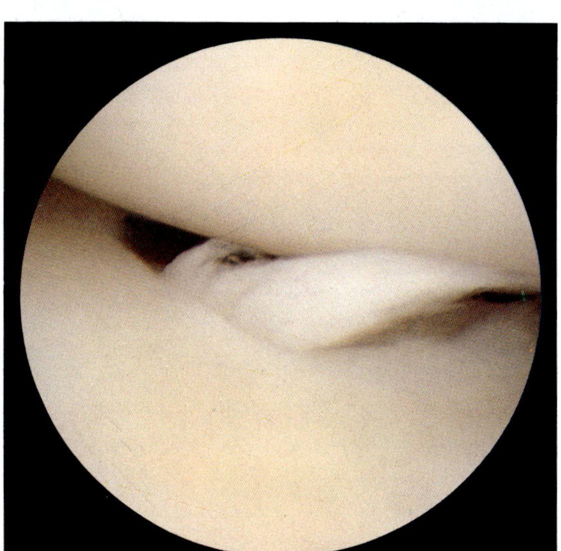

6.77

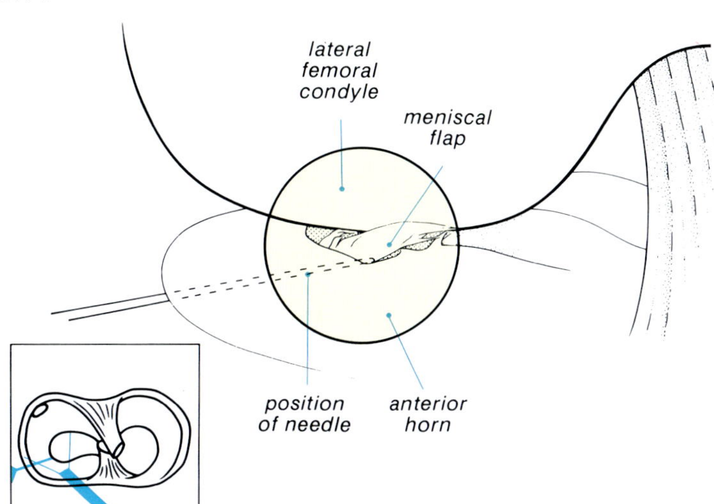

It sometimes happens that these tears do not reach the superior surface of the meniscus but extend laterally to the inferior meniscosynovial junction. It is then possible for the fragment to slip laterally and present as a swelling on the lateral joint line just in front of the popliteus tendon. These nodules are most apparent when the knee is in midflexion and disappear when a varus strain is applied. Such swellings are often considered to be 'cysts' of the lateral meniscus but are, in fact, meniscal flaps that are protruding laterally, carrying with them a thin covering of synovium.

Fig.6.78 shows the site of such a flap after arthroscopic excision. The superior surface of the meniscus is intact, but only just. The flap has been removed from the undersurface and the defect beneath the meniscus can be seen.

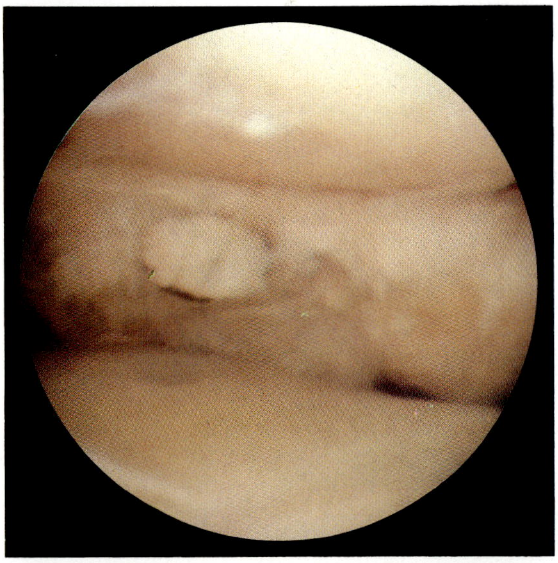

6.78

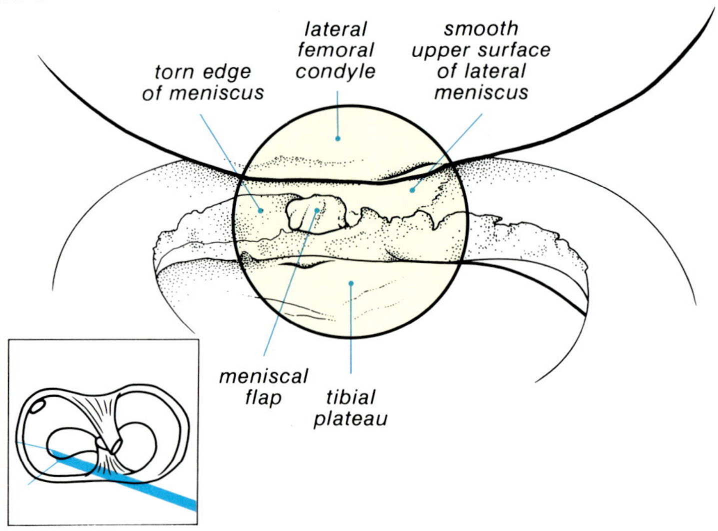

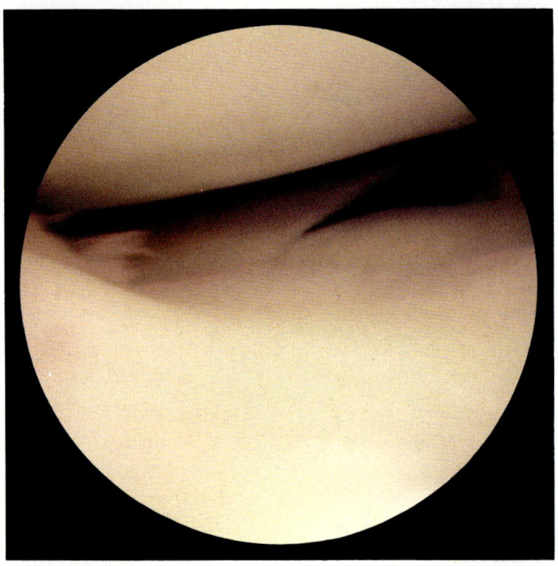

6.79

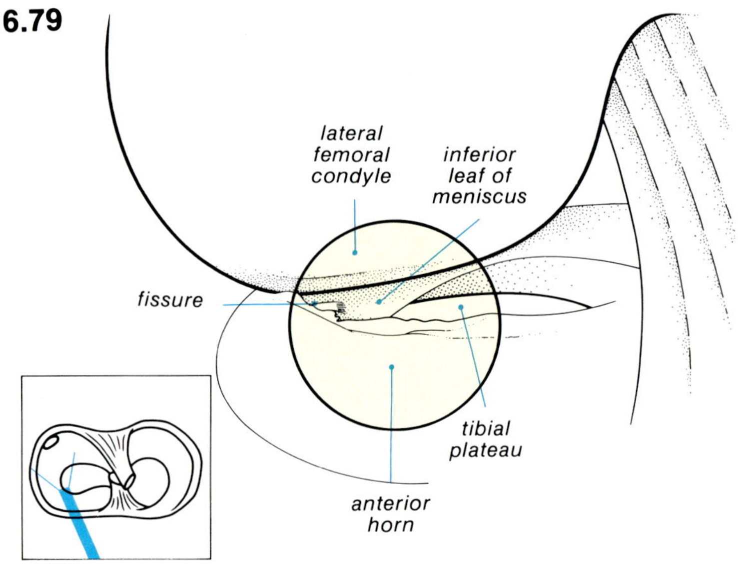

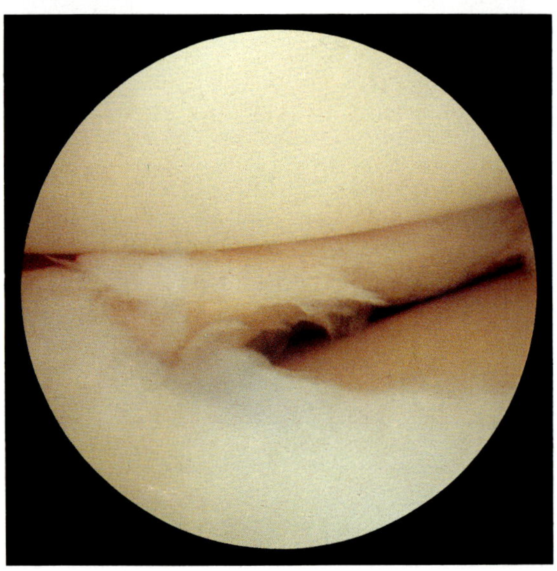

6.80

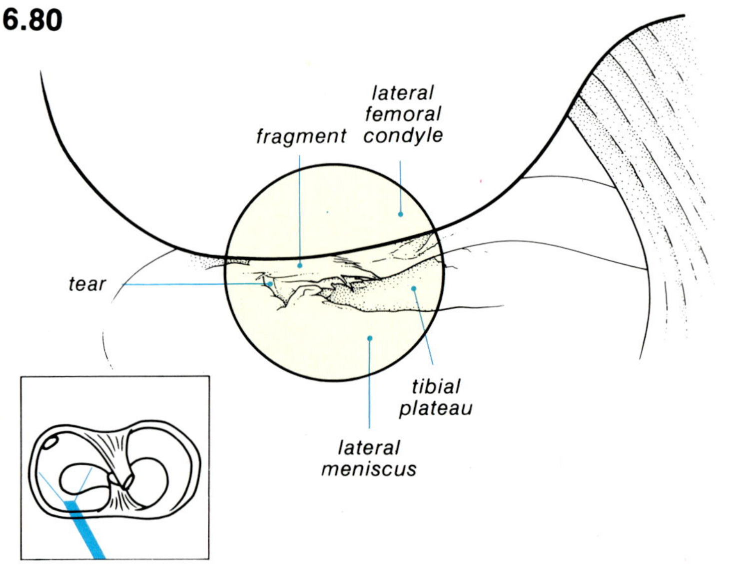

None of the oblique tears shown in Figs.6.75 to 6.78 enter the popliteus tunnel. Fig.6.79, however, shows a tear of the lateral meniscus in which the inferior tear enters the tunnel on its superior surface. The anterior part of the inferior flap retains its peripheral attachment and is therefore tethered. The fissure on the upper surface is clearly seen, but the inferior flap remains tucked beneath the meniscus. The upper and lower leaves of the meniscus were able to move upon each other when the knee was twisted under load and caused a painful click.

Because the tear in Fig.6.79 extends in front of the popliteus tunnel the flap is tethered, but in Fig.6.80 the anterior limit of the inferior tear is at the level of the tunnel and the flap is therefore mobile. The tip of the flap protrudes from beneath the femoral condyle and the tear on the upper surface curls away towards the popliteus tunnel. Because the fragment has retained some peripheral attachment, the mobile segment of meniscus is not large and much of the meniscus was preserved.

If the tear lies slightly more posteriorly than that shown in Fig.6.80, the whole of the meniscal flap will be mobile. Fig.6.81 shows such a flap protruding from beneath the meniscus. The flap was able to move into the centre of the joint because it was tethered only at its base, which lay behind the popliteus tunnel so that the lateral margin of the flap was not attached peripherally. The mobile fragment was therefore large and had to be removed completely. Because the tear was so large, the circumference of the meniscus was completely disrupted at the level of the popliteus tunnel and the meniscus was incompetent because it could no longer protect the articular surface when the joint was loaded. The prognosis for such a tear must be less satisfactory than for tears in which the peripheral attachments of the meniscus remain intact.

Moving a little further back in the knee, the tear on the superior surface may lie entirely behind the popliteus tunnel so that the posterior fragment presents as a mobile flap of meniscal tissue involving most of the meniscal thickness. The fragment seen in Fig.6.82 was very mobile and on inspection after its removal was found to include most of the inferior surface of the posterior third of the lateral meniscus.

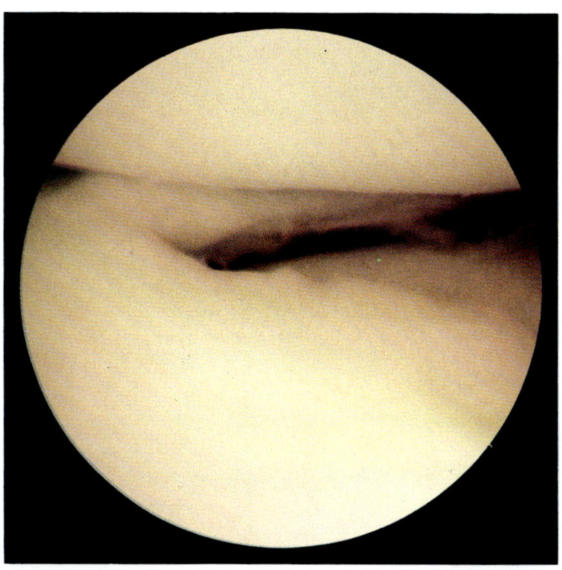

6.81

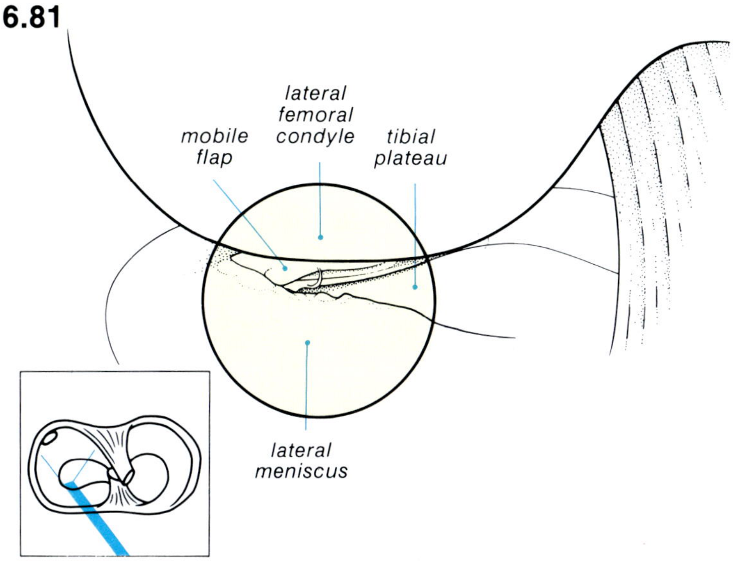

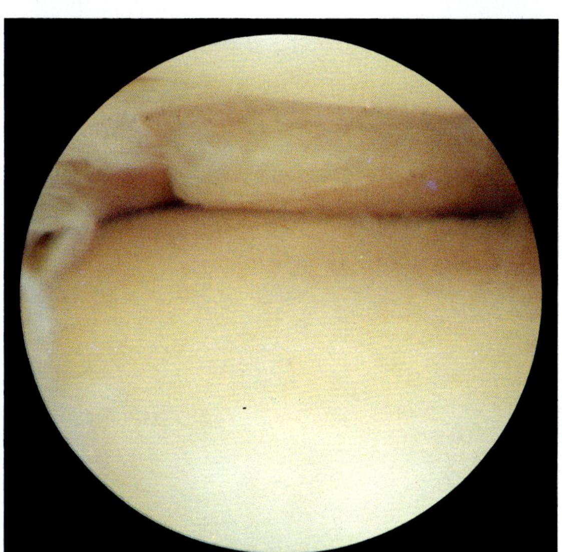

6.82

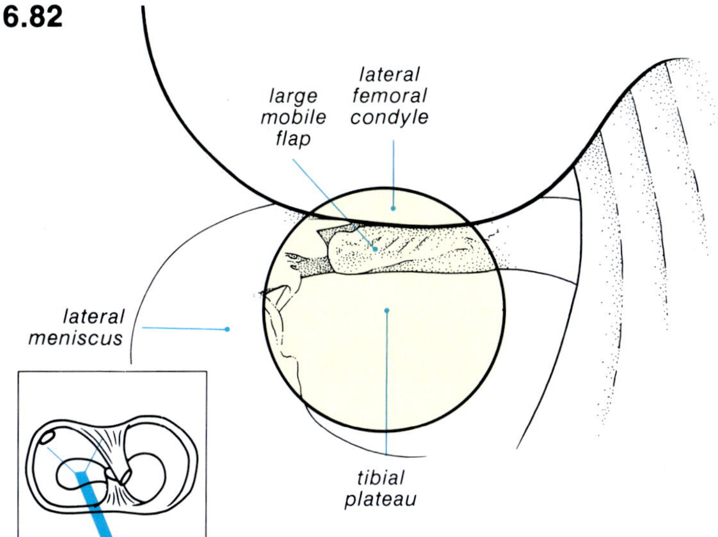

Although complex oblique tears vary in the position of the tear and its relationship to the popliteus tunnel, the lesions are almost always solitary. Fig.6.83, however, shows a double tear with two oblique flaps. One of the flaps had arisen from the posterior half of the meniscus and had come to lie on top of the anterior part of the meniscus, the opposite of the usual anatomy. The patient whose knee is illustrated was a vigorous semi-professional athlete who also had a rupture of the anterior cruciate ligament and a long history of ligamentous instability of the knee. The meniscus was grossly disrupted and had probably been torn on more than one occasion. Shattered menisci such as this are most commonly found in patients with ligamentous instability and often bear so many different tears that it is quite impossible to categorize them precisely.

Radial tears

True radial tears of the lateral meniscus also occur. Many of the radial tears that have been reported may have happened at meniscectomy when the anterior horn was pulled forward while the dissection was carried backwards along the meniscosynovial junction, but not all radial tears arise in this way. Fig.6.84 shows a radial tear of the midportion of the meniscus extending approximately halfway through the meniscal body.

The significance of radial tears is unclear. Although they are often discovered as an incidental finding in patients who have no symptoms referrable to the lateral compartment of the knee, the tear is well placed to propagate towards the popliteus tunnel and become a complex oblique tear, or even to act as a natural endpoint for a circumferential tear extending from either

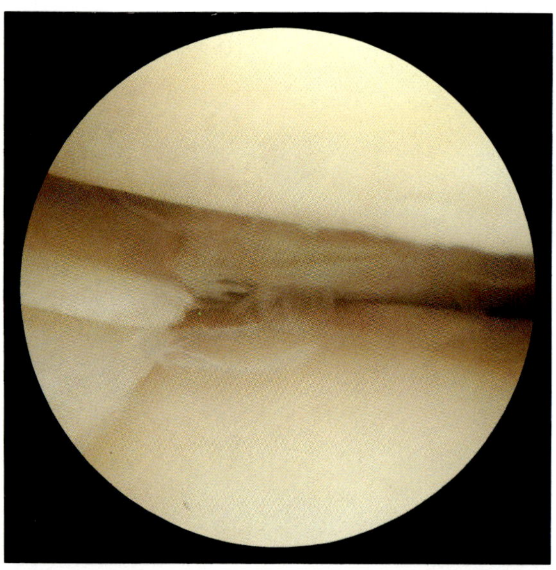

6.83

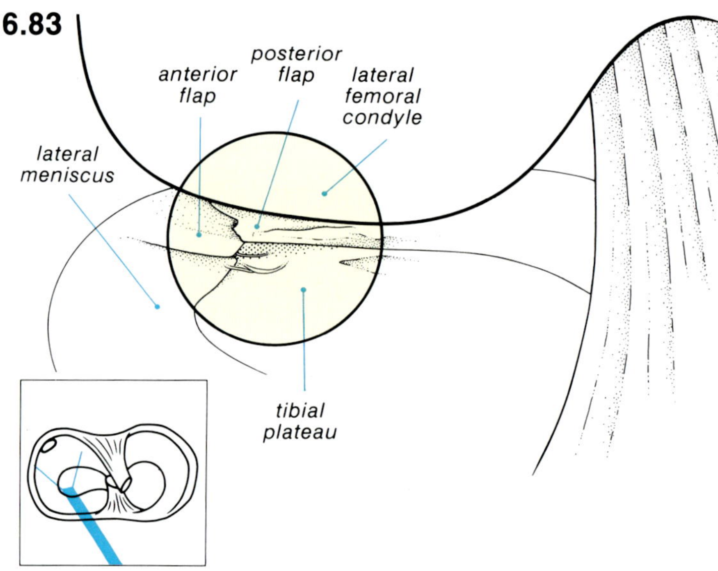

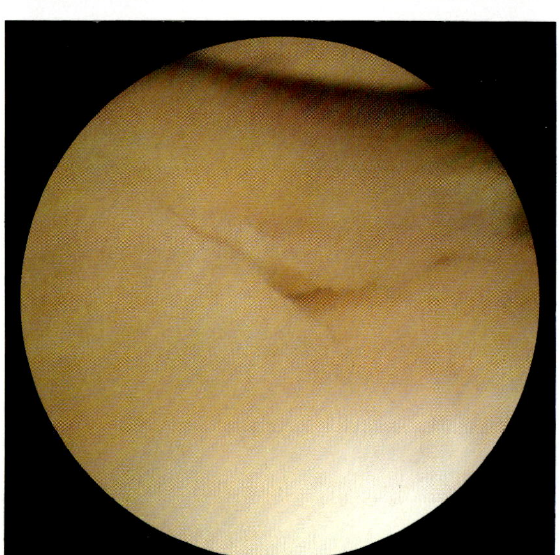

6.84

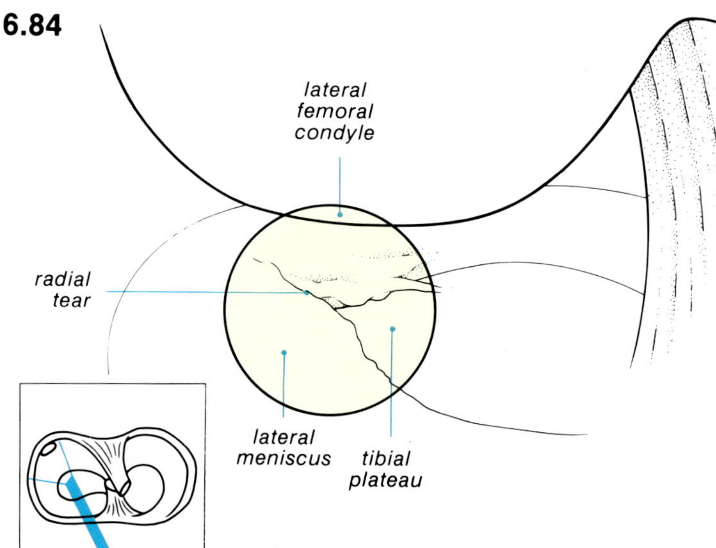

end and may account for the anterior tags seen in Figs.6.70 and 6.71 and the posterior tag seen in Fig.6.64. The correct management of such radial tears is unclear. If they do not cause symptoms, total meniscectomy would seem unnecessarily drastic; but if they are likely to propagate and cause an unpleasant complex oblique tear, prophylactic excision of the damaged area may be appropriate. Cautious excision of the tear down to healthy tissue is probably the treatment of choice.

POPLITEAL BRIDGE

The bridge of meniscus crossing the popliteus tendon is important not only in dictating the pattern of tears that occurs in the lateral compartment but also in protecting the articular cartilage. If the bridge is completely ruptured, the meniscus loses its protective function, the load on the articular surface is increased, and articular cartilage degeneration can be expected to proceed more rapidly than with the bridge intact.

Fig.6.85 shows a particularly wide and satisfactory bridge over the popliteus. The patient had undergone a lateral meniscectomy for removal of a partial-thickness bucket handle tear two years previously. The femoral condyle was entirely normal but the tibial surface had patches of articular cartilage irregularity. The meniscus crossing the popliteus tunnel has rounded off well.

Fig.6.86 shows the lateral compartment of a professional footballer whose lateral meniscus had been removed six months earlier. The bridge across the popliteus tendon is very narrow and the patient had continued to play football after his operation. There is extensive articular cartilage damage on both the femoral and tibial surfaces and the presence of articular cartilage debris and marked synovitis throughout the joint. Comparison of the articular surfaces in Figs.6.85 and 6.86 might suggest, but cannot prove, that the integrity of the popliteus bridge is important in preserving the articular surface.

6.85

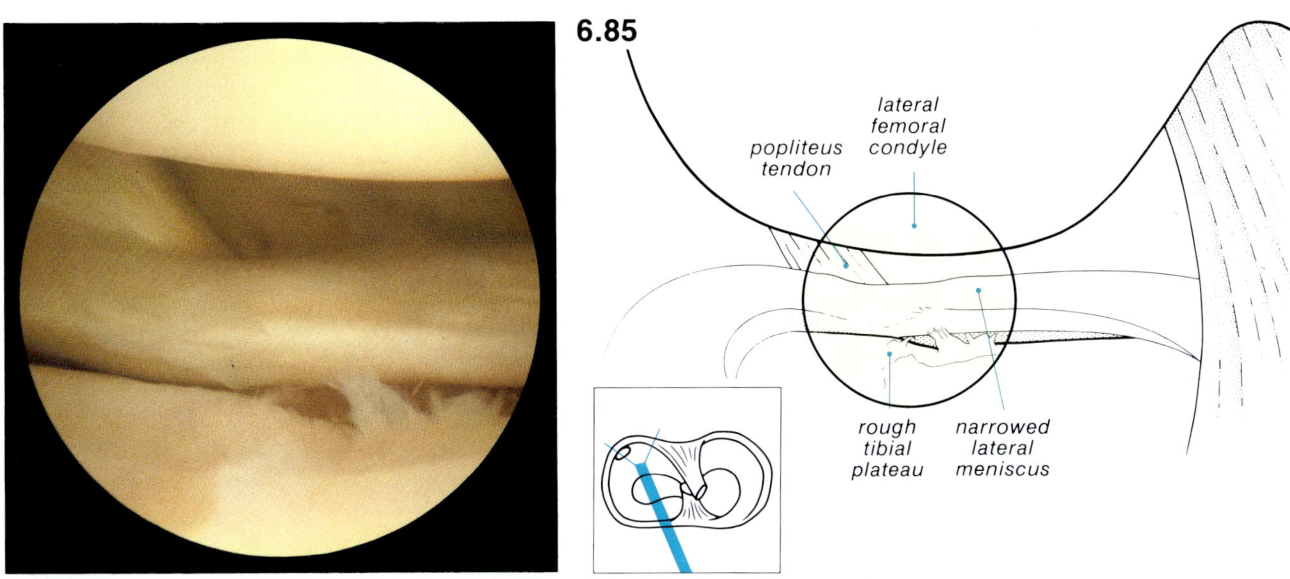

6.86

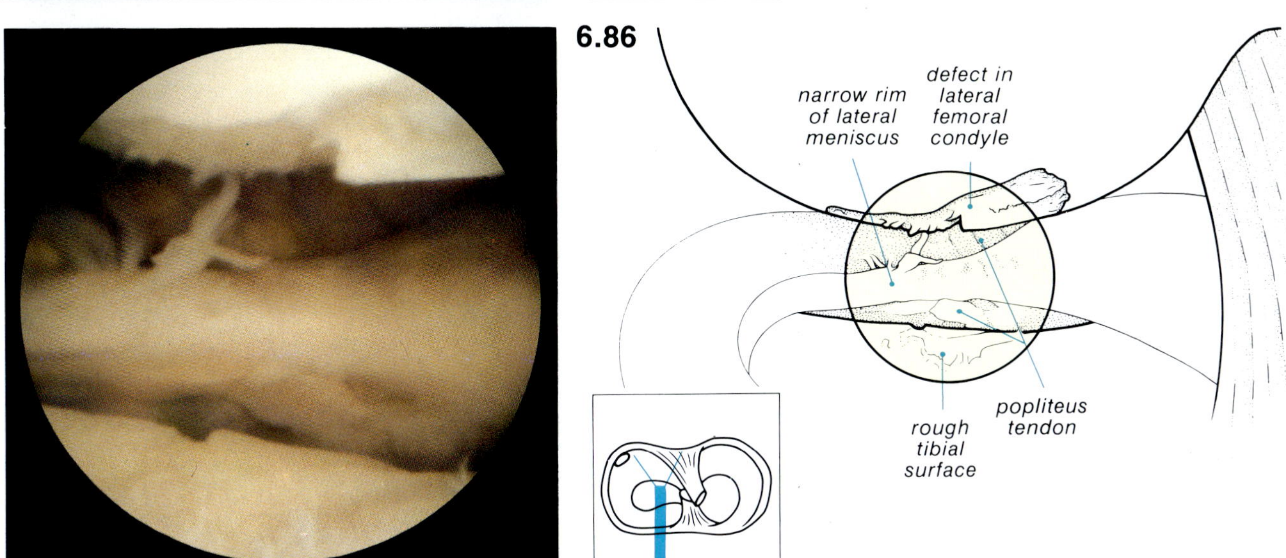

One disadvantage of leaving a stout meniscal bridge is that it may tear, particularly if the patient continues the activities that led to the original lesion. Fig.6.87 shows a meniscus following a partial lateral meniscectomy done three years earlier. A probing needle passed into the meniscal rim shows a tear extending as far forwards as the front of the popliteus tunnel and as far backwards as the posterior attachment of the meniscus to the tibia. After the original meniscectomy the patient had continued working as a physical education teacher until a second injury which was followed by recurrent locking of the knee in flexion.

As well as the tear in the meniscal rim, a defect is seen on the undersurface of the lateral femoral condyle opposite the popliteus tunnel, a lesion that will no doubt have progressed much more rapidly since the mobile

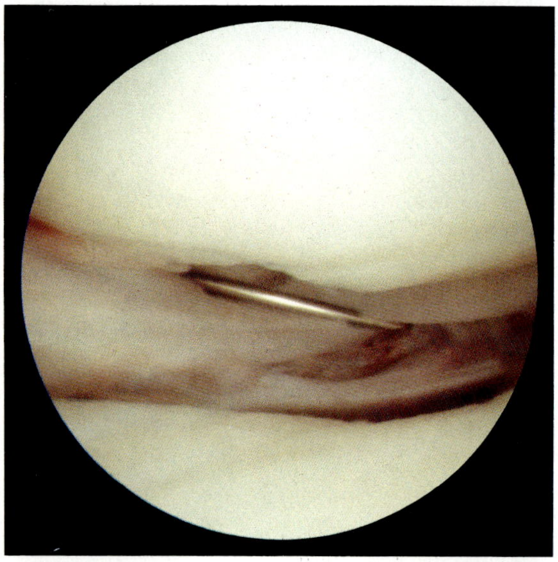

6.87

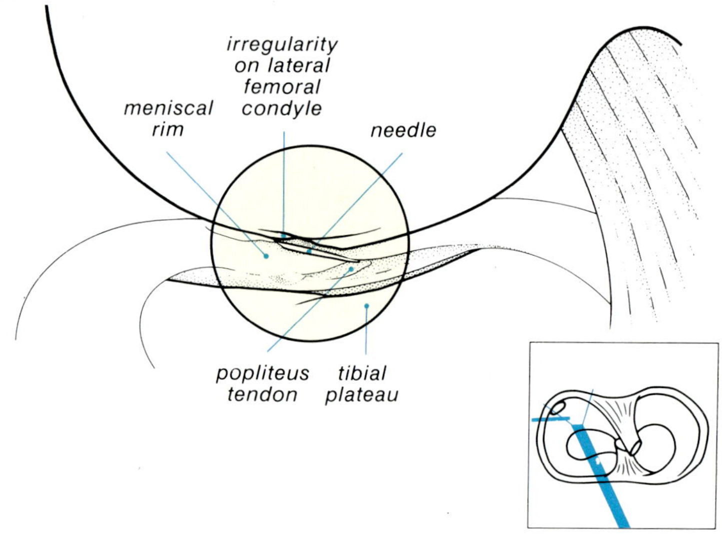

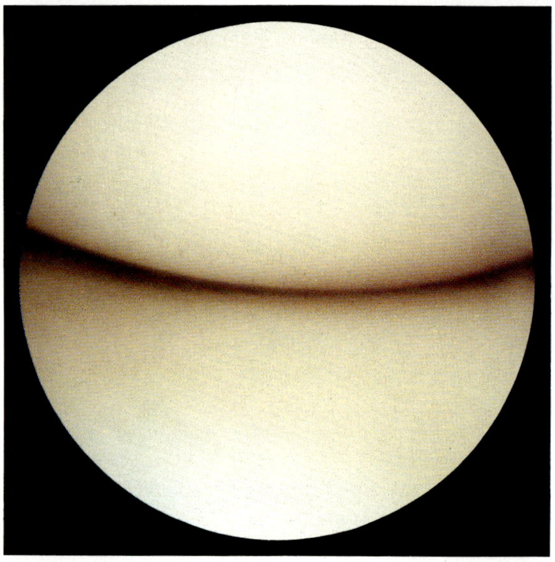

6.88

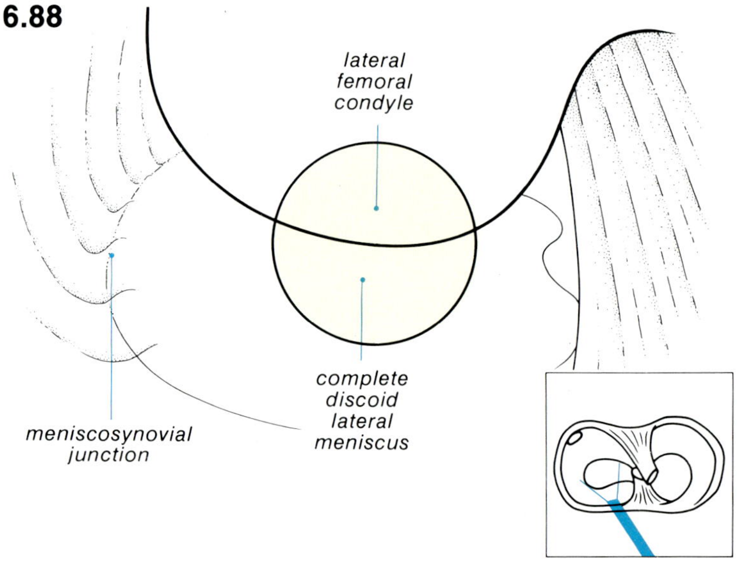

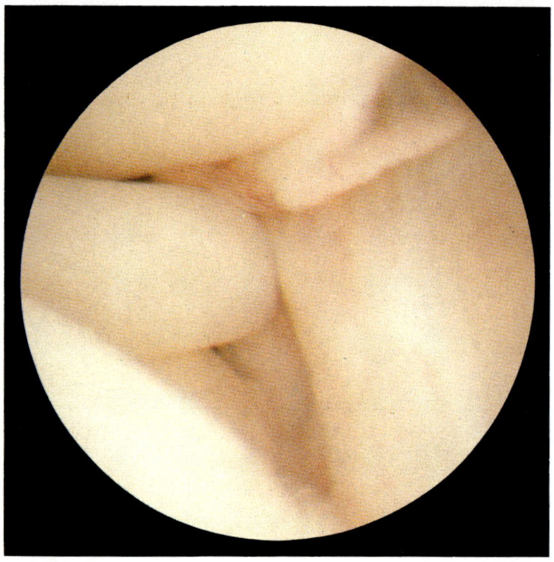

6.89

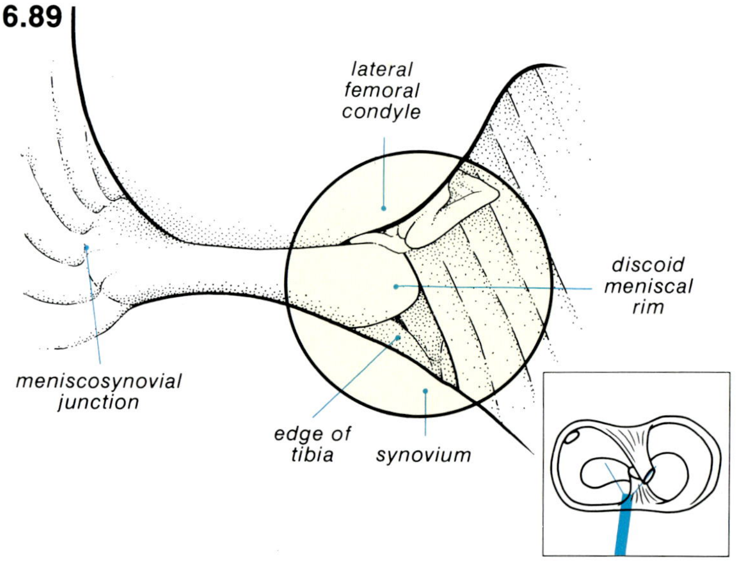

meniscal fragment was removed. It is tempting to speculate that the lesion would be even more advanced if a total lateral meniscectomy had been performed at the original operation.

Some degree of articular cartilage damage can usually be seen within two years of a lateral meniscectomy in almost any patient, and to find normal articular surface after this time is quite exceptional. The appearances are least satisfactory in heavy patients who have undergone a total meniscectomy with disruption of the popliteus bridge and in those who have continued with full participation in sporting activities. The results are most satisfactory in lightweight patients who have a good popliteus bridge and who place little stress upon their joints.

DISCOID MENISCI

Discoid lateral menisci do not always cause symptoms and are usually encountered as incidental findings in patients with other conditions. Their incidence in the normal population depends largely upon the point at which the meniscus is considered to be discoid. Discoid menisci can conveniently be classified according to the amount of tibial plateau covered by the meniscus.

A discoid lateral meniscus which covers one hundred percent of the tibial surface is seen in Fig.6.88. No meniscal margin can be seen and both the femoral and meniscal surfaces are smooth and intact. Because the margin of the lateral meniscus is such a useful landmark during arthroscopy, its absence can be disorientating and misleading.

The meniscal margin of a truly discoid lateral meniscus will be found in the intercondylar notch (Figs.6.89 & 6.90). In Fig.6.89 the meniscal margin is thickened and rounded and presents an appearance similar to a locked bucket handle fragment involving the full width of the meniscus. The appearance may indeed be so like a torn lateral meniscus that attempts may be made to remove the meniscal fragment before discovering that it is in fact the thickened margin of an intact and complete discoid lateral meniscus.

Not all discoid menisci have such thick margins. Fig.6.90, the same knee as in Fig.6.88, shows the edge of another truly discoid lateral meniscus with its margin lying in the intercondylar notch. This margin, however, is thin and could not possibly be confused with a locked bucket handle meniscal fragment.

Fig.6.91 shows a meniscus that covers much more of the lateral tibial plateau than normal but it is not truly discoid because the meniscus is not circular in shape. Its margin extends more than halfway across the lateral tibial plateau but does not reach the intercondylar notch and could be said to cover three-quarters or seventy-five percent of the tibial plateau. A crude estimate of the amount of tibial surface covered is helpful in the description and classification of discoid lateral menisci.

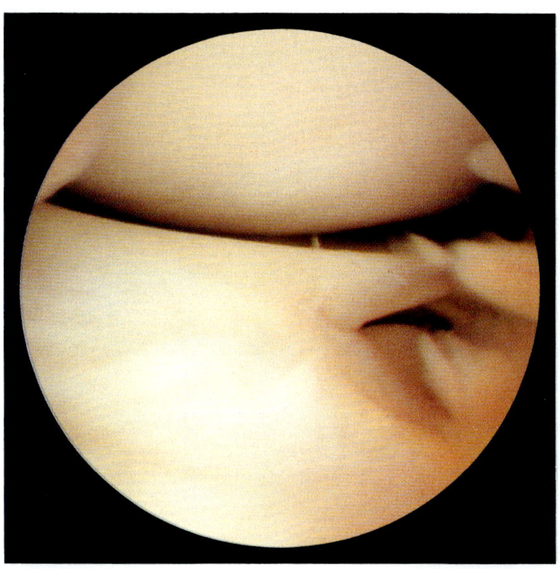

6.90

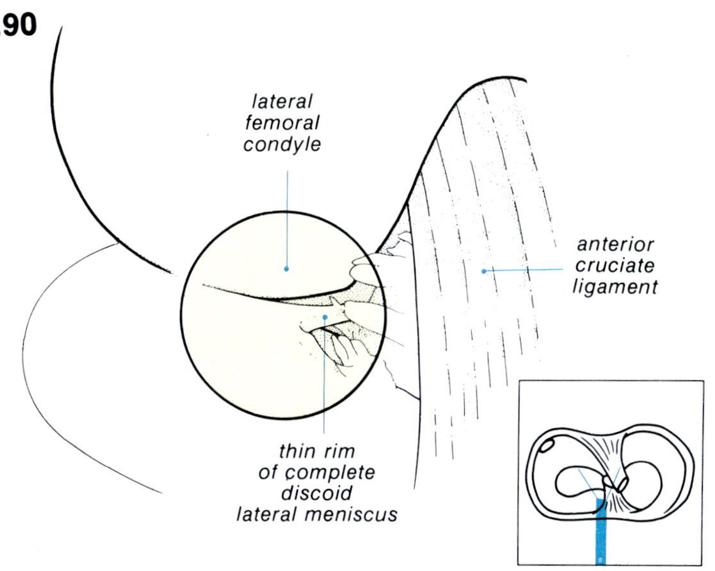

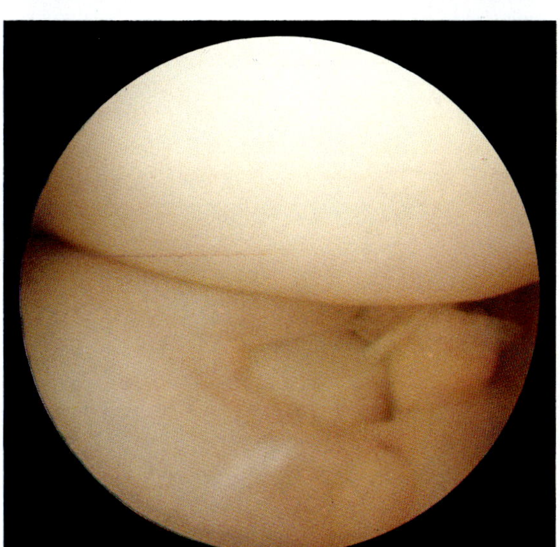

6.91

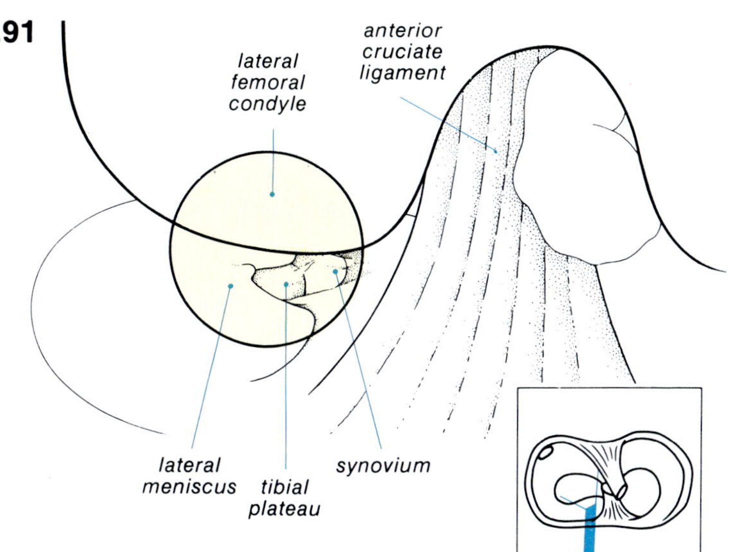

Fig.6.92 shows another lateral meniscus which is broader than normal but covers only one-half of the tibial plateau. The meniscal margin falls exactly under the centre of the femoral condyle and could be described as a fifty percent discoid lateral meniscus. The meniscus is intact and not causing symptoms. The articular surface is also intact and the knee is normal in every way except that the lateral meniscus is wider than usual. It is, however, of some concern that the meniscal margin lies at the point of closest contact between the femoral condyle and the tibial plateau, a position that must place unnatural stress upon the meniscus and probably renders it more susceptible to injury.

Although most discoid lateral menisci are intact and found as incidental observations at arthroscopy, tears of such menisci do occur. The central portion of a discoid lateral meniscus is usually its thinnest part and it is at that point that tears are most frequently seen. In Fig.6.93, the meniscal fragment has been displaced into the intercondylar notch and the defect is easily seen. The mobile fragment of meniscus was removed arthroscopically as if it were a particularly thick bucket handle fragment.

The fate of the remaining rim following excision of the central portion of a discoid lateral meniscus is sometimes discussed. Fig.6.94 shows such a rim seventeen months after removal of the abnormal portion of the meniscus.

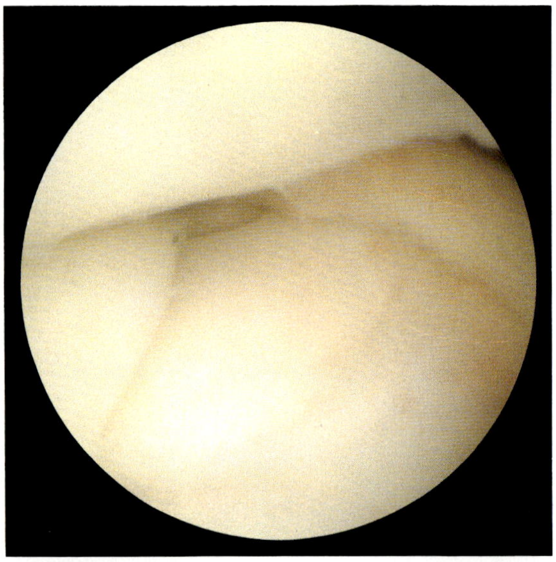

6.92

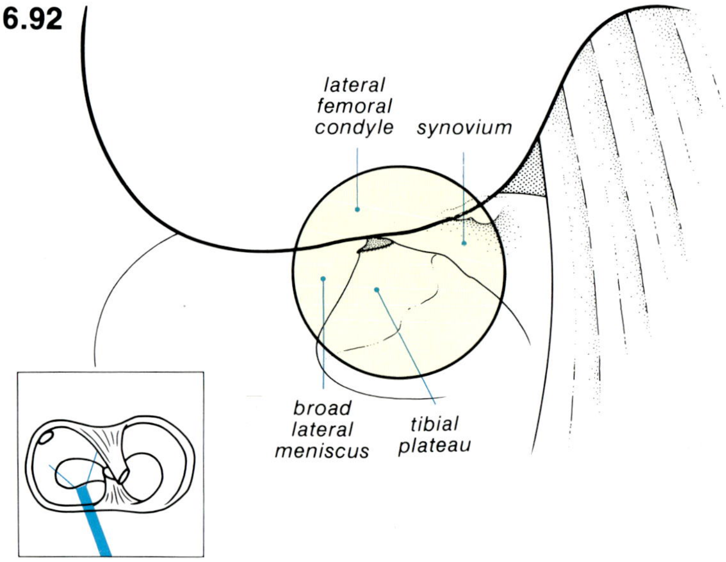

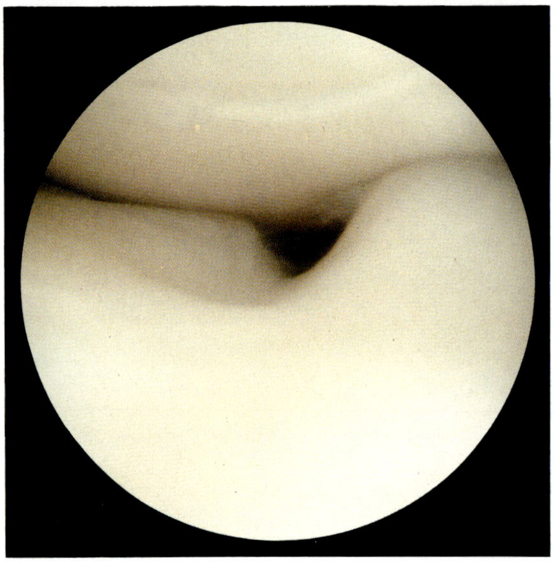

6.93

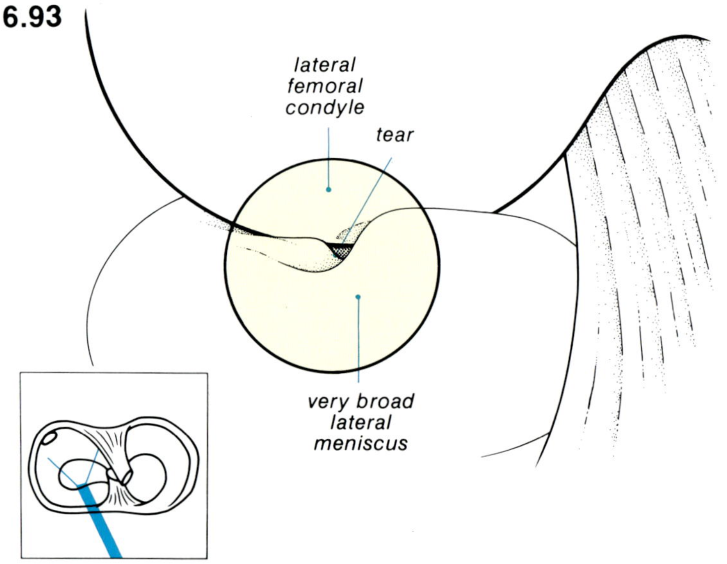

The meniscal margin is clean and sharp and the articular surfaces are normal.

Although the appearance of Fig.6.94 is satisfactory, it should not be assumed that removal of the central portion of normal asymptomatic discoid menisci is a procedure to be encouraged. Although the torn fragments of discoid meniscal tissue should be removed, as should any meniscal fragments, there is no reason to suppose that an intact discoid meniscus will give rise to problems. Indeed, it may be argued that the intact discoid meniscus protects the articular surface of the knee and that its removal could expose the articular cartilage to such abnormal stresses that it may develop degenerative change. It is also worth noting that the central portion of the tibial plateau is particularly vulnerable to scuffing by arthroscopic instruments during operation.

CYSTIC DEGENERATION

Although the most common lesion of the lateral meniscus is a tear that generates a mobile fragment which causes mechanical symptoms, cystic degeneration of the lateral meniscus also occurs. In Fig.6.95, the meniscus is bloated, split and swollen. Although no separate cysts can be seen, the meniscus is soft and friable in consistency. Examination of the meniscectomy specimen showed a few small cysts in its substance but no single large mucoid cavity.

The condition of cystic degeneration must be distinguished from isolated mucoid cysts found at the periphery of the meniscus, which may be regarded as ganglia at the knee rather than a disorder of the meniscus, and from the meniscal flaps that can protrude from beneath the lateral edge of the meniscus to produce joint line swellings covered by synovium (see Fig.6.78).

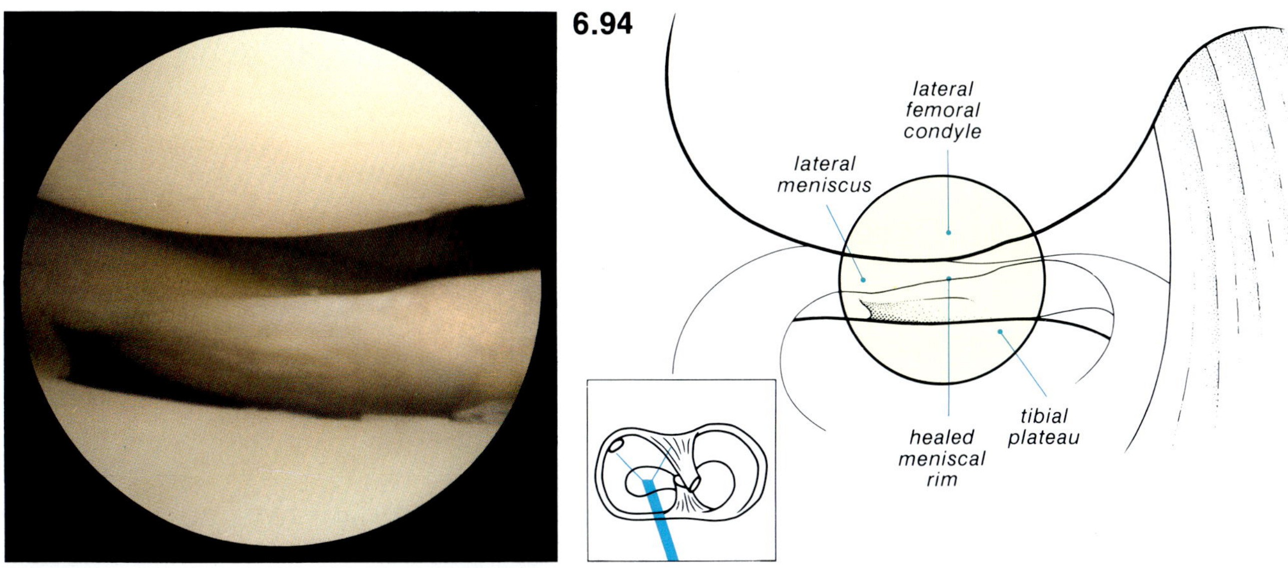

6.94

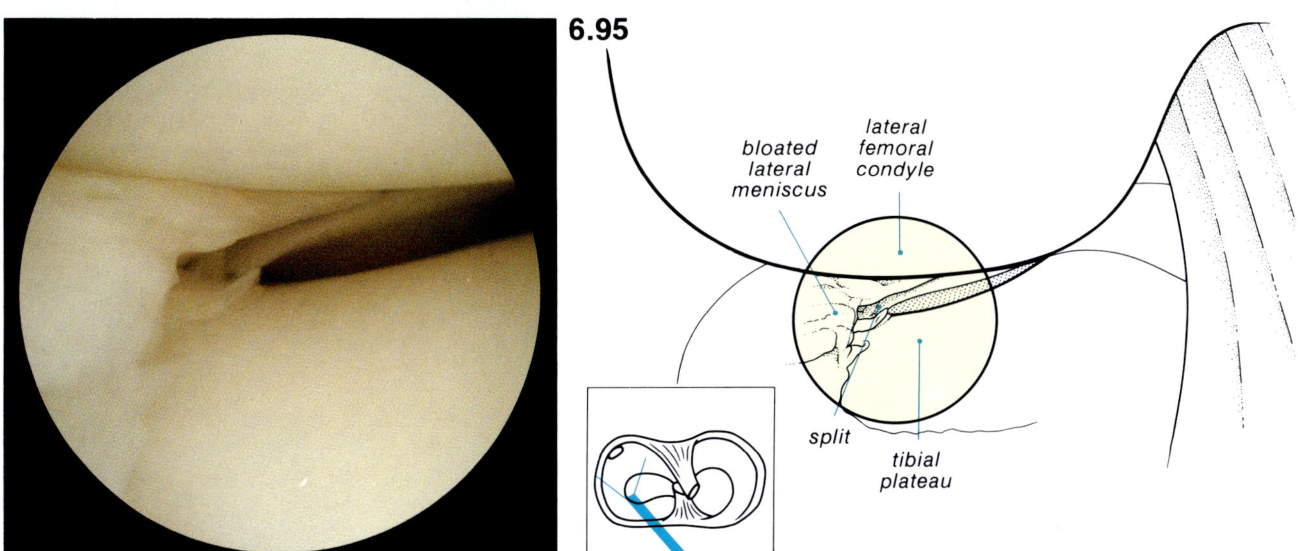

6.95

Index